This groundbreaking book makes the implicit explicit: Cognitive behavior therapy is grounded in a strong, respectful, and caring therapeutic relationship. The research is clear and compelling: Attention to the therapeutic relationship improves treatment outcome and decreases therapy drop out. If doubts linger, Dr. Wenzel's clinical experience and wisdom will convince you. And once convinced, you'll find in this book skills, strategies, and guidance that will add both power and compassion to the cognitive behavior therapy you provide.

—**Michael A. Tompkins, PhD, ABPP,** codirector, San Francisco Bay Area Center for Cognitive Therapy, Oakland, CA; faculty, Beck Institute for Cognitive Behavior Therapy, Bala Cynwyd, PA, United States

Dr. Amy Wenzel, a leading expert in cognitive behavior therapy (CBT), delivers a compelling and comprehensive guide for clinicians on therapeutic relationship processes in CBT, including those unique to the modality. Rich in theoretical concepts and empirical research synthesis, this guide offers clinicians practical insights they can immediately apply in their sessions.

—**Nikolaos Kazantzis, PhD,** Cognitive Behavior Therapy Research Unit, Melbourne, Australia, and author of *The Therapeutic Relationship in Cognitive-Behavioral Therapy: A Clinician's Guide*

W0229977

THERAPEUTIC RELATIONSHIP-FOCUSED COGNITIVE BEHAVIORAL THERAPY

THERAPEUTIC RELATIONSHIP-FOCUSED COGNITIVE BEHAVIORAL THERAPY

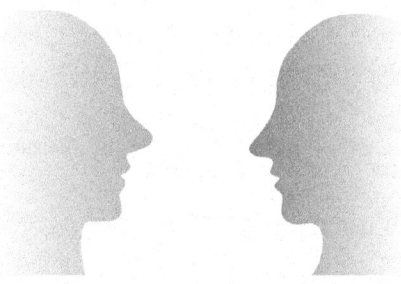

AMY WENZEL

AMERICAN PSYCHOLOGICAL ASSOCIATION

The opinions and statements published are the responsibility of the author, and such opinions and statements do not necessarily represent the policies of the American Psychological Association.

Published by
American Psychological Association
750 First Street, NE
Washington, DC 20002
https://www.apa.org

Order Department
https://www.apa.org/pubs/books
order@apa.org

Typeset in Charter and Interstate by Circle Graphics, Inc., Reisterstown, MD

Printer: Gasch Printing, Odenton, MD
Cover Designer: Beth Schlenoff Design, Bethesda, MD

Library of Congress Cataloging-in-Publication Data

Names: Wenzel, Amy, author. | American Psychological Association, issuing body.
Title: Therapeutic relationship-focused cognitive behavioral therapy /
   authored by Amy Wenzel.
Description: Washington, DC : American Psychological Association, [2025] |
   Includes bibliographical references and index.
Identifiers: LCCN 2024011518 (print) | LCCN 2024011519 (ebook) |
   ISBN 9781433835964 (paperback) | ISBN 9781433835971 (epub)
Subjects: MESH: Cognitive Behavioral Therapy--methods | Therapeutic
   Alliance | BISAC: PSYCHOLOGY / Clinical Psychology | PSYCHOLOGY /
   Psychotherapy / General
Classification: LCC RC489.C63 (print) | LCC RC489.C63 (ebook) |
   NLM WM 425.5.C6 | DDC 616.89/1425--dc23/eng/20240724
LC record available at https://lccn.loc.gov/2024011518
LC ebook record available at https://lccn.loc.gov/2024011519

https://doi.org/10.1037/0000424-000

Printed in the United States of America

10 9 8 7 6 5 4 3 2 1

*I dedicate this book to my long-standing childhood friends
of approximately 40 years, who taught me and still teach me to this day
about the healing value of positive regard, authenticity, and being known.*

Contents

Preface

Sarah[1] is a 28-year-old White woman who presented for psychotherapy for depression (carrying an "official" diagnosis of bipolar disorder) and distress associated with the dissolution of a unique romantic relationship situation. She had a distinctive appearance in that her hair was shaved on one side, she was dressed from head to toe in gothic style, she wore bracelets all the way up her arms and rings on every finger, and she had multiple piercings in her ears, nose, and lip. She was a self-proclaimed Wiccan and worked as a manager at a popular chain restaurant. She was referred by her general practitioner (GP), who had prescribed an antidepressant and a mood stabilizer.

Sarah had a long psychiatric history, with multiple psychiatric hospitalizations during adolescence for suicide attempts and what her parents labeled as defiant, belligerent behavior. They asked Sarah to leave home when she was still in high school, and she moved in with her best friend and her best friend's mother. Sarah and her parents continued family therapy with the hope of reunification, but they were unable to reach an agreement regarding household rules and expectations. She abruptly left her small Midwestern town at age 19 and moved to a large metropolitan area, where she met like-minded people and soon moved in with them. Although Sarah found great support in this small community of friends, she continued to have what she called "stress-induced breakdowns" and was hospitalized three times in her 20s for suicidal ideation or for making a suicide attempt of mild lethality.

---

[1]Client identity has been disguised to protect client confidentiality.

Sarah believed that she needed a "fresh start" with a new psychotherapist to acquire stress-management tools after the recent implosion of a complicated relationship situation, which she viewed as leaving her unable to function. When Sarah presented for treatment, she was in the midst of a 3-month leave of absence from work that was precipitated by this incident. She first described the incident as a breakup with her boyfriend of 1 year, with whom she had been living. She indicated that this man abruptly left her for another woman, claiming that this other woman was the "love of his life" and that he intended to marry her. Sarah was left reeling by this news, feeling understandably hurt, blindsided, and rejected. However, it became clear that the situation was more nuanced when Sarah indicated that she had been married to another man for the past 5 years. With no place to go after her boyfriend asked her to leave, she took up residence with her formerly estranged husband but slept in a separate room. Sarah was unsure whether she wanted to reconcile with her husband, focusing instead in the initial sessions on what she viewed as a "betrayal" by her former boyfriend.

People who provide psychotherapy undeniably encounter some very unique and unorthodox people and situations in their clinical practices. Psychotherapists are human beings; because of their human nature, many of these unique situations evoke internal reactions. Psychotherapy necessitates a relationship between the therapist and the client; as such, a culture develops between the two in which they get to know each other, negotiate these reactions to one another, and ultimately learn and grow from them.

Sarah was referred by her GP to a cognitive behavioral therapist for stress management. Many people (consumers and health care providers alike) view cognitive behavioral therapy (CBT) as an ideal therapeutic approach when clients need structure and tools that will help them manage distress. Indeed, Sarah's GP made this referral because she believed that Sarah desperately needed skills to manage depression and anxiety, improve functioning when faced with challenges, and prevent future suicidal crises. Sarah bought into this notion wholeheartedly: she expressed a desire for tools and for other tangible gains that she could make in therapy, and she mentioned that she did not view previous courses of psychotherapy as helpful in this regard.

I will disclose that I was the psychotherapist who treated the clients who form the basis for Sarah's case illustration (although I use the term *therapist* throughout the main chapters of the book for more generalized descriptive purposes). For context, I am a cognitive behavioral therapist who has a full-time practice (approximately 35 clients per week) focused on the delivery of evidence-based psychotherapy. I have held many academic appointments (including faculty appointments at the Dr. Aaron T. Beck Psychopathology Research Center at the University of Pennsylvania School of Medicine and at the Beck Institute for Cognitive Behavior Therapy), and I have trained and supervised thousands of clinicians across the globe in CBT. I have delivered CBT to many, many individuals with mixed clinical presentations characterized by multiple mental health diagnoses and the gamut of personality traits. I joke with my clients that I have "lived and breathed" CBT well over 40 hours per week across my clinical, training, and scholarly work for over 25 years.

In Sarah's case, I concurred that she would benefit from the acquisition of skills and principles to manage emotional distress. Indeed, in the 61 sessions in which I saw Sarah over the course of a 15-month period, I educated her about and practiced with her strategies such as cognitive restructuring, schema modification, behavioral activation, social problem solving, interpersonal effectiveness, distress tolerance, and mindfulness and acceptance (some of which are illustrated later in this book). I am not above admitting (sheepishly, though) that I was initially skeptical that Sarah would respond to my style of therapy. Between her history of defiance and her "alternative" style of self-presentation and my own ultra-organized style and (at times) overenthusiasm for the power of CBT, I wondered whether she would be interested in the psychoeducation I could provide for her and the specific homework exercises that I almost always encourage my clients to complete. Because Sarah had participated in so many courses of psychiatric and psychotherapeutic treatment in the past, I wondered about her commitment to treatment and about negative attitudes toward treatment that she might have developed over time (cf. Wenzel et al., 2008). I wondered whether her mental health issues were consistent with borderline personality disorder and, as such, I expected that at some point she would demonstrate belligerence toward me or other therapy-interfering behaviors. I wondered how long Sarah would be able to remain in treatment with me as an out-of-network provider who does not accept insurance, in light of the fact that she was employed in the restaurant industry and received no financial (or other) support from her family-of-origin. In addition, I wondered about her insight, as she was distraught about the unfairness of the way in which her boyfriend "discarded" her, when the entire time she was married to someone who (by her report) is kind, gentle, and supportive.

I can now say that I, unequivocally, was incredibly wrong in my initial impressions of Sarah and her capacity to respond to CBT and my style of psychotherapy. And being wrong in these impressions taught me invaluable lessons as a mental health provider. To take that notion one step further, it taught me invaluable lessons about life. I fully believe that I learned just as much from my work with Sarah as she learned from me.

The reason I make these declarations is that I experienced something powerful with Sarah, and my subjective sense is that this element was transformative in her healing and in both of our growth. As she and her GP had hoped, Sarah indeed acquired a vast array of cognitive behavioral strategies and skills, disproving my speculation that she would reject psychoeducation and homework. She never once demonstrated any therapy-interfering behavior. She arrived early for sessions, canceled well in advance if she needed to miss a session, scheduled several sessions out to ensure that she had protected time on my calendar, completed her therapy homework, and (on occasion) reached out to me in between sessions only in a judicious and appropriate manner. Thus, she disproved my hypothesis that she would demonstrate borderline personality behavior toward me and our work during the course of treatment. Sarah admitted that she was on a tight budget, but she expressed that she truly valued quality mental health treatment and made a special point to save money wisely in order to cover her sessions (and she never missed or was late for a payment). And the depth and insight that she displayed about her choices, her past, her family-of-origin, her complex relationship situation, and (as time went on, from a cognitive behavioral perspective) the core beliefs that formed the basis for her maladaptive schemas were among the most sophisticated of any clients with whom I have worked, despite the initial lack of insight that I observed.

There was something special that even went beyond these observations. Although I have a genuine liking of almost every client I see and genuine care for every single client I see, I found that I especially liked and cared for Sarah. She was an artist who did amazing work with everyday objects, and I admired her talent and ingenuity. In fact, she viewed her clothing, jewelry, makeup, and hairstyles as living works of art themselves. We stumbled upon the fact that aspects of our taste in music overlapped, so we often informed one another of bands that were playing at local venues. She was committed to her Wiccan practice in a way that I rarely saw among my own friends who were active in their mainstream spiritual communities. I was humbled by Sarah's extensive knowledge of art, design, music, and religion. She held personal relationships in very high regard, and I felt like I intimately knew her husband and a few of her close friends. Perhaps most profoundly, through our ever-evolving case formulation, we realized that she had been given the message from adolescence that she is "mentally ill" and is a perpetual "patient," which contributed to a lack of confidence that she could manage stress and disappointment through healthy means rather than destructive ones. Sarah worked toward shifting her core belief of being the patient to one of someone characterized by strength and centeredness, concurrently eliminating problematic coping behaviors that served to reinforce unhealthy beliefs. At the end of treatment, she gave me the feedback that I was the only mental health provider who believed in her and who did not dismiss her as mentally ill with little hope of being a good citizen who makes meaningful contributions to their community.

Put another way, Sarah and I did tremendous cognitive behavioral work together, and I believe it was the many aspects of the therapeutic relationship that made it so memorable. Specifically, we had an exceptionally strong therapeutic alliance in which we agreed fully on the goals and tasks of treatment; our therapeutic alliance was further enhanced by the incredible bond that formed the foundation of our care for one another. When we had reactions toward each other on the basis of our own histories, we discussed them openly and used them to inform our work. Moreover, we had a genuine connection (called the *real relationship*) that made us both look forward to our sessions together. I believe that we harnessed the power of the therapeutic relationship to elevate the CBT work in which we were engaged together. I learned quickly not to "judge a book by its cover," to see the beauty of human individuality, and to channel that beauty into a customized approach to help others.

In all, the totality of the course of treatment with Sarah was much more than the standard application of CBT techniques and the coaching of clients in the use of tools. I believe that every course of CBT can and should be conducted in this manner (even if I am manifesting the dreaded "should" statement, a classic cognitive distortion that many cognitive behavioral therapists teach their clients to avoid). Some people (consumers and health care providers alike) perceive CBT as so structured and technique driven that it leaves little room for emotional experiencing and the cultivation and use of a deep and meaningful therapeutic relationship. In this volume, I hope to show the reader how close attention to the therapeutic relationship—and even reverence of it—can elevate the delivery and experience of CBT, for both the client and therapist.

THERAPEUTIC RELATIONSHIP-FOCUSED COGNITIVE BEHAVIORAL THERAPY

INTRODUCTION

The Therapeutic Relationship and Its Relevance to Cognitive Behavioral Therapy

Cognitive behavioral therapy (CBT) is a powerful, efficacious approach to psychotherapy for a host of mental health and adjustment issues. It is an active, problem-focused, and time-sensitive approach to treatment in which therapists (a) form a sophisticated case formulation of the cognitive, emotional, behavioral, and environmental factors that contribute to, maintain, and exacerbate pathology; and (b) collaborate with the client to apply strategic interventions meant to reshape one or more aspects of this system. CBT has transformed the lives of countless individuals, facilitating healing that, for so many, had been elusive. And yet, it is not without controversy. One topic that receives much debate among scholars and providers within the mental health field is the role of the therapeutic relationship in the delivery and efficacy of CBT.

Allow me to illustrate this observation with an anecdote. When I am training mental health professionals who hope to obtain advanced supervision in CBT, they often pose a scenario like this: "I'm having a reaction to my client, probably based in my own 'stuff.' It feels like countertransference. I think this is off-limits in CBT. Right?" Here is another example: "My client just experienced a significant loss, and I thought it would be off-putting to implement

https://doi.org/10.1037/0000424-001

a CBT strategy. I just focused on providing care and support. But this means that I was no longer doing CBT. Right?" I always find the insertion of the simple question of reassurance ("Right?") to be fascinating because therapists, in certain instances, seem to have an intuitive draw toward attending directly to the therapeutic relationship, but they fear that by doing so, they would be stepping outside of protocol and, therefore, would be out of compliance. In other words, many therapists have the sense that a focus on what is happening in the therapeutic relationship is part and parcel of other types of psychotherapies (e.g., psychodynamic psychotherapy) and that to be "doing" CBT with fidelity, they must be limited to the technical application of strategies that promote cognitive and behavioral change.

My response in these and similar circumstances is, without question, "Wrong!" These assertions could not be further from the truth. I contend that the highest-quality CBT is delivered when simultaneous attention is given to the cultivation, nurturance, and enhancement of the therapeutic relationship and to the strategic and responsive delivery of cognitive behavioral therapeutic interventions (cf. Kohlenberg & Tsai, 1991; Safran & Segal, 1990). Part of the cultivation, nurturance, and enhancement of the therapeutic relationship is intuiting and listening to our clients' needs for empathy, support, validation, and care, especially after experiencing a significant loss, disappointment, or taxing challenge. Furthermore, attention directed to the therapeutic relationship itself may provide an important learning experience that prompts cognitive change about the self and relationships as well as behavioral changes in the way in which clients manage their relationships. I also contend that some of the very best CBT occurs when a pivotal issue has arisen in the therapeutic relationship, and cognitive behavioral principles and strategies are used to understand it, work through it, learn from it, and generalize it to other relationships outside of therapy. These contentions essentially form the thesis of this book on what I call *therapeutic relationship-focused CBT* (TRF-CBT).

Unfortunately, a stereotype exists about cognitive behavioral therapists, which is that they have ignored or minimized the importance of the therapeutic relationship on therapy process and outcome. This stereotype could have emerged because CBT is, indeed, a fairly structured therapy with treatment goals and an agenda that is set for each session and because there are, indeed, a vast array of techniques that are delivered with technical precision. Nevertheless, I believe the stereotype to be false. For instance, in their seminal book on behavior therapy, Goldfried and Davison (1976) emphasized the utmost importance of delivering behavioral techniques in a warm and empathetic manner of interaction with the client, making the provocative statement, "Any behavior therapist who maintains that principles of learning and social influence are all one needs to know in order to bring about behavior change is out of contact with clinical reality" (p. 55). Wilson and Evans (1977) regarded the therapeutic relationship as being a catalyst of behavioral change strategies, such as by providing reinforcement to increase desirable behaviors (e.g., appropriate interpersonal behaviors that enhance relationships), improving the likelihood of client response to therapist intervention, and establishing therapeutic expectancies (e.g., optimism that therapy can improve their symptoms). Arnkoff (1983) observed that the therapeutic relationship allows therapists to observe, in real time, aspects of clients' interpersonal functioning and to help clients adjust their interpersonal behavior within the relationship in a way that will generalize to relationships in their lives. Fast forwarding 40 to 45 years later, a consensus of 32 expert cognitive behavioral therapists regarded the development and maintenance of a good therapeutic alliance (a component of the therapeutic relationship, as described in Chapters 1 and 2 of this volume) as a core effective component of good CBT (Taylor et al., 2020).

Aaron T. Beck, who is regarded by most as the father of CBT, was heavily inspired by the writing of client-centered therapists who assigned a central role of the therapeutic relationship in psychotherapy, most notably Carl Rogers. Dr. Beck devoted a chapter to the therapeutic relationship in his seminal volume on cognitive therapy of depression (A. T. Beck et al., 1979), although his assertion in that chapter—that a strong therapeutic relationship is "a necessary but not sufficient agent of change" (p. 45)—often provokes strong reactions in therapists who practice from other theoretical orientations. Furthermore, observing Dr. Beck harness the power of the therapeutic relationship in real time was particularly striking for those of us fortunate enough to witness him conduct role plays and client consultations. I witnessed participants in workshops at the Beck Institute for Cognitive Behavior Therapy who watched Dr. Beck in action and were consistently awed by his kindness, empathy, sense of humor, and uncanny ability to connect with clients who were from very different backgrounds than himself. In the post-demonstration discussions that I often led, workshop participants concurred that they had expected Dr. Beck to demonstrate the masterful application of CBT strategies and techniques; what they had not expected was how "human" Dr. Beck came across to his clients and how it was the quality of the therapeutic relationship, rather than any specific CBT strategy he implemented, that stood out most.

Another insight about Dr. Beck's views of the therapeutic relationship became evident in a question-and-answer session in which I participated with him in 2019, approximately 2 years before his death in 2021 at age 100. In that session, Dr. Beck remarked that he made an important error in his early writings about cognitive therapy (which elicited a gasp from the audience). Specifically, Dr. Beck remarked that he assumed that clinicians learning CBT would have already had training in basic counseling skills and would have a great appreciation for ways to build the therapeutic relationship, so he focused his writing on the application of cognitive and behavioral principles, strategies, and techniques that were meant to be delivered in the context of a strong therapeutic relationship. Unfortunately, over time, this assumption morphed into a stereotype that cognitive behavioral therapists are uninterested in or inattentive to the therapeutic relationship (or both), which Dr. Beck lamented. This stereotype is beginning to loosen with the publishing of full volumes devoted to the therapeutic relationship in CBT (Gilbert & Leahy, 2007; Kazantzis et al., 2017), conceptual peer-reviewed manuscripts on the importance of the therapeutic relationship (K. S. Dobson, 2022; Kazantzis, Dattilio, et al., 2018; Lejuez et al., 2005), and empirical investigations into the role that components of the therapeutic relationship play in outcome in CBT (some of which are referenced in Chapter 2 of this volume). Nevertheless, criticism continues to be directed toward or implied about CBT with regard to the assumption that cognitive behavioral therapists assign a minimal role to the therapeutic relationship (e.g., Shedler, 2010) or do not fully appreciate distinctions among essential ingredients in the therapeutic relationship (Gelso, 2011).

I do, however, believe that cognitive behavioral therapists could stand to learn from and adapt the scholarship outside of the strict cognitive behavioral framework (e.g., from the psychodynamic literature, from the humanistic literature) that has great relevance to psychotherapy process and outcome (cf. Goldfried, 2013). Although CBT experts do a fantastic job of conducting empirical research to validate relevant constructs and quantify their association with treatment outcome, they do so almost exclusively within the cognitive behavioral framework (although there are some notable exceptions, such as collaborations at the University of Pennsylvania between Dr. Beck and renowned psychodynamic researchers such as Lester Luborsky, Paul Crits-Christoph, and Jacques Barber; cf. Crits-Christoph et al., 1998). With the publication of important books on CBT and the therapeutic relationship (Gilbert & Leahy, 2007; Kazantzis et al., 2017) in the past decade and a half, the time is ripe to integrate insights from outside of the cognitive behavioral framework to maximize the therapeutic relationship in the delivery of CBT. I believe cognitive behavioral therapists can learn a great deal from these insights that will only strengthen the efficacy of the approach.

The purposes of this book are (a) to provide a broad conceptualization of the therapeutic relationship by consulting and integrating literature that cuts across theoretical frameworks and (b) to apply this broad conceptualization to illustrate the way in which the therapeutic relationship can be used as both a facilitator of change as well as a central agent of change within the cognitive behavioral framework. In addition to acknowledging important theoretical and empirical scholarship on the therapeutic relationship that has been advanced by renowned CBT scholars, this book highlights and integrates important insights from scholars who operate outside of the cognitive behavioral framework. In addition, it provides specific clinical guidance for developing, maintaining, and enhancing the therapeutic relationship throughout the course of CBT, and it provides illustrations to support the notion expressed in the previous paragraph—that some of the very best CBT occurs in the context of an issue that is happening in real time in session within the therapeutic relationship (cf. Kohlenberg & Tsai, 1991; Safran & Segal, 1990). What is expected to emerge from this volume is a description of a TRF-CBT that brings together key scholarly advancements on the therapeutic relationship, translates them into clinical guidance, and sets up a foundation for future empirical research and clinical practice.

TRF-CBT is not yet another new manifestation of CBT. Instead, it is a framework that can be applied to any CBT protocol, approach, or delivery, in which the cognitive behavioral therapist is especially mindful of the following:

(a) Cultivating the therapeutic relationship, as early as during the very first contact with the client;

(b) Paying relatively equal attention to the therapeutic relationship and cognitive behavioral strategies and techniques as the course of a client's CBT progresses;

(c) Delivering CBT strategies and techniques from a client-centered framework;

(d) Applying CBT strategies and techniques in real time when issues arise within the therapeutic relationship to repair any potential rupture to the relationship and create a corrective learning experience that can be applied to relationships in clients' lives outside of session (cf. Alexander & French, 1946; Eubanks & Goldfried, 2019);

(e) When relevant, cultivating a therapeutic relationship that provides a fundamental learning experience for clients who have had damaging relationships with key figures, such as a parent, a significant romantic other, or another person who played an important role in their lives (cf. Young et al., 2003);

(f) When relevant, relying on the strength of the therapeutic relationship to weather any temporary plateaus or impasses that occur during the course of treatment (i.e., even in moments in which it seems that the cognitive behavioral interventions are not exerting their desired effects, the therapist and client are still cultivating and coexperiencing their therapeutic connection as they continue on their path to see the client through to recovery); and

(g) Using elements of the therapeutic relationship strategically, or in a way that facilitates the successful implementation of CBT strategies and techniques, as well as serving as an active agent of important cognitive, emotional, and behavioral change (cf. Zilcha-Mano, 2017, 2021).

I contend that delivering CBT with a focus on the therapeutic relationship pays homage to the history of psychotherapy scholarship, discourse, and research; enhances the therapeutic experience for both client and therapist; and, importantly (when verified by empirical research), has the potential to enhance engagement, retention in treatment, and ultimate outcome. Moreover, it is not difficult to surmise that when a client has a positive experience in psychotherapy attributed to a strong therapeutic relationship, they will readily return to treatment if they notice signs of relapse or are facing another major challenge in their life, and they would even speak highly of psychotherapy to others and encourage their loved ones to seek it out themselves.

Many psychotherapy research scholars differentiate between the relational and technical aspects of psychotherapy. There are an abundance of CBT texts that focus on the important technical aspects of the delivery of CBT, including fundamental strategies such as cognitive restructuring, behavioral activation, exposure, problem solving, and relapse prevention. This volume takes a different perspective in that I focus on the relational aspect that can be harnessed both in its own right and during implementation of the technical side of CBT.

STRUCTURE OF THIS VOLUME AND FINAL THOUGHTS

This volume is divided into two parts. Part I on contextual foundations describes theory, discourse, empirical research, and some clinical applications of general aspects of the therapeutic relationship. Chapter 1 considers various definitions of the therapeutic relationship as well as three components of the therapeutic relationship that pervade the psychotherapy literature in general and the psychodynamic literature in particular: (a) the therapeutic alliance, (b) transference and countertransference, and (c) the real relationship. In Chapter 2, I describe the common or generic factors that are applicable in any type of psychotherapy, highlighting research on their relation to outcome, referencing their application in CBT-specific research, and suggesting ways to facilitate them in treatment. I illustrate the dynamic unfolding of many of these constructs with the case of Sarah first presented in the Preface of this volume. Chapter 3 takes the same approach with CBT-specific factors that contribute to the therapeutic relationship, with much dialogue between Sarah and her therapist to demonstrate specific ways to apply these factors in conjunction with the common or generic factors described in Chapter 2. After reading Part I, it is expected that the reader will come away with a broad overview of factors at work in the cultivation of the therapeutic relationship.

Part II of this volume summarizes clinical guidance for the implementation of TRF-CBT. Collectively, these clinical chapters illustrate ways to be mindful of the common and specific therapeutic relationship-enhancing elements described in Chapters 2 and 3 in nurturing a real, genuine therapeutic relationship. They also describe ways in which relationship-enhancing elements and CBT strategies and techniques can address a potential rupture in the therapeutic alliance. In Chapter 4, I describe principles of which therapists can be mindful even in the very first contacts with a client inquiring about CBT and scheduling a first session, as well as ways that cognitive behavioral therapists can build a therapeutic alliance with their clients in the first several sessions. Chapter 5 focuses on the use of the therapeutic relationship in the delivery of cognitive restructuring, a fundamental strategic intervention in CBT. Chapter 6 considers social problem solving, including the solving of problems that emerge within the therapy arrangement. Chapter 7 highlights the importance of a strong therapeutic relationship as a foundation for undertaking exposure interventions, and it discusses ways in which the therapeutic relationship itself can serve as an agent of exposure. Chapter 8 turns to schema modification, or the shifting of painful fundamental beliefs and associated affective and behavioral patterns that emerge from clients' past experiences. It is here that cognitive behavioral work is especially ripe for transference and countertransference to occur (Leahy, 2012). Finally, Chapter 9 focuses on the ending of treatment, including reflecting on the therapeutic relationship as treatment ends and working through any reactions that clients might have. The volume concludes with Chapter 10, reiterating the main premises of TRF-CBT and proposing a rich framework for conceptualizing the therapeutic relationship within the practice of CBT.

I leave the reader with the following sentiment as they embark on critical evaluation and thoughtful reflection on the therapeutic relationship in CBT. As stated eloquently by psychoanalyst Ralph Greenson (1978), "Technical errors may cause pain and confusion, but they are usually repairable; failure of humanness is much harder to remedy" (p. 377). Above all, this volume is about being human as one delivers CBT (cf. J. S. Beck, 2021). And humanness comes with "warts and all"—in being human, sometimes therapists inadvertently do things that are not received well by the client. These are opportunities for therapists to grow as professionals and, more importantly, for clients to grow in their handling of the nuances of close interpersonal relationships. More generally, the gift of humanness has the potential to provide clients the opportunity to shift unhelpful and upsetting beliefs about their capacity for relationships, their own desirability in relationships, and the degree to which relationships are warm and trustworthy. From my standpoint, there is no greater experience that we can provide our clients in need.

PART **I** CONTEXTUAL
FOUNDATIONS

1
THE THERAPEUTIC RELATIONSHIP
Definition and Components

A logical starting point for the illustration of therapeutic relationship-focused cognitive behavioral therapy (TRF-CBT) is with an in-depth understanding of the therapeutic relationship itself. In this chapter, I consider various definitions of the therapeutic relationship that have been posed in the psychotherapy literature. Then, I turn to three standard components of the therapeutic relationship that have been highlighted in the psychotherapy literature, only one of which (i.e., the therapeutic alliance) has routinely been considered and evaluated in the CBT literature specifically. I chose this tripartite model because of its historical significance in the psychotherapy literature, fully realizing that it may not be embraced by all in the CBT community. It is my hope that the reader will entertain this expanded conceptualization of the therapeutic relationship; think critically about ways to recognize the components described in this chapter and utilize them during the course of CBT; and, perhaps, broaden their view of the relational processes at work in CBT.

https://doi.org/10.1037/0000424-002
Therapeutic Relationship-Focused Cognitive Behavioral Therapy, by A. Wenzel

THERAPEUTIC RELATIONSHIP: DEFINITIONS

Most therapists have an innate sense of what is meant by the term *therapeutic relationship*. In my proposal for this volume, I stated that I had hoped to supply a range of definitions of the therapeutic relationship, comparing and contrasting commonalities among them as well as distinct features (perhaps as a function of theoretical orientation). Much to my surprise, I found that there were far fewer explicit definitions of the therapeutic relationship than I had anticipated. It seemed almost as if the notion of the therapeutic relationship is so ubiquitous that people who study and deliver psychotherapy intuitively know what it means. Nevertheless, it is important to consider some definitions that have, indeed, been published to serve as a backdrop for the material in this volume.

John Norcross and Michael Lambert (2019) referred to the psychotherapy relationship as the "healing alliance between client and clinician" (p. 2). The word "alliance" suggests that an association exists in which both parties have mutual goals and experience mutual benefits. The notion of the therapeutic alliance is a cornerstone in the structural components of the therapeutic relationship, although the Norcross and Lambert definition is broader than the therapeutic alliance that is discussed in the next section of this chapter. The word "healing" suggests that much of what takes place in the therapeutic relationship is associated with the client becoming healthy, achieving wellness, and fostering self-growth. Although this definition is quite broad and general, it paints the therapeutic relationship as one that is benign and nurturing, as well as one in which both the therapist and client are invested in the outcome of treatment.

Another oft-cited definition was proposed by Gelso and Carter (1985), stating that the therapeutic relationship is "the feelings and attitudes that therapist and client have toward one another and the manner in which they are expressed" (p. 159). This definition indicates that cognition, emotion, and behavior are essential components of the therapeutic relationship. Cognition could include views of one another's character (e.g., "My client is a strong person," "My therapist is a kind individual"), concern for their well-being (e.g., "I hope my client is doing okay in the midst of these contentious divorce proceedings," "I hope my therapist is feeling well after being out sick last week"), expectations for their work together (e.g., "I truly believe that I can help this client," "I like that my therapist can teach me tools for stress management"), and evaluations of their ongoing relationship (e.g., "I am proud of this client after last week's breakthrough," "My therapist really seems to care about me"). Emotions include the vast array of feelings that we have toward people when we think of them in general (e.g., a sense of warmth, a sense of dread), as well as feelings that we experience in particular situations (e.g., joy when a client reports that a session has been helpful, frustration when it seems as if the therapist has forgotten an important detail). Behavior (or the way cognition and emotion are expressed) can be verbal (e.g., a statement of pleasure with therapeutic work, a statement of frustrated disagreement with the therapist's missed session policy), nonverbal (e.g., a smile, a frown), or action oriented (e.g., a therapist proactively reaching out to the client's psychiatrist to maximize coordination of care, a client missing a session without notice).

In addition to these cognitive, emotional, and behavioral components, Gelso and Carter's (1985) definition emphasizes the fact that the relationship is reciprocal; in other words, both the therapist and client hold their own unique cognitions, emotions, and behaviors about one another and their work together. Although this point might seem self-evident, it is worth highlighting because many approaches to understanding the therapeutic relationship emphasize therapist behavior (e.g., empathy) without considering what the client brings to the relationship (Gelso, 2011; Safran & Segal, 1990). The therapeutic relationship is a fluid, dynamic entity that is shaped by the interactions between a therapist and a client, expectations they have for one another and the work in which they are engaging, and their own personal histories (Barrett-Lennard, 1985).

Kazantzis et al. (2017) supplied a similar definition of the therapeutic relationship, defining it as "an exchange between therapist and client that develops for the purpose of sharing intimate thoughts, beliefs, and emotions in an endeavor to facilitate change" (p. 17). The reference to "sharing" further emphasizes the reciprocal relationship between the therapist and client and hints at a partnership of equals who both contribute to the interactions that take place between them. Moreover, the reference to facilitating change suggests that the therapeutic relationship is purposeful and can prompt important changes that clients make in their own lives, perhaps "healing" as Norcross and Lambert (2019) suggested. Kazantzis et al. (2017) further delineated generic therapist behaviors and goals of the therapeutic relationship that are evident in psychotherapies conducted across theoretical orientations (e.g., empathy, positive regard) and CBT-specific therapist behaviors and goals (e.g., collaborative empiricism, Socratic dialogue). Elaboration of these generic elements of the therapeutic relationship is considered in Chapter 2 of this volume, and discussion of CBT-specific elements of the therapeutic relationship is contained in Chapter 3.

The three specific definitions discussed in this section offer a welcome foundation to guide our consideration of this construct. Moreover, an understanding of the components discussed in the next section can help guide therapist behavior in any one moment with a client to achieve an ongoing cultivation of the therapeutic relationship.

THERAPEUTIC RELATIONSHIP: COMPONENTS

Scholars within the psychoanalytic/psychodynamic tradition have long regarded the therapeutic relationship as a tripartite model consisting of three components: (a) the therapeutic alliance, (b) transference and countertransference, and (c) the real relationship (i.e., the "human" connection between the therapist and client; cf. Gelso, 2014; Gelso & Samstag, 2008; Greenson, 1965, 1967; Meissner, 2007). The notion of the therapeutic alliance has been welcomed by the CBT community, and assessment of the therapeutic alliance is frequently included in CBT process research, some of which is noted in Chapter 2 of this volume. In contrast, transference and countertransference and the real relationship are referenced much less in the CBT literature and during CBT trainings. However, it is possible that greater consideration of these constructs would have the potential to strengthen the relational component of our cognitive behavioral therapeutic work with clients. Throughout the volume, I consider ways in which all three constructs—the therapeutic alliance, transference and countertransference, and the real relationship—can manifest in CBT to both facilitate the application of cognitive behavioral strategies and techniques and to be the focus of corrective learning themselves.

Component 1: Therapeutic Alliance

In a seminal paper that still has great influence over research and practice of psychotherapy today, Edward Bordin (1979) identified three facets of the *therapeutic alliance* that facilitate the work of therapy: (a) an agreement between the therapist and client on the goals of therapy, (b) an agreement between the therapist and client in deciding upon the tasks of therapy, and (c) the bond between the therapist and client. Thus, the therapeutic alliance captures the essence of a successful working relationship between the therapist and client, such that they are aligned in what they are hoping to accomplish in psychotherapy and how they would go about doing so (Gelso & Carter, 1994). This means that they are "on the same page" with their work and are operating together collaboratively to achieve well-defined goals. Moreover, this alliance keeps clients engaged in therapy and maintains their commitment to the work that has been proposed (Hatcher, 2010).

The therapeutic alliance has received so much attention in the psychotherapy literature that it has been referred to as the quintessential integrative variable (Wolfe & Goldfried, 1988), and it is regarded as the most frequently studied process of change (Castonguay et al., 2006). It is not surprising that of the three components of the therapeutic relationship, the therapeutic alliance has received the most attention from CBT scholars, as two of its components (i.e., agreement on the goals of therapy and agreement on the tasks of therapy) are consistent with what are typically espoused as fundamental tenets of CBT (i.e., collaboration and goal setting; see Chapter 3 of this volume).

According to the Third Interdivisional APA Task Force on Evidence-Based Relationships and Responsiveness (Norcross & Lambert, 2018), there is "demonstrable evidence" that the therapeutic alliance is an efficacious element of the therapeutic relationship in its relation to outcome, with much empirical research supporting this association (e.g., Barber et al., 2000; Klein et al., 2003). Authors of meta-analytic work have calculated correlations with r values ranging from .22 to almost .28 between the therapeutic alliance and outcome across a number of different types of psychotherapies (Flückiger et al., 2018, 2020; Horvath & Symonds, 1991; Horvath et al., 2011; Martin et al., 2000), which accounts for roughly 5% of the variance in outcome. These results mean that there is a small but consistent association between the strength of the therapeutic alliance and outcome and that the therapeutic alliance accounts for a small but meaningful contribution to treatment outcome. Moreover, research examining session-by-session assessments of the therapeutic alliance and symptom severity demonstrates that increases in the therapeutic alliance detected in one session are associated with symptom reduction in the subsequent session and delayed effects on symptoms that are detected in the session thereafter (Falkenström et al., 2016). Conversely, poor alliance is associated with early dropout (Constantino et al., 2002; Sharf et al., 2010).

A strong early therapeutic alliance can improve ultimate treatment outcome in several ways, such as by engaging clients in treatment, instilling hope, and providing a scaffolding for the remainder of the course of therapy (Gaston, 1990; Horvath & Luborsky, 1993; Whisman, 1993). Many of my clients have expressed at the commencement of treatment that they would like an overview of therapy, including the course, procedures, and expected outcome, to understand more fully what they are undertaking. Collaboration and explicit agreement on the goals and tasks of therapy emerge as these reasonable requests are addressed in the early sessions of psychotherapy. Moreover, a strong bond can be inviting, such that it keeps the client coming back for sessions even when the work is difficult to face. The therapeutic alliance, then, gives a "human touch" to the proactive and productive work that has been tasked by the client and therapist.

Alliance Ruptures

When one consults the literature on the therapeutic alliance, they will see references to both the "therapeutic alliance" and the "working alliance," and, at times, the terms are used seemingly interchangeably. According to Hatcher (2010), experts who use the term therapeutic alliance rather than working alliance are expanding the construct to include not only the collaborative work and agreement on goals but also the acts of developing, maintaining, and repairing the alliance as important activities in and of themselves. In this way, the therapeutic alliance is viewed as a dynamic entity that evolves between the client and therapist, requiring attention and effort to cultivate, shape, and refine. This broad view of the therapeutic alliance incorporates a focus on repair as a central feature, suggesting that instances in which the therapeutic alliance is compromised are relatively common in courses of psychotherapy (Safran et al., 1990). There is a rich line of research and scholarship that has examined this very issue. It is considered briefly here because much contemporary research has been devoted to disruptions in the therapeutic alliance, and because a central premise of TRF-CBT is that these disruptions can be viewed as opportunities for growth, skill development, and good outcome at the end of treatment.

According to Eubanks-Carter et al. (2010), a *rupture* is a "deterioration in the alliance, manifested by a lack of collaboration between patient and therapist on tasks or goals, or by a strain in the emotional bond" (p. 74). A rupture can be a major breakdown in the relationship, an instance of minor tension that might not be fully evident to the therapist or client, or a "vicious cycle" of push and pull between the therapist's beliefs and the client's beliefs and behavioral responses (Muran et al., 2010). When the therapeutic alliance is measured quantitatively, a rupture is defined as an instance in which alliance ratings decrease by at least 20% between the first third and the second third of the session (Safran et al., 1990). Between 19% and 37% of clients and between 43% and 56% of therapists report the presence of ruptures during the course of treatment (Eames & Roth, 2000; Muran et al., 2009), and neutral observers identify ruptures in up to 75% of sessions (Eubanks-Carter et al., 2010). Results from qualitative research suggest that the two most common reasons cited by clients for ruptures were therapist behaviors that were not received well and the absence of therapist behaviors that were wanted or expected (Hill, 2010; Rhodes et al., 1994). There are two main types of ruptures: (a) *withdrawal ruptures*, when the client moves away from the therapist (i.e., disengages, becomes silent); and (b) *confrontation ruptures*, when the client moves against the therapist (i.e., expresses anger or dissatisfaction). Muran et al. (2010) described these types as follows:

> . . . withdrawal and confrontation markers can be understood as reflecting different ways of coping with the dialectical tension between two fundamental human motivations: *the need for agency versus the need for relatedness.* Ruptures mark a breakdown in the negotiation of these needs with another. Thus, a withdrawal rupture could be understood as the pursuit of *relatedness* at the expense of the need for *self-agency*, and a confrontation rupture the expression of *self-agency* at the expense of *relatedness.* (pp. 321–322; italics in original)

Indeed, within the CBT literature, it has been found that in the context of client resistance (i.e., client behaviors that oppose the direction set by the therapist), therapist responses characterized by affiliation and reinforcement of client agency are associated with better outcome than responses characterized by hostility and directiveness (Hara et al., 2022). I believe that resistance can be a precursor to, but is not necessarily the equivalent of, a rupture; nevertheless, a shift toward a focus on the therapeutic relationship in the here-and-now in instances in which a client is not receptive to the therapeutic intervention can be helpful in maintaining a collaborative working relationship characterized by respect for client autonomy.

Most therapists (understandably) find the prospect of a rupture in the therapeutic alliance to be daunting. After all, most therapists enter the field with the hope that they can be a positive influence in their clients' lives, and a rupture often means that their client is having a negative reaction to something the therapist did. In actuality, ruptures can serve as opportunities both for increasing the bond between the therapist and client as well as for ultimately improving outcome. This is the case because the rupture is addressed before clients decide to disengage and drop out of treatment. Moreover, repair of the rupture serves as an important corrective learning experience that clients can apply to relationships outside of session that might be characterized by some sort of difficulty. In fact, meta-analyses have found a moderate relation between rupture resolution and positive outcomes in treatment ($r = .24–.29$; Eubanks et al., 2018; Safran et al., 2011). Ruptures that are successfully repaired can facilitate sudden gains in the therapeutic alliance in subsequent sessions (Zilcha-Mano et al., 2019), bringing the therapeutic alliance to greater heights than if a rupture had not occurred. Conversely, ruptures that are not accompanied by repair are associated with inferior outcomes (Haugen et al., 2017). Much attention has been devoted to clinical guidance for the repair of therapeutic alliance ruptures (Muran

& Eubanks, 2020; Safran & Muran, 1996, 2000; Safran et al., 2001), which has important implications for TRF-CBT (e.g., Okamoto & Kazantzis, 2021).

Research by Hara et al. (2015) raised the possibility that cognitive behavioral therapists are not always adept at identifying signs of ruptures. In this study, therapist ratings of resistance were unrelated to client ratings of the therapeutic alliance, homework compliance, and posttreatment worry, unlike observer ratings of resistance. These results suggest that cognitive behavioral therapists could use guidance in conceptualizing ruptures and identifying when ruptures are happening. In the clinical chapters of this volume (Chapters 4–9 in Part II), in-session instances in which potential ruptures are beginning are described, along with dialogue illustrating the manner in which therapists can address and repair them. These illustrations will demonstrate that a focus on the relationship is the foundational factor in repairing potential ruptures, and that cognitive behavioral strategies and tools can be used for repair through that focus on the relationship.

Component 2: Transference and Countertransference

The second main component of the therapeutic relationship involves the reactions that clients have to their therapist on the basis of their own personal histories, as well as therapists' reactions to clients based on their own personal histories. According to Gelso (2019), *transference* is "the patient's experience and perceptions of the therapist that are shaped by the patient's own psychological structures and past, involving carryover from and displacement onto the therapist of feelings, attitudes, and behaviors belonging rightfully to and originating in earlier significant relationships" (p. 11; cf. Gelso & Hayes, 1998). Research by Gelso and Bhatia (2012) suggested that transference occurs in all types of psychotherapy, not only in psychodynamic approaches that view the resolution of transference as a primary goal of successful treatment, although Gelso (2011) asserted that it is largely ignored by cognitive behavioral therapists unless it interferes with the work of therapy (a notion for which I hope to pose an alternative viewpoint with this volume). Moreover, transference is a phenomenon that is cocreated by both the client and the therapist, as opposed to something for which the client is solely responsible, as the client is reacting to something that the therapist has done (Gelso & Hayes, 1998).

Countertransference, as defined by Gelso (2019), is "the therapist's internal or external reactions to the patient shaped by the therapist's unresolved past or present emotional conflicts or vulnerabilities" (p. 25). Countertransference is not simply a strong reaction to a client; it is a reaction that has roots in the therapist's own "baggage." In fact, Gelso and Hayes (2007) are well-known for advancing the idea that viewing countertransference as all therapist reactions to a client is essentially useless because it encompasses everything. Thus, for a therapist reaction to be considered countertransference, it must be linked to a therapist's own belief system that stems from their own unique past experiences, a proposition called the *countertransference interaction hypothesis* (cf. Gelso et al., 1995; J. A. Hayes & Gelso, 1993). Countertransference can be acute, such as in response to a specific set of circumstances with specific clients, or chronic, stemming from a fundamental aspect of a therapist's personality (Reich, 1951). Examples of countertransference behaviors include (a) withdrawing from the client (e.g., remaining silent, daydreaming), (b) becoming overly involved with the client (e.g., excessive reassurance), and (c) expressing hostility (Gelso & Hayes, 2007). Although it is commonly thought that the most seasoned therapists do not demonstrate countertransference, research by J. A. Hayes et al. (1998) determined that countertransference occurred in 80% of sessions across a range of therapists with diverse levels of experience and psychotherapy orientations.

Transference can be negative, such as the client expressing anger at the therapist for behaving in a manner that reminds the client of someone who mistreated them in the past, or positive, such as the client idealizing the therapist for having qualities like a significant other from the client's past. Both types of transference have the potential to influence the course of therapeutic work, and both have the potential to bring issues to the forefront that, when worked through, bring about significant change in the client's life.

The following is a simple but powerful example of negative transference and countertransference reactions. I will never forget an instance in graduate school when I had begun to see clients in a training clinic, and I was assigned an extremely complicated case of a client with numerous psychiatric diagnoses. I was trying my darndest to connect with the client and to communicate an eagerness to build a relationship with her because I so badly wanted to be of service to her. However, she had a distinctive transference reaction to me, saying, "You remind me of my sister." I responded with a tentative "Oh really?"—hoping beyond hope that the reminder of her sister meant that she experienced a sense of warmth and belongingness in my presence. No such luck. The client continued, "Yeah, she was a blonde bimbo too." The admission, in turn, activated insecurity in me, as I recalled shame-inducing instances in my own past when I was dismissed as lacking in intelligence and insightfulness because of my long, blonde hair. Stunned and unsure of how to respond, I continued blandly with whatever therapeutic task had been the focus of that session, avoiding her statement altogether. Not surprisingly, this client failed to report for her subsequent session, and the clinic never heard from her again.

Had I been a more seasoned therapist, expecting transference reactions from clients because they are part of human nature and having the confidence to quickly conceptualize what was happening and work with them, I could have given the client space to say more about it. We could have had a rich conversation about the assumptions she was making about me, on the basis of her experiences with her sister, and the underlying beliefs that were activated when she found herself in that place. I could have allowed her space to talk more about the way she felt in the presence of her sister and how that was affecting her comfort level with me. The question remains as to whether this client would have continued with me in therapy, and ultimately had a growth experience in therapy, had we directly addressed and worked through this transference reaction and had I overcome the avoidance behavior induced by my countertransference reaction. However, the reader can be assured that I would handle this situation very differently at this stage of my career, with the utmost appreciation of the processes at work in the therapeutic relationship.

Positive transference and countertransference reactions are, in some ways, trickier to navigate because on the surface, they behave in a way that enhances aspects of the therapeutic relationship (e.g., the bond between the therapist and client), but they can, nevertheless, disrupt therapeutic work. Take, for example, a young adult client whose mother passed away prematurely; the client very much misses her mother and feels nurtured and even "held" (cf. Winnicott, 1955, 1963) by an older female therapist who reminds her of her mother. Certainly, the connection this client feels with the therapist would likely contribute to consistent attendance and a high level of engagement in therapy. However, it is possible that there could be unintended consequences of this identification, such as the client becoming increasingly dependent on the therapist for support and nurturance without learning how to obtain both from her other close relationships. The client could unwittingly obtain secondary gain from her symptoms by continuing with therapy indefinitely, rather than acquiring the mindset and tools she needs to function in life outside of session. I once knew of a situation in which a female client in this type of circumstance became so close with her therapist that she spent holidays with her therapist and her therapist's family—clearly an overstepping of clinical boundaries on the therapist's part, no matter how much the client's situation activated a rescuing and nurturing response in the therapist! Thus, it is essential for the therapist to identify instances of positive transference and carefully examine its function to ensure that it is not interfering with the ultimate goals and tasks of therapy or reinforcing unhelpful beliefs clients have about their own autonomy and independence, their capability of functioning in the world, and the role of healthy relationships.

Transference and countertransference can overlap with the therapeutic alliance because such reactions can cause ruptures in the alliance, and successful repair of the rupture to establish the therapeutic alliance can involve resolving the transference–countertransference process. In fact, it has been posited that alliance ruptures are essentially enactments of a transference–countertransference process (Safran & Kraus, 2014). Empirical research indicates that early expectations for the therapeutic alliance are determined in large part by projecting representations of significant others onto the therapist, although the impact of these representations changes over time as the client has the opportunity to get to know the therapist's personality and style (Zilcha-Mano et al., 2014). Moreover, there is empirical evidence that therapists impose their own representations with significant others, particularly parental figures, that can contribute to or detract from the repair of a rupture (Tishby & Wiseman, 2022). Thus, therapists are encouraged to be keenly aware of ways in which aspects of one therapeutic relationship component can affect, and are affected by, another.

Unlike the therapeutic alliance, transference and countertransference receive much less attention in the CBT literature (although for important exceptions, see A. T. Beck et al., 1979; J. S. Beck, 2021; Leahy, 2012). As will be illustrated in various capacities in this volume, I believe that it is important to attend to these constructs in our cognitive behavioral clinical work in order for clients to achieve powerful core belief change. Interestingly, A. T. Beck et al. (1979) suggested that the very nature of CBT helps to minimize the types of behaviors that can create a ripe context for transference and countertransference (e.g., passivity, lack of initiative) due to CBT's active, problem-focused nature. However, as many contemporary cognitive behavioral therapists can attest, CBT's active, problem-focused nature certainly does not eliminate the possibility of transference, as clients can have reactions to their perception that the therapist has high expectations for them, much like key figures in their past.

Component 3: Real Relationship

The *real relationship* between the therapist and client is defined as "the personal relationship existing between two or more persons as reflected in the degree to which each is genuine with the other and perceives the other in ways that befit the other" (Gelso, 2011, pp. 12–13). This term might strike many cognitive behavioral therapists as odd, as we are not typically taught about the "real relationship" in graduate school or in CBT trainings. The word "real" was chosen to distinguish this aspect of the therapeutic relationship from its other aspects that are influenced by transference and countertransference—which, by definition, distort the way in which the relationship is perceived. The therapist elements of genuineness and congruence (Rogers, 1957) are key contributors to the cultivation of the real relationship. The real relationship pertains both to the therapist and client as individuals experiencing one another, as well as to the communication between them (Couch, 1999) in a dynamic context in which each is responsive to the moment-by-moment unfolding of the session (Stiles et al., 1998).

Gelso's long line of scholarship has further divided the real relationship into (a) *genuineness*, or being authentic in the presence of the other; and (b) *realism*, or viewing the other in a way that transcends the viewer's need to impose their wishes, needs, or fears on the other (Gelso, 2011). Genuineness relies on both the therapist's ability to recognize their authentic experience and on their ability and willingness to communicate that authentic experience to the client (cf. Greenberg, 2002). According to Gelso (2011),

> [If a therapist] proceeds to be deeply immersed in the therapy experience, and shows the patient in numerous indirect ways that the patient is cared about and understood and if the therapist's indirect disclosures, as well as his or her direct therapeutic responses do not suggest any phoniness to the patient, this therapist is likely to be experienced as genuine, perhaps deeply so. (p. 33)

Realism, in contrast, refers to the accurate perception of the other. From a psychoanalytic perspective, the resolution of clients' transferences is replaced by the real relationship. Gelso (2011) made the provocative statement that cognitive behavioral therapists are concerned with neither the genuineness or realism aspects of the real relationship, instead focusing on developing a "good enough general relationship, oftentimes used synonymously with the word *rapport*, to facilitate the use of CBT techniques" (p. 22). This is another notion that I hope to dispel in this volume.

Furthermore, the nature of these components of the real relationship can be understood in terms of (a) *magnitude*, or the degree of genuineness and realism evident at any one time; and (b) *valence*, or the feelings and thoughts about one another and the relationship that can range from positive to negative. Gelso (2011) speculated that magnitude and positive valence correlate with outcome, in that the more genuineness and realism that occur in the context of positive thoughts and feelings evident in the therapeutic relationship, the better will be the outcome. That said, the ways in which ruptures in the therapeutic alliance (which involves at least temporary negative thoughts and feelings about the therapeutic relationship) can facilitate a corrective learning experience were highlighted earlier in this chapter. Thus, the idea is that a positive-valenced real relationship can provide the scaffolding for clients to express any negative thoughts and feelings that arise in the therapeutic alliance so they can be addressed in session.

Some have speculated that the bond factor within the therapeutic alliance is, in fact, the real relationship (e.g., Wampold & Flückiger, 2023). However, Gelso and Kline (2019) disagreed and instead suggested that the bond is evident in both the therapeutic alliance and the real relationship. They divided the bond into the *working bond*, which is part of the therapeutic alliance, and the *person-to-person bond*, which is part of the real relationship. According to Gelso and Kline (2019), the working bond consists of the following:

> . . . connecting that comes from the therapist and patient doing their jobs well, the patient trusting that the therapist can be counted on to conduct the treatment wisely and efficiently, the therapist's motivation to do the work of therapy, and the patient's sense that the therapist understands him or her. In contrast, the personal or person-to-person bond that constitutes the real relationship is not directly related to the work of therapy, but instead is a function of two human beings coming together, where each appreciates the person of the other, and in its most positive rendering, each enjoys and likes the other. (p. 143)

Gelso also extended the notion of ruptures—which had been examined exclusively within the context of the therapeutic alliance—to problems that can arise in the real relationship. In fact, Gelso and Kline (2019) advanced the notion that ruptures in the real relationship are different than ruptures in the therapeutic alliance. Specifically, they stated,

> A real relationship rupture may be seen as a failure on the part of the therapist to appreciate or demonstrate caring or empathy for the person of the patient at particular times when caring and empathy are called for, such that the patient consequently experiences painful affects tied to the therapist response. (pp. 147–148)

Whereas a rupture in the therapeutic alliance pertains to disagreement about (or a client's negative reaction to) the work being done in therapy, a rupture in the real relationship pertains to the client's sense that they are not receiving care and empathy from the therapist. Thus, ruptures in the real relationship have the potential to be even more damaging and difficult to repair than ruptures in the therapeutic alliance. These ruptures emerge when the client has the sense that the therapist does not like or respect them. It is not difficult to imagine thoughts and beliefs to which the client is prone that could facilitate this conclusion (e.g., anticipation of rejection, core beliefs of unlikability or unlovability). However, therapist behaviors could certainly contribute as well, such as taking a phone call during the session, multitasking during a telehealth session, or responding blandly to clients' reports of significant events in their lives (e.g., a promotion, death of a loved one).

Although there is much less quantitative research on the real relationship than there is on the therapeutic alliance, the studies conducted to date demonstrate that the real relationship overlaps with but is distinct from the other therapeutic relationship constructs in the tripartite model. For example, in a study in which practicing psychologists and psychology trainees completed measures of their perception of the therapeutic relationship, Gelso et al. (2005) found a correlation of $r = .47$ between the self-reported strength of the real relationship and a therapist measure of the therapeutic alliance. This association is to be expected because a positive therapeutic alliance stems from a strong and genuine human connection but, at the same time, is distinctive from the real relationship because it is geared only to the "work" of psychotherapy. In addition, Gelso et al. reported an inverse relation of $r = -.29$ between the therapist perception of negative transference and the quality of the real relationship. Again, this result was expected because transference is a "distorted" view of the therapeutic relationship based on the client's personal history, and the real relationship captures the realism in the relationship. A subsequent study by Kelley et al. (2010) with clients (rather than therapists) as participants found more overlap between the real relationship and the therapeutic alliance ($r = .79$), which the authors suggested had stemmed from the theoretical notion that the therapeutic alliance emerges from the real relationship (cf. Greenson, 1967) and that these dimensions are less distinguishable from clients' points of view than from therapists' points of view. Moreover, empirical research has demonstrated an association between the strength of the real relationship and clients' and therapists' perception of progress in treatment ($r = .36$ and .47, respectively; Fuertes et al., 2007), and that it predicts posttreatment symptoms above and beyond the severity of pretreatment symptoms and the strength of the therapeutic alliance (Marmarosh et al., 2009). In a meta-analysis examining the association between the strength of the real relationship and outcome, Gelso et al. (2018) found a correlation of $r = .38$ (95% CI [.30, .44], $d = .80$), regardless of the manner in which outcome was defined (e.g., session outcome, treatment progress, end-of-treatment outcome) or whether the client or therapist served as the subject who rated the real relationship. Collectively, this body of research indicates that the nature of the real relationship can be quantified and that it contributes something unique beyond the therapeutic alliance to psychotherapy outcome.

CONCLUDING THOUGHTS

As is evident in this overview, the therapeutic relationship is an entity that is extraordinary in its purpose and meaning. It involves two people—the client and therapist—who come together with the explicit aim of joining together in reducing the client's suffering. Along the way, the client and therapist get to know each other as fellow human beings, negotiate the ups and downs of their collaborative work together, recognize and resolve instances in which their interactions bring up issues from their past, and celebrate the client's triumphs that result from their work together. The three components of the tripartite model of the therapeutic relationship—the therapeutic alliance, transference and countertransference, and the real relationship—operate in a fluid manner, such that the relative prominence of each component continually changes as a function of the dynamic unfolding of therapy (Gelso, 2011).

I propose that cognitive behavioral therapists can and should actively attend to each of these three aspects of the therapeutic relationship to maximize the client's experience in CBT. TRF-CBT calls for therapists to (a) be intentional and mindful of the therapeutic relationship throughout the course of therapy to facilitate optimal conditions (e.g., a sense of warmth, respect, safety) for clients to engage in difficult therapeutic work and (b) seize opportunities to use aspects of the therapeutic relationship as agents of change in the client's life. In other words, the therapeutic relationship can be used as a technique unto itself (Goldfried & Davila, 2005) and can provide an important backdrop for the sophisticated application of cognitive behavioral strategies and techniques. There is an entire (and extremely impressive) system of cognitive behavioral psychotherapy—functional analytic psychotherapy (FAP)—devoted to this powerful notion (Kohlenberg & Tsai, 1991). FAP is one specific contextual behavioral approach in which therapists attend to client behaviors in session in order to shape clients' interpersonal behavior and encourage generalization to relationships outside of session. Here, I propose that this focus can be integrated into the delivery of any type of CBT, beginning with the therapist being mindful and intentional of cultivating the therapeutic alliance, recognizing and addressing transference and countertransference, and balancing the real relationship with the technical delivery of cognitive behavioral principles and strategies.

Some of the most common questions asked by trainees are, "How do we do this? What specific skills are needed to establish, fortify, and maintain a strong therapeutic relationship characterized by these components?" The next chapter describes some of the specific therapeutic relationship-facilitating constructs and therapist skills that have been identified in the psychotherapy literature as contributing to outcome.

2 COMMON THERAPEUTIC RELATIONSHIP-FACILITATING ASPECTS OF PSYCHOTHERAPY

Cognitive behavioral therapy (CBT) is one of many systems of psychotherapy. As such, CBT can benefit tremendously from theory and research on the factors that make psychotherapy generally effective regardless of the specific ingredients delivered. When the average person is asked to contemplate what makes psychotherapy special, unique, and inviting, they often point to relationship factors, such as having the attention of someone who listens intently or being in the presence of someone who is empathetic and nonjudgmental and who truly values them. I argue that these factors are just as important in CBT as in any system of psychotherapy. They not only facilitate the effective application of CBT strategic interventions, but I believe that they also serve as an agent of change in and of themselves by providing a corrective learning experience that can ultimately be generalized to a reduction in symptoms and an improvement in quality of life. Therapeutic relationship-focused CBT (TRF-CBT) maximizes these factors.

This corrective learning experience can take place in the form of learning by therapist modeling, as therapists conduct themselves in a way that maximizes these relationship factors. However, because the psychotherapy relationship is just that—a relationship—it allows clients the opportunity to practice being open to and receiving these factors as well as reciprocating.

https://doi.org/10.1037/0000424-003

It also teaches clients something important about their capacity to give and receive in relationships. In this chapter, I consider some of the most commonly theorized and researched of these factors that have relevance to the therapeutic relationship and therapist behaviors, broadly summarizing research on their association with outcome and contemplating their applicability to CBT and ways to maximize them in the context of the delivery of CBT.

COMMON FACTORS FRAMEWORK

The factors that I highlight in this chapter are typically regarded as representative of the *common factors* of psychotherapy, or factors that are evident in any course of therapy and are thought to enhance the therapeutic experience and even contribute to outcome (referenced by Kazantzis et al., 2017, as *generic factors*). The notion of common factors that cut across schools of psychotherapy was first introduced by Saul Rosenzweig (1936), who advanced the *dodo bird argument* about the relative equivalence of psychotherapies. The notion of the dodo bird stems from the story, *Alice's Adventures in Wonderland and Through the Looking-Glass*, when the dodo bird commented on the results of a caucus race by saying, "Everybody has won, and all must have prizes" (Carroll, 2010, p. 16). Rosenzweig (1936) posited that it might very well be these common factors of psychotherapy that can account for this purported dodo bird effect. Examples of common factors with the potential to be powerful forces in psychotherapy outcome include the instillation of hope, positive expectations for outcome, the opportunity to have corrective experiences, and a strong relationship with the therapist (Wampold & Imel, 2015). From this framework, one would view a strong therapeutic relationship as being an important component that contributes to good outcome in psychotherapy because it directly and indirectly achieves many of the aims of these common factors.

This is not to say that specific ingredients, such as the numerous ingredients of CBT highlighted in the clinical chapters of this volume (Part II), are unimportant. In fact, Wampold and Imel's (2015) contextual model of psychotherapy—a rich and thoughtful common factors approach to understanding psychotherapy process—posits three pathways that work together to produce good outcome in psychotherapy, after an initial therapeutic bond has been established. These pathways include (a) the real relationship (described in Chapter 1 of this volume) that forms a sense of belongingness and connection, (b) the establishment of positive expectations for treatment, and (c) the delivery of specific therapeutic ingredients that lead to healthy behavior. Regarding the first pathway, Wampold and Imel stated that empathy is the key factor in forming the real relationship. Because much research has been devoted to examining the degree to which empathy predicts psychotherapy outcome, empathy is one common factor considered in this chapter. Regarding the second pathway, expectations go beyond hope and relief associated with the mere act of contacting a therapist for treatment. For a client to truly develop positive expectations for treatment, they must buy into (a) a credible explanation for their clinical condition and (b) the corresponding therapeutic interventions that can help them overcome their symptoms and the effects of these symptoms on their life. Both requirements are met in CBT; thus, the cultivation of positive expectations for treatment is also considered in this chapter. Regarding the third pathway, Wampold and Imel implied that there could be a range of specific therapeutic ingredients that are curative depending on the particular school of psychotherapy; but what is consistent across schools is the client's implementation of something healthy that results in the changes for which the client had been hoping when they presented for treatment. Stated in this manner, both positive expectations formed by a cogent rationale and accompanying treatment plan, and implementation of the treatment plan itself, are common factors associated with good outcome in psychotherapy.

There has been great debate between Wampold (and proponents of the contextual model; Laska et al., 2014) and others who believe that specific schools of psychotherapy, such as CBT, are unique and superior for particular mental health disorders (e.g., Asnaani & Foa, 2014; Hofmann & Barlow, 2014). I do not evaluate the merits and drawbacks of the model here. Instead, I take the stance that (a) cognitive behavioral therapists can learn much from scholars and clinicians who advocate for a common factors approach, such that they can hone and maximize their delivery of CBT's specific ingredients when they do so in a way that harnesses the common factors; and (b) it is important to be mindful of common factors that are especially relevant to cultivating the therapeutic relationship because they can set the stage for corrective interpersonal learning experiences (cf. Safran & Segal, 1990).

THERAPEUTIC RELATIONSHIP-ENHANCING COMMON FACTORS

In the remainder of this chapter, I discuss some of these therapeutic relationship-enhancing common factors, with the idea that cognitive behavioral therapists who practice from a TRF-CBT framework keep these factors top of mind. This aim, however, begs the question as to the criteria I used to include or exclude the particular common factors described in greater length. When I began writing this portion of the volume as someone who was not expert in the common factors of psychotherapy, I searched for an elusive list of common factors that I hoped would be regarded as comprehensive, exhaustive, and authoritative. At the time of the writing of this chapter, I am still not sure that such a list exists. In their seminal volume on the contextual model of psychotherapy, Wampold and Imel (2015) highlighted the therapeutic alliance, empathy, goal consensus/collaboration, positive regard/ affirmation, congruence/genuineness, expectation in therapy, and cultural adaptation on the basis of meta-analyses that had calculated effect sizes of the association between these variables and outcome.

Perhaps the most authoritative source on these factors comes from the fruits of the tireless labor of the American Psychological Association Division of Psychotherapy Task Force on Empirically Supported Therapy Relationships. This task force was commissioned in 1999 to gather, evaluate, and disseminate information on empirically supported therapy relationships in the midst of great dissension over the definition and application of evidence-based practice in psychology (see American Psychological Association, 2006). The results of this comprehensive analysis were published in Norcross (2002). Division 12 (Clinical Psychology) joined forces with Division 29 on a second task force 10 years later to update the database and clinical guidelines that emerged from data analysis (Norcross, 2011). More recently, the Third Interdivisional APA Task Force on Evidence-Based Relationships and Responsiveness yielded yet another iteration of this work, separating discussion into two volumes focused on evidence-based healing qualities of the therapeutic relationship (Vol. 1; Norcross & Lambert, 2019) and ways to adapt the therapeutic relationship on the basis of individual client characteristics (Vol. 2; Norcross & Wampold, 2019). Many of the therapeutic relationship-facilitating common factors described in this chapter are examined in detail in these volumes.

With guidance from Wampold and Imel (2015) and the Third Interdivisional APA Task Force on Evidence-Based Relationships and Responsiveness, I focus on the following common factors in this chapter: (a) the therapeutic alliance, (b) empathy, (c) positive regard, (d) congruence and genuineness, (e) cultivation of positive outcome expectations, and (f) cultural adaptation and responsiveness. For all of the factors considered in this chapter, I describe a cursory summary of the empirical research on their association with psychotherapy outcome, often in the form of results from meta-analysis. I also consider their relevance in CBT and ways in which attention to these factors can maximize outcome in CBT.[1]

---

[1]The astute reader might be wondering why goal consensus and collaboration are considered together as an important construct identified by the Third Interdivisional APA Task Force on Evidence-Based Relationships and Responsiveness but not included in this chapter. Because collaboration and goal consensus are such fundamental and central tenets of CBT, I consider them at greater length in the subsequent chapter on specific aspects of CBT that contribute to the cultivation of the therapeutic relationship.

Therapeutic Alliance as a Common Factor

As mentioned in Chapter 1 of this volume, the therapeutic alliance consists of three components, including (a) agreement between the therapist and client on the goals of therapy, (b) agreement between the therapist and client on the tasks of therapy, and (c) the bond between the therapist and client. In other words, the therapeutic alliance is the working relationship between the therapist and client, and it is a cornerstone in the characterization of the greater therapeutic relationship. The therapeutic alliance contributes meaningful variance to psychotherapy outcome, and instances in which ruptures in the therapeutic alliance occur can actually be crucial opportunities for the therapeutic relationship to strengthen through repair of the alliance and to serve as an important corrective learning experience.

The majority of research on the therapeutic relationship and CBT focuses on the association between the therapeutic alliance and outcome. As mentioned in Chapter 1 of this volume, it is sensible that CBT researchers would gravitate to the therapeutic alliance, as this component has the most empirical research to link it to outcome, and there are many reliable and valid assessment tools of the therapeutic alliance and its components. Moreover, two of the three alliance components (agreement on goals of therapy and agreement on tasks of therapy) are themselves fundamental tenets of CBT that are strongly emphasized in even the most basic CBT trainings.

The association between the strength of the therapeutic alliance and outcome in CBT, as measured by a reduction in symptoms, has been demonstrated across an array of mental health disorders and issues. Examples include posttraumatic stress disorder (Cloitre et al., 2002), panic disorder (Huppert et al., 2014), obsessive compulsive disorder (Maher et al., 2012; Simpson et al., 2011), social anxiety disorder (Kivity et al., 2021), specific phobia (Pan et al., 2011), health anxiety (Weck, Richtberg, et al., 2015), bulimia nervosa (Accurso et al., 2015), borderline personality disorder (Bedics et al., 2015), and Cluster C personality disorders (Strauss et al., 2006).

The relation between the therapeutic alliance and outcome in CBT for depression, however, has received perhaps the greatest and most systematic attention in the literature. In a meta-analysis, Cameron et al. (2018) calculated an association of $r = .26$ between the therapeutic alliance and outcome in CBT for depression, which is similar to the association found by other scholars in their examination of psychotherapy in general. Nevertheless, there is variability across studies, depending on the methodological approach used. For example, several studies found that an association between the strength of the therapeutic alliance and depressive symptoms at the end of treatment became nonsignificant after prior symptom change was controlled, raising the possibility that a strong therapeutic alliance is more a consequence than a cause of symptom change (DeRubeis & Feeley, 1990; Feeley et al., 1999; Strunk et al., 2012) or is very small after methodological and statistical variables are accounted for (Whelen et al., 2021). In contrast, other researchers concluded that the strength of the therapeutic alliance indeed precedes symptom change (Schwartz et al., 2018). Results from a study conducted by Lorenzo Lorenzo-Luaces and colleagues (2017; cf. Lorenzo-Luaces et al., 2014) raise the possibility that the number of previous depressive episodes moderates the association between the strength of the therapeutic alliance and outcome, with the effects of the therapeutic alliance being greatest for individuals with no prior episodes, moderate for those with one prior episode, and small for those with two or more prior episodes.

More nuanced measurements of the therapeutic alliance and its components, as well as additional ways of conceptualizing outcome, may be needed to fully disentangle the picture of the association between the therapeutic alliance and outcome in CBT for depression. For example, Webb et al. (2011) found an intriguing pattern of results in which the component of the alliance focused on agreement of the goals and tasks of therapy predicted depressive symptoms even when prior symptoms were controlled, whereas the component of the alliance focused on the bond was associated with outcome but not when prior symptoms were controlled. The findings of Webb et al. emphasize the importance of agreeing on the goals and tasks of treatment at the beginning of therapy and suggest that the bond emerges with continued work, especially as early gains in therapy are observed, thereby creating momentum in the therapeutic relationship that further propels outcome. Moreover, others have found that a stronger alliance is associated with a reduced risk of premature dropout, even when pretreatment predictions of the alliance are controlled (Murphy et al., 2022).

Rupture–repair episodes have also been examined in the context of CBT. In an eloquent study of clients with avoidant and obsessive compulsive personality disorder, Strauss et al. (2006) found that 56% of the client–therapist dyads experienced a rupture, and an additional 27% of clients experienced a rupture that was not repaired. All but one of the clients (93%) who experienced a rupture–repair episode reported a 50% or greater reduction in symptoms, relative to 27% of those who did not have a rupture–repair episode. As seen in the psychotherapy process literature at large, the presence of a rupture in the alliance was actually desirable for outcome, rather than being detrimental. Interestingly, results from this study also indicated that the strength of the overall therapeutic alliance predicted outcome even when early symptom change was controlled, leading the authors to speculate that the therapeutic alliance is particularly important in the treatment of clients with personality disorders.

An issue that has been the subject of much debate is whether the therapeutic alliance exerts its influence in CBT as a facilitator of the successful application of specific techniques and an agent of change in and of itself. For example, Castonguay et al. (2010) proposed, specifically within cognitive behavioral frameworks, that "the main purpose of the therapeutic alliance is to foster engagement in the specific techniques of therapy, and a collaborative relationship is ideally suited for this purpose" (p. 153). Raue and Goldfried (1994) crafted the following illustrative metaphor:

> From a cognitive-behavioral vantage point, the alliance plays an important role in the change process in much the same way that anesthesia is needed during surgery. The implementation of certain surgical procedures requires an adequate and appropriate level of anesthesia. Great care is taken to ensure that an effective anesthesia is in place before surgery begins. Once surgery is underway, the primary concern is with the effective implementation of the surgical procedures—the primary reason the patient entered the treatment setting. (p. 135)

From this standpoint, the therapeutic alliance provides a strong foundation from which cognitive behavioral therapists can deliver therapeutic interventions.

Conversely, Zuroff and Blatt (2006) analyzed data from the National Institute of Mental Health Treatment of Depression Collaborative Research Program to demonstrate that the therapeutic alliance measured early in the course of treatment predicted symptom reduction and adaptive functioning throughout an 18-month follow-up period, even after controlling for a variety of client characteristics and prior symptom change. This pattern was observed in each of four conditions: Beckian cognitive therapy (which most scholars in the field now refer to as the CBT condition), interpersonal psychotherapy, imipramine plus clinical management, and placebo plus clinical management. The authors concluded that the data argued against the alliance being a facilitator of specific treatment techniques, as there were no specific treatment techniques in the clinical management condition beyond the provision of care and support. Instead, they speculated that a positive therapeutic alliance contributes to a shift in clients' views of themselves and others in relationships—a curative factor in and of itself (although not unique to any one therapeutic approach).

Recent theoretical and empirical work has the potential to address this distinction between the therapeutic alliance as a facilitator versus agent of change. Sigal Zilcha-Mano (2017, 2021) advanced the notion that there are traitlike and statelike components to the therapeutic alliance and that this framework can capture both stances. The traitlike feature of the therapeutic alliance represents clients' and therapists' ability to form strong relationships with others, which could serve as a precursor to good treatment that facilitates the successful application of specific therapeutic techniques. In contrast, the statelike component of the therapeutic alliance emerges over time in a dynamic manner and has the potential to be curative in and of itself, as it reshapes negative representations of the self and others in close relationships and improves the quality of relationships outside of session. Zilcha-Mano raised the possibility that a strong traitlike therapeutic alliance is most important in CBT, where there are other mechanisms of action (e.g., cognitive change) that are more central to the basic foundations of treatment. In contrast, Zilcha-Mano indicated that a strong statelike therapeutic alliance is most important in other types of therapy (e.g., brief relational therapy; Safran & Muran, 2000), in which negotiation of the therapeutic relationship is the core mechanism of action itself.

I contend that when it is cultivated thoughtfully and when therapists remain mindful of it throughout the course of therapy, the therapeutic alliance can both facilitate the successful application of cognitive behavioral techniques and serve as an agent of change. I pose the possibility that the efficacy of CBT can be maximized when cognitive behavioral therapists recognize and harness both these traitlike and statelike features of the therapeutic alliance, meaning that they keep top of mind the ways in which the agreement on the goals and tasks of therapy and the bond can serve as a catalyst for engagement in treatment, and when these elements serve as corrective learning experiences in and of themselves. This idea is not new. For example, Castonguay et al. (2010) stated the following:

> Several authors have suggested that therapists would be wise to foster strong alliances not just as an indirect facilitation of but also as part of a theoretically cohesive system of CBT designed to achieve a direct path toward changing cognitive, changing interpersonal behavior, and providing corrective learning experiences to clients. (p. 163)

Moreover, when there is potential for a rupture in the therapeutic alliance, I contend that cognitive and behavioral principles and techniques can facilitate repair and enhance ultimate outcome in treatment.

Let us consider various scenarios in which both factors would be at work in CBT. Take, for instance, Client A. This client has a straightforward clinical presentation, like a specific phobia, and is otherwise psychologically healthy, has the ability to form strong relationships with others, and is eager and ready to take on the work of CBT. He quickly forms a therapeutic alliance with the therapist as they shape the goals and tasks of therapy, the treatment (i.e., exposure-based CBT) is delivered across the course of eight sessions, and therapy ends when the severity of Client A's specific phobia has decreased to a minimal to mild level. In this example, the therapeutic alliance serves as a facilitator of change, as the agreement on the goals and tasks of therapy serves as the foundation from which the therapist delivers exposure, and there is no need for a shift in self-representation or for application to other relationships in the client's life.

Now take Client B, who has the same straightforward clinical presentation—a specific phobia—but is ambivalent about treatment and is hesitant to embark on a course of exposure-based CBT despite the impressive body of literature supporting its efficacy (Wolitzky-Taylor et al., 2008). In this case, the therapeutic alliance would begin on a tenuous note because there would likely be an initial lack of agreement on the goals and tasks of therapy. On the basis of research conducted in the first 2 decades of this century, the therapist might very well use motivational interviewing (Westra, 2012) with Client B before moving forward with CBT in order to allow the client space to identify reasons for change and cultivate a firmer commitment to treatment. Motivational interviewing harnesses many client-centered principles of the psychotherapy relationship (e.g., empathy, positive regard), so it is possible that, generally, the role of the therapeutic relationship would be more central in successful outcome with Client B, relative to Client A who presents for treatment with eagerness and readiness to commence exposure-based CBT. More specifically, it could be said that motivational interviewing may enhance the therapeutic alliance, which may in turn facilitate outcome. In other words, the therapeutic alliance would still be a facilitator of change rather than an agent of change, but its facilitator role would be more central in a positive outcome with Client B relative to Client A.

Consider, however, the impact of a positive outcome in exposure-based CBT for Client B who is initially ambivalent about treatment. Say, for instance, that Client B has two specific phobias: (a) a dog phobia that is the target of exposure-based CBT and (b) a vomit phobia that is more impairing and also more resistant to treatment. Before participating in CBT, Client B refuses to consider addressing her vomit phobia using exposure. However, after resolving her ambivalence and successfully completing a course of exposure-based CBT to treat her dog phobia, the client reconsiders her unwillingness to address her vomit phobia in therapy, and she now agrees to take on exposure for this issue in a second phase of treatment. When Client B completes this phase of treatment, she states that the rationale for exposure-based therapy and her experience with the systematic planning and execution of exposure have instilled hope and confidence that she can resolve her vomit phobia as effectively as she did her dog phobia. Moreover, she remarks that the therapist's warmth and support are incredibly helpful and very much appreciated as she takes on new exposures. In this case, the therapeutic alliance also serves as an agent of change in that the goals and tasks of therapy, as well as the bond between the client and therapist, create a mindset shift that allows Client B to view a problem that she once previously regarded as too difficult to address to one that she can now take on.

Most clients do not have such straightforward clinical presentations as a specific phobia without other behavioral, adjustment, or interpersonal issues to address in therapy. Moreover, most therapists would likely agree that the majority of clients on their caseload exhibit some deficits in goal setting, systematic implementation of problem solving, or interpersonal effectiveness (or all three). This observation raises the possibility that the therapeutic alliance can function as the agent of change to some degree across a range of clients, as cultivating a therapeutic alliance can give these clients much-needed practice with goal setting, problem solving, and interpersonal effectiveness. The astute cognitive behavioral therapist then can be versed in mobilizing the therapeutic alliance for this purpose, in addition to cultivating it for the more general purpose of facilitating the strategies and techniques of CBT.

In sum, points for cognitive behavioral therapists to keep in mind about the therapeutic alliance are as follows. First, the therapeutic alliance is the foundation that underlies the collaborative work done in therapy. It is essential for all therapists, including cognitive behavioral therapists, to ensure explicit agreement between themselves and their clients on the work on which they will embark during the course of treatment. Second, cognitive behavioral therapists should be alert for signs of ambivalence about the goals or tasks of therapy or resistance. Examples of such signs include hesitant speech, lack of eye contact, off-topic conversation, expressions of doubt about whether therapy will be helpful or about their ability to engage in it, references to participating in therapy to satisfy the wishes of others rather than their own wishes, and overt disagreement (cf. Westra et al., 2012). When these signs are detected, motivational interviewing can be used to resolve ambivalence and reinforce a commitment to change (Norouzian et al., 2021). More generally in these instances, the cognitive behavioral therapist can focus first and foremost on cultivating a strong therapeutic relationship, including a developing bond with their client, to create a safe, nondefensive environment that invites the client to consider with an open mind all that therapy has to offer.

Finally, cognitive behavioral therapists are encouraged to identify ways in which the development of a sound therapeutic alliance can itself make a difference in clients' lives. A sound therapeutic alliance demonstrates the power and benefits of collaboration with another person. It models how to set goals and develop a specific plan to meet them. It also focuses clients' attention on goal-directed behavior, which is particularly helpful for clients who describe feeling lost or overwhelmed. Clients who have difficulty setting and enacting goals can then acquire a new skill as the therapeutic alliance is established. Moreover, regardless of whether a particular client comes to therapy with a deficit in goal-setting skill, most clients develop a sense of hope and confidence as the work of therapy is established, which can generalize to other areas of their lives. Thus, establishment of the therapeutic alliance might very well be the first of many opportunities for clients participating in CBT to experience meaningful cognitive and behavioral change.

Empathy

According to Watson and Kalogerakos (2010), "Therapeutic empathy works to track the moment-by-moment unfolding of the client's experience," and "Empathic responses consist of reflections of feelings, cognitions, and behaviors as well as metaphors to capture and evoke the poignant aspects of clients' phenomenological experience" (p. 193). In other words, empathy helps clients to feel known by their therapist. In their report on the role of empathy as an evidence-based therapeutic relationship component, Elliot et al. (2019) differentiated among three types of therapist empathy, which they aligned with three distinct theoretical frameworks. Specifically, they indicated that humanistic psychotherapists demonstrate empathy by being in tune with clients' moment-by-moment emotional and phenomenological experience, whereas psychodynamic psychotherapists demonstrate empathy by making great effort to understand the historical and current forces that help explain clients' current situations. Cognitive behavioral therapists, they stated, emphasize rapport and support, exhibiting "a benevolent compassionate attitude toward the client" and demonstrating that they "understand the client's experience, often to set the stage for effective treatment" (Elliot et al., 2019, p. 247).

It is true that cognitive behavioral therapists have emphasized rapport in their writings. For example, in their writing on the therapeutic alliance in CBT, Castonguay et al. (2010) defined rapport as "an interactive experience between therapist and client involving a secure, comfortable, sensitive, and empathic exchange" (p. 155). A. T. Beck et al. (1979) certainly emphasized rapport in their chapter on the therapeutic relationship in their seminal volume on cognitive therapy of depression. However, in their groundbreaking volume on an interpersonal approach to delivering CBT, Safran and Segal (1990) encouraged readers to go well beyond rapport and mere reflection, stating that empathy "involves the process of immersing oneself in the patient's inner world so as to articulate tacit experience" (p. 85). Ultimately, empathy reflects what Safran and Segal called *affective attunement*, because empathy allows the therapist to get the subjective feel of a client's inner experience in addition to the meaning that the client's experience holds for them. Importantly, Safran and Segal emphasized that empathy and cognitive interventions are not separate activities; rather, they are entirely interdependent. This premise anticipates one of the main messages of this volume, as mentioned previously in Chapter 1: CBT can (and should) be delivered from a client-centered framework even when a specific and strategic cognitive behavioral intervention is being executed.

Psychotherapy process research on empathy demonstrates that it is an important determinant of clients' experience in therapy and in outcome. Results from qualitative research indicate that clients attribute the change that occurs from their participation in psychotherapy to being listened to and understood (Myers, 2003; Myers & White, 2010). Moreover, quantitative research has demonstrated that therapist empathy is associated with a reduction in attachment insecurity (Watson et al., 2014). A meta-analysis conducted by members of the Third Interdivisional APA Task Force on Evidence-Based Relationships and Responsiveness yielded a weighted r of .28 between empathy and psychotherapy outcome, or a medium effect size that accounts for 9% of the variance in outcome (Elliot et al., 2019). A trend emerged (described as "tantalizing" by Elliot et al., 2019; p. 266) for the empathy–outcome association to be stronger in CBT ($r = .30$) than in experiential/humanistic psychotherapy ($r = .24$) and psychodynamic psychotherapy ($r = .21$). Although the reason underlying this trend is unknown, it certainly behooves cognitive behavioral therapists to attend carefully to expressions of empathic understanding to their clients because it might ultimately enhance outcome.

Empathy has been examined in a small number of CBT outcome studies. Burns and Nolen-Hoeksema (1992) found that therapist empathy had a significant effect on depression scores when controlling for homework compliance but, conversely, the effect of depression severity on empathy was quite small. This finding is notable because it separated the effects of an aspect of the therapeutic relationship on symptom change from the effect of symptom change on an aspect of the therapeutic relationship (however, in a criticism of this study, it was noted that the therapeutic relationship measure used by Burns and Nolen-Hoeksema confounded empathy with other positive relationship qualities; Elliot et al., 2019). Moreover, in the cognitive behavioral treatment of clients with generalized anxiety disorder, clients who rated their therapists higher in empathy in the first five sessions of treatment reported lower levels of anxiety posttreatment (Hara et al., 2017), and greater levels of empathy after an incident of therapy resistance at either session 3 or 5 were associated with reduced posttreatment anxiety as well (Hara et al.,

2018). However, clients' perception of therapist empathy was unrelated to outcome in the cognitive behavioral treatment of panic disorder (Hoffart & Sexton, 2002) and social anxiety disorder (Hoffart et al., 2009); even in the treatment of generalized anxiety disorder, the relation between perceived therapist empathy and outcome was nonsignificant when a resistance variable was included in analyses (Constantino, Westra, et al., 2019).

Empathy is another construct, like the therapeutic relationship itself, about which most people intuitively know what it means and what it feels like, but for which there are few contemporary operational definitions or guidelines (cf. Bachrach, 1976; Thwaites & Bennett-Levy, 2007). Elliot et al. (2019) described five types of empathy responses: (a) *empathic reflection* (i.e., a statement that demonstrates an understanding of the client's experience), (b) *empathic affirmation* (i.e., a statement that validates the client's experience or viewpoint), (c) *evocative reflection* (i.e., a statement that uses powerful language to capture the client's experience), (d) *empathic conjecture* (i.e., a statement that reflects a reasonable inference about the client's experience that goes beyond what has been communicated in session), and (e) *communicative attunement* (i.e., a statement that conveys the therapist's felt understanding of what it would be like to be in the client's shoes). In my experience, a therapist knows when an empathic statement (particularly an evocative reflection, an empathic conjecture, or communicative attunement) has been well-received by a client when the client perks up in response to the statement and says something like, "Yes! That's exactly it." I have one client who repeats my empathic conjectures when I make them, which is validating to me that I am in tune with her in real time, reflective of the synergy that unfolds and builds in the therapeutic relationship.

Collectively, this body of scholarship and research has abundant implications for CBT. Although it is true that some studies have detected no association between therapist empathy and outcome in CBT, other studies have indeed found this association, and results from the most authoritative meta-analysis conducted to date raise the possibility that the empathy–outcome association is even stronger in CBT than in other forms of psychotherapy (even in humanistic psychotherapy, for which empathy is viewed as a central agent of change). Consistent with the recommendation of Safran and Segal (1990), I suggest that cognitive behavioral therapists be mindful of delivering specific cognitive behavioral interventions while simultaneously communicating empathy. An empathic observation can be made prior to the delivery of an intervention (e.g., a heartfelt statement like, "I appreciate how difficult some of these changes in your life have been to make for you. [Then provide an astute example from the client's life.] I wonder if it would be helpful to try . . ."). Or empathy can be communicated nonverbally while an intervention is delivered (e.g., through an empathic facial expression) or expressed following delivery of an intervention (e.g., a heartfelt statement like, "I appreciate how difficult things have been for you, and I share in your readiness to see some change. I am hopeful that the implementation of . . . will help you to achieve that change"). Above all, I suggest that cognitive behavioral therapists prioritize empathy over the rigid application of a cognitive behavioral intervention (cf. Castonguay et al., 1996; Piper et al., 1999), as my clinical experience suggests that expressions of empathy are particularly salient to clients when they think back to what was most meaningful for them in therapy.

Positive Regard

Carl Rogers (1957) introduced the notion of positive regard within his client-centered therapy framework. He referenced characteristics of positive regard such as "warm acceptance," "no conditions of acceptance," and "prizing of the person" (p. 101). *Positive regard* is an attitude that "signals to clients that their experience is accepted fully and valued without judgment" (Watson & Kalogerakos, 2010, p. 193). In their essential volume on positive regard, Farber et al. (2022) described it as follows:

> the therapist's support and acceptance of the client regardless of how the client may behave in the present moment. It is not about specific words or behavioral gestures but a consistent attitude—a nonjudgmental and caring attitude, with a touch or more of warmth. (p. 26)

Positive regard is thought of as an agent of change in psychotherapy because it communicates a sense of worth, which is particularly important for clients who have experienced being dismissed by others or have endured a great deal of criticism (Watson & Kalogerakos, 2010). According to Rogers (1959), the sense of acceptance that clients feel from their therapist begins to translate to self-acceptance of their experiences, restoring a person to a place of wholeness. Research by Suzuki and Farber (2016) found that positive regard consists of three main factors: (a) supportive/caring statements (i.e., affirmations of clients' qualities and work they are doing in therapy), (b) unique responsiveness (i.e., clients' sense that they are heard and responded to as unique individuals by the therapist), and (c) intimacy/disclosure (i.e., physical proximity or self-disclosure).

A small body of research supports Rogers' assertion that positive regard plays an important role in therapy success. Farber et al. (2019) calculated an aggregate effect size of $g = .28$ between positive regard and outcome, suggesting that positive regard has a small but significant impact on psychotherapy outcome. The Third Interdivisional APA Task Force on Evidence-Based

Relationships and Responsiveness deemed positive regard to be a "probably effective" evidence-based element of psychotherapy relationships (Norcross & Lambert, 2018, 2019). In a unique study of positive regard, Suzuki et al. (2021) compared perceptions of positive regard in 540 clients who participated in one of four therapy types: psychodynamic, cognitive behavioral, eclectic, and humanistic/existential. Their results indicated that clients receiving psychodynamic therapy reported a greater sense of positive regard from their therapists than clients who received CBT, after controlling for client demographics, therapist demographics, client perceptions of the therapeutic alliance, and client self-esteem. In contrast, on a scale measuring clients' estimation of the likelihood that their therapist would make supportive and caring statements, clients who received CBT scored higher than clients who received psychodynamic and eclectic therapy. Suzuki et al. (2021) reasoned,

> One way to view the apparent PR [positive regard] advantage of CBT relative to psychodynamic and eclectic therapies is that the combination of therapist's direct focus on change, and his or her supportive comments and positive reframes, forms an especially positive synergy. (p. 140)

Within the framework of CBT, positive regard has the potential to create a context for a fundamental shift in core beliefs of worthlessness, unworthiness, unlikability, undesirability, and one's capacity for intimacy. However, this notion remains to be tested using empirical research. In a systematic review of elements of the therapeutic relationship in CBT for anxiety disorders, Luong et al. (2020) failed to find one study examining the impact of positive regard on outcome. Nevertheless, because positive regard is a fundamental common factor that enhances psychotherapy regardless of theoretical orientation, cognitive behavioral therapists are encouraged to be mindful of positive regard as they deliver cognitive behavioral interventions. As I stated in the previous section on empathy, cognitive behavioral interventions can be delivered in a way that they simultaneously achieve their aim that is based in theory and research and communicate positive regard to the client. Positive regard can be communicated with (a) a statement indicating that the therapist clearly knows the client, (b) an intervention with components that are specifically tailored to the client's unique clinical presentation or life circumstances, and (c) in the context of a metaphor that utilizes details from the client's life.

Congruence and Genuineness

According to Rogers (1957), *congruence* occurs when the therapist interacts and behaves with the client in a way that is authentic and an accurate representation of the therapist's internal state. Thus, there are two key components of congruence: (a) the therapist has an awareness of their internal state and (b) the therapist has the ability to convey this in a skillful and accurate manner to the client (Kolden et al., 2019). *Genuineness*, in contrast, overlaps with congruence but is a broader construct in that it encompasses authenticity, sincerity, openness, and honesty in both the therapist and client as well as in the relationship (Gelso, 2002; Gelso & Hayes, 1998). In many examinations of psychotherapy process, congruence and genuineness are used interchangeably (Kolden et al., 2019). Rogers (1957) viewed congruence as an agent of change because he reasoned that many clients come to psychotherapy in a state of incongruence, such that they experience their worlds through the lens of fear and avoidance instead of with openness and authenticity. When therapists behave in a congruent manner, they are modeling authenticity for their clients.

Kolden et al. (2019) conducted a meta-analysis of 21 studies examining the correlation between congruence and psychotherapy outcome for the Third Interdivisional APA Task Force on Evidence-Based Relationships and Responsiveness. They obtained a weighted aggregate effect size of $r = .23$, or Cohen's d of .46 (95% CI [.13, .32]), which accounts for approximately 5.3% of the variance in outcome. However, they acknowledged that there were factors at work that could account for both an overestimation and underestimation of effect sizes (i.e., publication bias and exclusion of studies that reported a global relationship score, respectively). These results mean that there is a small to medium effect for the impact of congruence on psychotherapy outcome. The size of this effect is somewhat lower than those observed for the therapeutic alliance, empathy, and positive regard; nevertheless, it is not insubstantial, and it is indicative of another common factor dimension for therapists to harness with their clients.

The provision of congruence and genuineness can be a welcome reprieve to clients struggling with interpersonal relationships fraught with uncertainty and even deceit or manipulation. Many clients comprising my caseload torture themselves with the importance or meaning underlying various exchanges with others in their lives, such as text messages and messages through social media, or their observation of the social behavior of others (e.g., through activity on social media). For example, a client I saw the day before writing this paragraph told me that it was easier to conclude that a romantic interest "hated his guts" than to risk further perceived rejection after he saw that she had opened a message on social media but did not respond to it. He expressed this sentiment after several sessions in which he agonized over how quickly he should respond to her previous messages, or what it meant when she responded with a single emoji. Their back-and-forth interactions seemed like a chess match, with both responding to one another obtusely rather than making it clear where they stood in the relationship. Together, the client and I considered what it would be like to have mutual interactions with this young woman that were characterized by genuineness and authenticity and ways to begin to enact that stance on his end. What better grounds for understanding, cultivating, and practicing genuineness than within the therapeutic relationship? Through this discussion, the client was able to develop an operational definition of the behaviors that constitute genuine interaction, identify contexts in which to enact those behaviors, and entertain a healthy view of the benefits of relationships characterized by genuineness, congruence, and authenticity—all important behavioral and cognitive changes that emerged from the work done in session.

To my knowledge, there has been no empirical research on the association between genuineness/congruence and outcome in CBT, although Jung et al. (2015) reported that perceptions of genuineness (as well as other therapist characteristics such as empathy, positive regard, competence, and convincingness) were associated with a stronger therapeutic alliance in CBT for psychosis. As with many of these common factors, not only would it be logical for genuineness and congruence experienced in therapy to be associated with good outcome for the reasons stated previously, but one could also expect genuineness and congruence to be associated with retention in treatment, return after relapse, and overall satisfaction with treatment. Moreover, as with empathy and positive regard, the provision of genuineness and congruence has the potential to shift unhelpful beliefs about clients' ability to exist and participate in relationships.

Cultivation of Positive Outcome Expectations

When clients present for treatment, they are usually struggling. They might believe there is no hope for a better future, they are incapable of making necessary changes in their lives, or they are so flawed that they have made a mess out of their lives. A critical component of psychotherapy, then, is that the client believes they can benefit or improve from it (Frank, 1961). This notion is operationalized as a positive *outcome expectation*, which is defined as the client's anticipation of how they will respond to the course of treatment on which they are embarking (Constantino, Vîslă, et al., 2019).

Much empirical research has been devoted to the association between outcome expectation and actual treatment outcome. In a close examination of the National Institute of Mental Health Treatment of Depression Collaborative Research Program, Sotsky et al. (1991) found that a positive outcome expectation measured before commencement of treatment was associated with lower depression posttreatment as well as a greater likelihood of complete response in each of the four treatment conditions (i.e., Beckian cognitive therapy, interpersonal psychotherapy, imipramine plus clinical management, and placebo plus clinical management). In their updated meta-analysis on the association between positive outcome expectation and outcome for the Third Interdivisional APA Task Force on Evidence-Based Relationships and Responsiveness, Constantino, Vîslă, et al. (2019) calculated an overall r of .18 (95% CI [.14, .22]), or a Cohen's d of 0.36 (signifying a small effect size). This finding means that positive outcome expectation indeed affects psychotherapy outcome, albeit to a lesser extent than some of the other factors described in this section, such as the therapeutic alliance. It is possible that a positive outcome expectation works in conjunction with other variables to produce good outcome in treatment, as research has found that clients' perception of therapist competency improves outcome expectations, which in turn is related to good outcome (Westra et al., 2011) and that a stronger therapeutic alliance facilitates positive outcome expectation, which reduces the frequency of interpersonal problems (e.g., sensitivity, ambivalence, aggression) in treatment (Vîslă et al., 2018).

Many practices of good CBT emerge from this body of research. Because there is such an abundance of research examining the efficacy and effectiveness of CBT, cognitive behavioral therapists can share compelling results from outcome studies using understandable language. Knowledge of such an outcome can instill hope in clients that their clinical issues can be addressed and that there are solutions to their life problems. In addition, cognitive behavioral therapists can share vignettes of successful cases (Kazdin & Krouse, 1983). Such vignettes can humanize CBT outcomes beyond the aggregate data that are typically yielded by outcome studies. Clients may recognize aspects of themselves in the vignettes, which can provide another layer of optimism for good outcomes in CBT.

Conversely, cognitive behavioral therapists can talk frankly about any negative attitudes toward psychotherapy in general or CBT in particular that have the potential to decrease positive outcome expectations. Oftentimes, these attitudes are based on erroneous beliefs about psychotherapy or CBT; in these cases, the therapist can ask permission to share data and observations to soften these misperceptions, thereby creating the opportunity for the client to revise their viewpoint. Of course, this should be done in a way that is open and nondefensive on the therapist's part in order to model that the therapist welcomes skepticism and even negative feedback, takes the client's concerns seriously, and is willing to entertain views different than their own. Any negative experiences with psychotherapy, and CBT in particular, should be validated, and a gentle discussion about ways in which this new course of psychotherapy could be different may ensue. When done skillfully, such a conversation could be conducted in the spirit of the very cognitive behavioral principles and strategies that are expected to create shifts in mindset and behavior in other areas of the client's life, outside of the therapy session.

Cultural Adaptation and Responsiveness

A client's cultural experience and background has the potential to influence the development of the therapeutic alliance and the unfolding of the greater therapeutic relationship, which in turn could have implications for treatment engagement, outcome, and satisfaction (Casas et al., 2016; La Roche & Christopher 2008). Two variables that have been considered in the psychotherapy process literature include *cultural adaptation*, or the degree to which therapists modify therapeutic interventions on the basis of their clients' cultural backgrounds, and *multicultural competence*, or a therapist's ability to work effectively with people of different cultural backgrounds (Soto et al., 2019). Cultural adaptations are evident when therapists match the language, content, metaphors, and methods used with clients' cultural backgrounds (Bernal et al., 1995; Hinton & Jalal, 2019; Hinton & Patel, 2017; Rathod et al., 2019). Therapists demonstrate multicultural competence when they have the following: awareness of their own background and the background of their clients, as well as the way in which their own perspectives or biases might affect their work with clients of different cultural backgrounds; knowledge of the experiences of specific cultural groups; and skill in engaging clients of different cultural backgrounds and adapting treatment to them (Arredondo et al., 1996; Sue, 1998). Moreover, therapists who demonstrate multicultural competence are attuned to the many psychotherapy process variables described in this chapter (e.g., therapeutic alliance, outcome expectations) and adjust accordingly with humility (Goodwin et al., 2018).

Soto et al. (2019) conducted a comprehensive meta-analysis examining the association between these variables and outcome for the Third Interdivisional APA Task Force on Evidence-Based Relationships and Responsiveness. Across 99 studies examining cultural adaptations to treatment, the treatment was delivered in the client's preferred language in 75% of instances; cultural values were mentioned in 75% of instances; the racial or ethnic backgrounds of the client and therapist were matched in 55% of instances; cultural adaptations were developed in consultation with people from that cultural background in 48% of cases; and the mental health staff had received training in cultural adaptations in 28% of instances. The effect size capturing the magnitude of the association between cultural adaptations and outcome was $d = .50$ (95% CI [.42, .58]), indicating that interventions incorporating cultural adaptations were more effective than interventions that did not. Moreover, when specific treatment characteristics were considered, the effects were greater when treatments were conducted in clients' preferred languages, when assessments were presented in clients' preferred languages, when treatment goals were based on cultural values, when culturally relevant metaphors were used, and when treatment methods were modified in a culturally appropriate manner. In addition, multicultural competence was associated with client participation ($r = .26$, 95% CI [.05, .44], $d = .54$) and with outcome ($r = .24$, 95% CI [.10, .37], $d = .50$), meaning that client engagement in treatment is greater when therapists demonstrate multicultural competence.

There are a multitude of ways in which cultural adaptation and responsiveness can enhance CBT. As demonstrated in greater detail in Chapter 3 of this volume, cognitive behavioral therapists respect and embrace individual differences as they work with their clients to develop the case formulations of their clients' clinical presentations. Not only does this stance contribute to the development of a customized treatment plan, but it is hoped that clients experience therapy as being characterized by nonjudgmental curiosity, respect, and care for them as individuals. In addition, if clients have experienced microaggressions and discrimination, it is hoped that cultural adaptation and responsiveness will provide a safe environment free of such challenges as well as an opportunity to experience a different type of interaction. If a misunderstanding that has relevance to culture or ethnicity occurs and results in a rupture in the therapeutic alliance (cf. Chang et al., 2021), this provides a forum for the therapist and client to work through it using a cognitive behavioral framework and its associated strategies and techniques.

Above all, I encourage cognitive behavioral therapists to cultivate sophisticated awareness of their cultural and ethnic biases and perspectives, recognize when those biases and perspectives are operating in the course of psychotherapy, and, when relevant, do the work to seek additional knowledge or supervision to optimize work with clients of different cultural backgrounds. In my experience, the effort devoted to learning about the client's culture (and then, perhaps, crafting a compelling metaphor on the basis of that knowledge) goes a long way in cultivating a strong therapeutic relationship and demonstrating genuine investment to clients. Moreover, asking questions from a curious perspective as the opportunity arises demonstrates genuine interest in clients' experiences, which contributes to a host of these relational factors (e.g., empathy, positive regard).

APPLICATION TO CASE

The ways in which Sarah's[2] therapist applied many of these factors, especially in the first several sessions of her course of treatment, are demonstrated in Chapter 3 on specific CBT factors that enhance the therapeutic relationship and in Chapter 4 on the initial contacts with the client. As will be demonstrated throughout this volume, every interaction that a therapist has with a client within the CBT approach can be had from a client-centered stance. In this section, a few examples of the ways in which Sarah's therapist intentionally cultivated the therapeutic relationship from the common factors framework are illustrated.

> Sarah repeatedly lamented the fact that she was "pathetic" for having such a pronounced reaction to the ending of her relationship with her boyfriend. When she made statements of this nature, her therapist said things like, "This relationship was extremely important to you; after all, you viewed him as your 'soulmate.' Most people I know would be devastated if the world as they knew it were suddenly pulled out from underneath them." Moreover, the therapist would communicate this sentiment with a vocal tone and facial expression that communicated warmth and acceptance. Such statements and presentation provide validation. Although the therapist might not necessarily know exactly what it is like to be in Sarah's shoes, she can certainly appreciate and normalize the emotional reaction that Sarah would have under these circumstances. Because the therapist could imagine what it would be like to have her own world suddenly pulled out from under her, her response to Sarah communicated empathy. Further, the therapist accepted Sarah and her situation without judgment, fully focusing on Sarah's needs and the pain she was experiencing, she was operating from a stance of positive regard. Finally, because the therapist's responses to Sarah were from her heart and filled with care for Sarah's well-being as well as concern about her suffering, the therapist was demonstrating genuineness and congruence.
>
> As therapy progressed, Sarah's unique appearance often played some sort of role in session. At times, she proudly displayed a new hairstyle, piercing, or piece of clothing. Her therapist genuinely admired Sarah's creative self-expression, so in these instances, she would comment on an intimate aspect of Sarah's new self-expression (e.g., "Your necklace is striking"), or she would express a warm comment about the meaning that the self-expression held for Sarah (e.g., "I know how much you have been wanting that new piercing. I am so heartened that you are able to enjoy it"). In other instances, Sarah would succumb to self-flagellation about her appearance, referring to herself as a "freak" or a "misfit." Because her therapist genuinely admired Sarah's self-expression, she would respond with statements like, "Sarah, it strikes me that not many people would have the courage to express themselves like you do.

---

[2]Client identity has been disguised to protect client confidentiality.

I applaud you for being true to yourself and presenting yourself to the world in a way that feels right to you."

Sarah's therapist genuinely felt true admiration for Sarah, so the expression of these statements was congruent with the way she thought and felt about Sarah. Moreover, Sarah's therapist knew that Sarah had a history of estrangement from her family-of-origin as well as a recent rejection by her boyfriend whom she had considered her soulmate. Thus, Sarah's therapist took great care in prizing Sarah for her strengths and giving her the message that she is deserving of care, acceptance, and even admiration—all part of positive regard.

Sarah's therapist had a genuine liking of her, making it natural for her to extend empathy, authentic interest, and positive regard. Therapists will undoubtedly encounter clients in their practice toward whom they would not naturally gravitate and may not even necessarily like. When I have found myself in the latter scenario, I dig deep to remind myself of my core professional and relational values, such as providing the highest quality of care to all clients (I call this bringing my "A+ game" to each session) and to truly honor each person because they are a human being. I also remind myself that clients who come to therapy are hurting in some way; as such, it is quite likely that I am not seeing them at their best and that I can play an important role in their healing and growth. Moreover, I challenge myself to find something about these clients that I appreciate and am sure to incorporate it into my interactions with them so that I truly exude genuineness and congruence with regard to the warm affect that I am expressing. With this mindset, more often than not, I find that I develop a new way of relating to the client and genuine liking emerges over time.

CONCLUSION AND FUTURE DIRECTIONS

The therapeutic relationship has curative properties in itself, even in the absence of the delivery of specific intervention factors. The common factors described in this chapter, and others that have been described in the literature, set into motion important shifts in beliefs about the self and others and templates for approaching life's challenges in an adaptive manner. The development of a strong therapeutic alliance allows clients the experience of being a collaborative team member as they agree on the goals and tasks of therapy in a caring manner. The provision of empathy communicates to clients that they are worthy of being known and provides validation of their personhood. Positive regard reinforces a sense of self-worth and allows space for clients to work through painful issues associated with shame and embarrassment. Congruence and genuineness provide an opportunity for clients to practice being their authentic selves (and, combined with positive regard, an opportunity for clients to be truly accepted by another person when they are their authentic selves). The cultivation of a positive outcome expectation instills hope, which could shift a client's pessimistic mindset of hopelessness, helplessness, and being trapped in their current life circumstances. Moreover, cultural adaptation and responsiveness validates and honors clients' unique cultural backgrounds, celebrating them and communicating that they are valuable. When cognitive behavioral therapists deliver whatever specific CBT approach they are using while keeping these common factors top of mind, they are practicing TRF-CBT.

Future research on many of these common factors and outcome within CBT is sorely needed. Although the therapeutic alliance is now routinely measured in clinical trials examining the efficacy and effectiveness of CBT, research on therapist provision of positive regard, genuineness, and congruence is lacking. Moreover, it will be important for future research to isolate the specific role that these factors play in successful outcome in CBT. For example, it is not difficult to imagine that the association between the delivery of a particular CBT intervention and outcome could be mediated (or partially mediated) by some of these common factors.

All of the common factors described in this chapter are those that can be delivered *in conjunction* with specific CBT relationship-building strategies (described in Chapter 3 of this volume) and the specific CBT intervention strategies for change (described in Chapters 5–9). In other words, cognitive behavioral therapists can achieve fidelity to the CBT approach while simultaneously cultivating the therapeutic relationship (de Felice et al., 2019; Tschacher et al., 2014). The bottom line is that CBT can and should be delivered within a client-centered framework (cf. Tursi & Cochran, 2006). We know that when therapists are trained in client-centered principles and they encounter client resistance, they demonstrate more affiliative behaviors (e.g., affirming, understanding) and fewer hostile behaviors (e.g., blaming), which is in turn associated with better outcome in follow-up periods after the end of therapy (Hara et al., 2022). It is for this reason that I view CBT, when delivered in this manner, as a client-centered psychotherapy.

Recall that in some instances, researchers pitted various schools of psychotherapy against one another (e.g., CBT versus experiential/humanistic psychotherapy versus psychodynamic psychotherapy) when they examined the role of a common factor in outcome. Much to the surprise of the researchers who conducted these studies, these relationship factors were found to be just as important in CBT as they are in the other theoretical traditions, and, if anything, the association between these factors and outcome was greater in CBT than in the other therapies. It is my hope that such data will defuse the notion that cognitive behavioral therapists do not attend to the therapeutic relationship. Much interpersonal skill is required for cognitive behavioral therapists to simultaneously form an emotional connection with their clients, truly listen to and hear their clients' concerns and life histories, provide psychoeducation so that clients can make sense of what they are experiencing, and deliver specific cognitive and behavioral change interventions. The next chapter describes some of the relationship-building strategies that are central in the delivery of CBT and that build on the common factors described in this chapter.

3 SPECIFIC THERAPEUTIC RELATIONSHIP-ENHANCING ASPECTS OF COGNITIVE BEHAVIORAL THERAPY

Although many people view cognitive behavioral therapy (CBT) as a technique-driven approach to psychotherapy, in reality there are several fundamental features of CBT that contribute directly to the development, maintenance, and enhancement of the therapeutic relationship (Safran & Segal, 1990). This chapter describes many of those features, including collaboration, feedback, goal setting, empiricism, guided discovery, and customized case formulation (cf. Kazantzis et al., 2017; Okamoto et al., 2019). All of these features place the utmost respect on the client's experience, both in their life in general as well as within the context of what happens during the course of psychotherapy. This chapter considers the specific ways in which these essential features of CBT contribute to the therapeutic relationship, illustrating with our clinical example and therapist–client dialogue that exemplifies the therapeutic relationship-focused CBT (TRF-CBT) approach.

COLLABORATION

Collaboration occurs when the therapist and client, together, actively determine the goals for therapy, create an agenda for the session, and decide which strategies and principles are most relevant to the client's life circumstances

https://doi.org/10.1037/0000424-004
Therapeutic Relationship-Focused Cognitive Behavioral Therapy, by A. Wenzel

at hand. Although cognitive behavioral therapists are sometimes referred to as "directive," in reality they work as equal members of a team with their clients, elicit and listen carefully to their clients' views, and modify their position when their clients express preferences or viewpoints that are different from their own. Collaboration is an active process (Kazantzis et al., 2015), and it enhances the therapeutic relationship because it often helps clients to feel valued, rather than talked down to, and that another person is on the journey with them and is very invested in their well-being.

Collaboration was an aspect of the therapeutic relationship that the Third Interdivisional APA Task Force on Evidence-Based Relationships and Responsiveness (Norcross & Lambert, 2018) found to be "probably effective" in improving treatment outcome. Results from one meta-analysis found a correlation of $r = .33$ between collaboration and psychotherapy outcome (Tryon & Winograd, 2011), suggesting that collaboration is a particularly potent relationship factor that is associated with outcome. To be clear, collaboration is certainly not a feature of psychotherapy that is unique to CBT. However, cognitive behavioral therapists emphasize collaboration as being a central tenet of CBT because of their strong desire to promote client autonomy, which is instilled over time when clients play as active a role in treatment as their therapist. Collaboration allows the client to achieve this aim because the client uses the therapeutic relationship and therapy structure as scaffolding to learn a new way of relating to the world, a skill they will hone to such a degree that they will eventually not need the assistance of therapy.

Collaboration is evident when the therapist and client work together to form the therapeutic alliance in that, together, they determine and come to agreement on the goals and tasks of treatment. However, this broad view of collaboration does not end when the treatment plan has been developed at the beginning of the session. Cognitive behavioral therapists periodically review the treatment plan with clients, seeking their input as to whether goals have been reached, whether goals need to be redefined or reshaped, and whether new goals should be considered. Moreover, they seek input as to whether clients believe they are moving in a direction consistent with the expectations they had about therapy at therapy's commencement. I view this as *macrolevel* or *big-picture collaboration*. I say more about this in the goal-setting section later in this chapter.

Collaboration also takes many forms in any one session, which I view as *microlevel* or *moment-to-moment collaboration*. It occurs near the start of the session when the therapist and client both decide what they hope to accomplish during their time together. Collaboration also occurs when the client is reviewing the homework they completed between sessions, such that the therapist demonstrates great interest in what the client did and what they learned from doing it and offers feedback that could refine the work that the client has done. Moreover, collaboration occurs when a clinical decision is to be made, such that more than one cognitive behavioral strategy or principle would be relevant to advance the treatment of a particular issue, and the therapist and client, together, decide which approach would be optimal in that moment (Wenzel, 2013). Finally, collaboration occurs at the end of the session when the therapist and client, together, summarize what was covered in the session and identify key take-home points that are important to remember as treatment advances.

The following dialogue illustrates collaboration with Sarah[1] in the third session. In the previous session, her therapist had introduced the notion of cognitive restructuring, and Sarah agreed that it would be a useful skill to acquire to reshape some of her most unhelpful thinking. For homework, Sarah had agreed to track situations that were associated with an uptick in upsetting emotions, key thoughts that she experienced, and the specific associated emotion, along with the intensity of that emotion.

THERAPIST: What were you hoping to focus on in our session today? [*This question aims to set the session agenda in a collaborative manner.*]

SARAH: I'm still having a really hard time with Andy moving on. I just don't know how to get over it.

THERAPIST: [responding with empathy] Of course, we can certainly continue to talk about that. I realize that this has been a very painful time for you. [pausing] I'm also wondering if you referenced this situation in your homework when you were recording the situation–thought–emotion sequence.

SARAH: Yes, almost everything I wrote was about the Andy situation in one form or another.

THERAPIST: How is this for a plan? Why don't we take a look at what you wrote down for homework, focusing first and foremost on the ones that were about Andy. And I can continue to work with you to practice some skills for reshaping the thoughts as we're going through those examples? [*This excerpt illustrates asking Sarah's permission to approach the session in this manner, rather than telling her that this is the way in which the session will proceed.*]

SARAH: [looking relieved] That sounds perfect.

---

[1]Client identity has been disguised to protect client confidentiality.

THERAPIST: Why don't you share with me the first Andy-related scenario that you wrote about?

SARAH: So, the situation was that I was looking at his Instagram. I know I shouldn't do that; we don't even follow each other anymore. But, of course, I do it just to torture myself! And guess what I see? All sorts of pictures of the two of them and memes about true love.

THERAPIST: [taking care to demonstrate nonverbal expressions of care and concern] I can just imagine how difficult it is to see posts like that. When you saw the photos and memes, what thought ran through your mind?

SARAH: [becoming tearful and speaking softly] That he's with her now.

THERAPIST: [recognizing that Sarah's thought was actually part of the situation and deciding to probe further for the meaning associated with the situation in a gentle manner] It does seem like he is with her right now, very unfortunately. If we take it one step further, what does it mean to you that he's gone in this direction?

SARAH: [crying] It means that I wasn't good enough for him!

THERAPIST: [continuing to demonstrate nonverbal expressions of empathy] What an upsetting notion that is, that you're not good enough for him. When you have that idea, tell me what emotion you feel.

SARAH: [continuing to cry] Sad. Awful. Dejected. Like a 10 out of 10.

THERAPIST: [speaking gently] It makes a lot of sense that you would be experiencing very intense negative affect when you carry the idea that you're not good enough for him. I wonder if that is most upsetting to you here?

SARAH: [nodding her head] Yes, I think it is.

THERAPIST: [speaking gently] Would it be worth it for the two of us to take a closer look at that thought? [*This question reflects collaboration because the therapist is asking for permission to focus on Sarah's thought that she was not good enough for her boyfriend, rather than dictating the course of their continued work together.*]

SARAH: Definitely. Not being good enough . . . that's been the real story of my life, what has come up over and over with all of my other therapists.

This dialogue illustrates the manner in which the cognitive behavioral therapist is cognizant of collaboration in nearly every exchange she has with the client. On the basis of research and their clinical experience, cognitive behavioral therapists often have a sense of a direction to go in session that would be beneficial for the client. However, in most cases, they do not move in that direction until they have evidence that the client also is interested in moving in the same direction. Sometimes, when cognitive behavioral therapists actively involve their clients in such decision making, they can be pleasantly surprised that the client has a different idea of what would be helpful. In my experience, adjusting the intervention and its target on the basis of this collaboration makes the therapy experience more engaging and meaningful for both the client and therapist.

Of course, Sarah was amenable to the therapist's suggestions in this example, making collaboration on the structure and work of therapy relatively seamless. Novice and seasoned therapists alike know all too well that collaborative work in session does not always proceed as the therapist anticipates. At times, suggestions for session structure or therapeutic intervention are not always well-received by clients; at other times, clients have a different idea than their therapist does about how they would like the session to proceed; at other times, clients have experienced upsetting events between sessions that increase demoralization; and at still other times, clients are holding onto upset about something that occurred in the previous session. In such instances, I suggest that therapists attend to the interactional process in the present moment, communicating positive regard and respect for the client's agency despite not being "on the same page" in terms of the work of therapy. Negotiation of the factors that are interrupting the (seemingly) collaborative work of therapy is collaborative in itself, as it is an example of the therapist responding to something important that the client is communicating. On the basis of this negotiation, the therapist and client, together, can adjust the type of therapeutic work that they are enacting and their shared expectations for the way in which the work will proceed.

FEEDBACK

The elicitation of feedback was identified by expert cognitive behavioral therapists as a core feature of good CBT (Taylor et al., 2020), although to date, there is a paucity of studies examining its association with outcome in CBT (Luong et al., 2020). There are two ways that feedback is elicited and used in CBT: The first occurs when the therapist checks in with the client on their preferences and reactions during the course of therapy, such as when the therapist asks the client to indicate the most important topic to focus on in therapy or if a certain line of questioning is okay for the client. The second occurs when the therapist obtains standardized feedback from the client that speaks to progress toward goals and ultimate outcome in therapy. Both aspects of client feedback are considered in this section.

The solicitation of feedback as the session progresses goes hand in hand with collaboration because client feedback is essential to obtain in collaboratively determining how to proceed with intervention. In fact, feedback was obtained on a few occasions in the previous dialogue, such as when the therapist asked Sarah whether the plan the therapist was devising was agreeable to Sarah, and whether they should focus on the notion of not being good enough for her boyfriend, rather than on the most simplistic (and largely factual) notion that he has moved on to another relationship. When cognitive behavioral therapists solicit feedback from their clients, it communicates a genuine interest in their views and the notion that their views and opinions matter, which can readily enhance the strength of the therapeutic relationship.

Two opportunities for client feedback are built into CBT session structure, which guides many cognitive behavioral therapists in conducting their sessions. Near the beginning of the session, cognitive behavioral therapists obtain a bridge from the previous session. The *bridge from the previous session* is a reference to the contents of discussion that occurred in the previous session, which can serve to orient clients to the work being done in therapy and establish a thread that runs across sessions. Rather than the cognitive behavioral therapist providing a summary of the session, the bridge is an ideal opportunity to obtain feedback from clients about what they learned from the previous session, what from the previous session ultimately made a difference in their lives in between sessions, and what distinctive reactions they had to the previous session. Not only do questions of this nature allow clients to consolidate the learning that they are acquiring in treatment, but they also allow them to express whether they believe that both client and therapist are "barking up the right tree," and, importantly, they also allow space for clients to express any positive or negative reactions to treatment.

The following dialogue illustrates the solicitation of feedback in the bridge from the previous session. This dialogue took place near the beginning of the fourth session, following the session captured in the previous dialogue that was focused on restructuring cognition indicative of the theme of not being good enough.

THERAPIST: What did you ultimately take away from last week's session?

SARAH: [pausing] Oh . . . I don't know exactly . . . I guess we were talking about the whole "I'm not good enough" tape that runs over and over in my head.

THERAPIST: Yes, that was a big focus of our session. What do you conclude from our conversation?

SARAH: [looking forlorn and avoiding eye contact] I guess . . . I mean . . . I guess you're trying to help me see a bunch of reasons why I am good enough? [pausing] It's hard to believe that, though. I've been told I'm not good enough all my life.

THERAPIST: [pausing] Am I right in sensing that perhaps our focus of the previous session was less helpful than we had hoped it would be? [*Here, the therapist picks up on subtle signs that Sarah might not be on board with the cognitive restructuring intervention and seeks additional feedback to verify this hypothesis.*]

SARAH: I don't know, maybe.

THERAPIST: I'm really glad to know this, Sarah. Feedback on your experience with therapy is really important to me, and if it seems like we're going in a direction that does not feel compelling to you, I'd like to hear more about that. [*Here, the therapist takes the opportunity to reinforce the importance of client feedback for the therapy experience as well as to remind Sarah that her feedback is welcomed and valuable.*]

Notice that Sarah's therapist was open to Sarah's feedback, framing it as natural and as a healthy part of the therapy process. Client disagreement does not always mean that the client is being difficult or resistant, and it does not mean that therapy is ineffective. In fact, I would postulate that, in many instances, a client expression of disagreement is a sign of effective therapy because it suggests that the client feels comfortable enough in the therapeutic relationship to speak their mind. Moreover, it offers an additional opportunity for collaboration because the therapist can refine the case formulation or plan for therapeutic intervention (or both) in light of client preferences. In this case, Sarah's therapist honored this feedback by pulling back from "traditional" cognitive restructuring and, instead, concentrating on helping Sarah to focus on her strengths and successes in her life (e.g., her artistic ability, her close friendships) to get her through a difficult time of disappointment and loss.

Another structured opportunity for feedback occurs near the end of the session with the *final summary and feedback*. In a similar manner as what was described with the bridge from the previous session, the final summary and feedback provides an opportunity for clients to share what they found to be meaningful from the session, as well as notable reactions they had to what was discussed. As with the bridge, this feedback allows clients to put their own words onto cognitive behavioral principles and strategies that they are learning and to reflect on the degree to which they anticipate that the work done in session will make a difference in their lives. During the final summary and feedback, cognitive behavioral therapists often ask clients whether they found anything in session to be upsetting to be sure they are not leaving with negative feelings about the events that transpired that day. This question has direct relevance to the therapeutic relationship, as it can help identify any potential sources of upset that could lead to a rupture in the therapeutic alliance. Moreover, if a client indeed has a negative reaction to something that occurred in session, the therapist has an opportunity to model the sensitive and effective handling of the transgression.

The following dialogue illustrates the final summary and feedback with Sarah, at the end of the same session in which Sarah communicated indirectly that she did not find it helpful to contemplate the notion of whether she was good enough.

THERAPIST: Sarah, we're almost out of time, and I'd like to summarize what we have done here today. What are you taking away from our session?

SARAH: [looking considerably brighter than she did at the beginning of the session] That maybe the whole question of whether I am really good enough is not even relevant. You know, like everyone is different, and different matches are better for different people. So, even if I'm not the best match for one person, it doesn't mean that I'm not good enough overall. It just means that I don't quite fit with that person.

THERAPIST: I couldn't have said that better myself. How do you expect, then, that your homework will reinforce this notion?

SARAH: I think by keeping that log of my successes in a bunch of areas of my life, you know, work, friends, my art . . . then I will be able to see actual evidence that I am doing pretty well in a lot of areas of my life.

THERAPIST: Yes, I think it will have that effect as well. I'm eager to see what you have come up with when we meet next week.

SARAH: [looking hopeful] Me too!

THERAPIST: Before we end, Sarah, I'm wondering how you are feeling about today's session. When we started, it seemed like you were a bit discouraged. How do you feel about today's work together?

SARAH: I feel really good about it! And I really appreciated our discussion about whether we should adjust our approach.

THERAPIST: I'm really glad that we were able to put our heads together and make some modifications.

SARAH: Yeah, me too. When I was in therapy, like endlessly as a teenager, it always seemed that every therapist implied that there was something wrong with me if whatever we were doing wasn't working. It really turned me off the therapy for a lot of years.

THERAPIST: That's important to know, Sarah. My philosophy is that if something doesn't seem quite right, it can be treated as information that can inform us as we adjust our strategy to meet your individual needs. [*This statement sets a foundation for work on any therapeutic alliance ruptures that might unfold in the future.*]

SARAH: [smiling] That's a much better way of putting it than I was told in the past. I just thought I was a bad patient!

THERAPIST: Honestly, Sarah, I find you to be a delight. You're hard working and thoughtful—not at all a bad patient in my book. [*This sentiment fosters the real relationship because it reflects the therapist's genuine thoughts and feelings about Sarah.*]

Sarah responded to the therapist by bringing her hands to her heart, a clear expression of being touched by the therapist's words.

The second major source of feedback for cognitive behavioral therapists is scores on self-report inventories that clients complete between sessions or at the beginning of the session to inform subsequent treatment (Lambert et al., 2003). In but one example, for many years, I served as a trainer-supervisor on a massive project to facilitate the dissemination of CBT for depression to clinicians who worked in Veterans Administration hospitals across the United States (Karlin et al., 2012). Clients who received CBT from therapists being trained in this project completed the Beck Depression Inventory–II (A. T. Beck et al., 1996), the Working Alliance Inventory–Short Revised (WAI-SR; Hatcher & Gillaspy, 2006), and the World Health Organization Quality of Life–BREF (World Health Organization, 1993). Notice that the battery of questionnaires did not just target symptoms; they also targeted clients' perceptions of the therapeutic alliance and quality of life. I strongly encouraged my supervisees to carefully review their clients' responses to the questionnaires, treat scores on those questionnaires as important feedback about the treatment process and the degree to which treatment was yielding its intended outcome, and discuss the information obtained in session to reconsider treatment goals and inform treatment moving forward. Moreover, I viewed responses on the WAI-SR as especially important to consider because any indications that clients viewed the therapeutic alliance in a less than favorable light would be particularly valuable to address in session. Empirical and meta-analytic research verifies that obtaining and adjusting one's psychotherapy practice on the basis of client feedback reduces the likelihood of deterioration and increases the likelihood of improvement at the end of treatment (Lambert et al., 2019).

At times, I have encountered supervisees who view the review of questionnaire data as a bit dry, and they wonder whether it detracts from the genuineness of therapeutic interaction. In my experience, review of questionnaire data is only as dry as the therapist makes it. When therapists explain what the questionnaire data mean in everyday language, comparing clients' scores to normative data and to their own data collected earlier in the course of therapy, I find that most clients are intrigued and appreciate tangible measures of progress. Moreover, it is extraordinarily gratifying to see the look on a client's face when they question whether they have made progress in therapy, only to absorb outcome data graphed over time demonstrating that their symptoms are decreasing and that positive outcomes are improving. Anecdotally, I have found that such a demonstration infuses renewed enthusiasm for treatment and enhances the therapeutic relationship.

GOAL SETTING

Because CBT is known as an active, problem-focused treatment, *goal setting* is a fundamental activity that takes place in the early stage of treatment as well as at the beginning of each session. Just as I demonstrated that collaboration and feedback go hand in hand, goal setting is also not mutually exclusive from either of those constructs, as collaboration and client feedback are integral to the establishment of meaningful goals for therapeutic work that facilitate motivation, commitment, and ownership. Goal setting helps the therapist and client remain focused on the most important issues to the client, allowing for sustained work on these issues that is expected to result in meaningful change. As mentioned previously, the setting of goals certainly enhances the therapeutic alliance because it allows the client and therapist to come to an agreement on the goals and tasks of therapy. Moreover, goal setting often instills hope and optimism for treatment, as it establishes an organized template for problems to be solved and corresponding pathways for doing so. Many clients report that they had been "spinning their wheels" prior to the commencement of therapy, and that it is a relief to have a safe place and trusted individual to sort out their problems, develop skills for coping with and addressing their problems, and cultivate solutions.

The establishment of treatment goals usually occurs within the first few sessions of CBT. Goal setting played a central role in clarifying the work that Sarah and her therapist were going to pursue in CBT, described more in Chapter 4 in the context of establishing a therapeutic alliance in the early sessions. For the purpose of this discussion about goal setting, it can be said that Sarah took the lead on identifying the major problem areas that she hoped to address; at the time of the subsequent session, Sarah and her therapist, together, translated those problem areas into tangible goals to work toward in treatment. Subsequently, the therapist provided psychoeducation as to strategies that CBT has to offer that would help Sarah to attain her goals and solicited feedback and agreement that she was on board for the plan of action. The fruits of this collaborative endeavor in goal setting are summarized in Table 3.1.

Although treatment goals are set in the early sessions during the course of CBT, it is important to realize that they are malleable and can be revisited and reshaped as treatment progresses. As mentioned in the section on collaboration earlier in this chapter, I suggest that the therapist and client periodically review the treatment plan to reflect on progress made, generalize these gains to other areas of the client's life, and identify additional problem areas and associated goals that become evident. Many times, as clients make progress in treatment, they realize that there are additional issues, perhaps not as immediate or pressing in nature, that they would like to address once they have found a therapist with whom they are comfortable working. I conceptualize this phenomenon almost as if clients are moving from Phase I of treatment, focused on addressing acute problems or emotional distress requiring immediate attention, to Phase II, focused on preventing future emotional distress, shifting unhelpful underlying beliefs and schema modification, and overcoming a more general lack of fulfillment and life satisfaction. When this occurs in treatment, we reconceptualize the treatment plan, formulating new goals, associated interventions, and ways to measure progress.

Just as goal setting is essential in developing a vision for the course of treatment, it is equally as important in clarifying the aims of each session. This corresponds to the basic session structure technique of *agenda setting*, which occurs when the client and therapist, together, determine what they

TABLE 3.1. Sarah's Treatment Planning Worksheet

Problem area	Manifestations of problem area	Measurement of progress	CBT strategy
1. Difficulty accepting ending of romantic relationship	1. Rumination 2. Spontaneous crying 3. Sitting around, scrolling on phone	1. Decreased rumination, as evidenced by self-report and engagement in goal-directed activities 2. Decreased crying, as evidenced by self-report 3. Free time spent on artistic expression, spiritual practice, and social engagement	Behavioral activation Cognitive restructuring Acceptance-based strategies
2. Emotion dysregulation	1. History of self-harm, suicidal ideation, and suicide attempts 2. Interpersonal instability in romantic relationships 3. Difficulty self-soothing	1. Prevention of future self-harm and suicidal acts 2. Maintenance of existing close, healthy relationships; improved decision making regarding the continuation of "toxic" relationships 3. Ability to tolerate distress without isolating or engaging in self-defeating behavior	Emotion regulation skills Distress tolerance skills Cognitive restructuring Acceptance-based strategies
3. Uncertain future	1. Indecision about marriage 2. Indecision about whether to move to her home state	1. Improved ability to make small decisions, which will serve as a template for making larger life decisions	Problem solving

Note. Distress tolerance skills, emotion regulation skills, and acceptance-based skills are fundamental skills taught in CBT that are not explicitly highlighted in this volume but are no less important. From *Cognitive Behavioral Therapy for Beginners: An Experiential Learning Approach* (p. 42), by A. Wenzel, 2019, Taylor & Francis. Copyright 2019 by Taylor & Francis. Reprinted with permission.

will cover in session. Thus, agenda setting is an opportunity for collaboration, as illustrated earlier in this chapter, as well as for within-session goal setting. Proponents of agenda setting believe that it helps the therapist and client make efficient and effective use of time in session, ultimately helping the client to meet their treatment goals. Critics of agenda setting believe that it is rigid and has the potential to damage the therapeutic relationship by stifling spontaneous emotional expressions and discussion of unanticipated topics.

It is my experience that, when applied flexibly and responsively to clients' concerns and spontaneous reactions in session, agenda setting can significantly enhance the therapeutic relationship. Psychotherapy is an investment of time, energy, and financial resources, and many clients find it heartening that their therapist expresses overt care and concern about using the time wisely. Further, many clients actually welcome an agenda, as well as a therapist who is mindful of the agenda throughout the session. It is my frequent experience that when clients veer from the agenda and I gently ask whether they would like to table the agenda and focus on the new issue that has arisen, they respond with a sentiment that is something like this:

> Oh gosh, no. The goals of the session that we had established before are most important. I appreciate that you asked, because this is something that happens to me often, and I don't finish what I start. I am grateful that you said something so that we can get back on track.

My philosophy, then, is that clients are always in the "driver's seat" and are the ultimate determiners of the agenda, but that I would not be doing everything that I could do to help them if I inadvertently reinforce or enable a disorganized, random, or haphazard way of approaching their life problems. When I communicate this in a warm, collaborative, and transparent manner, it almost always enhances all three components of the therapeutic alliance.

Thus, goal setting enhances the therapeutic relationship in many ways. It instills hope and optimism in clients that their life problems can be addressed. It also enhances the therapeutic alliance with the collaborative agreement on the goals and tasks of therapy, forming the foundation of a productive and caring working relationship. As sessions progress, it is hoped that clients see tangible conclusions, insights, and nuggets of wisdom from each session as a result of the focused work that emerges from a clear agenda. Instances in which clients veer from the established goals of each session are opportunities for enhancement of the therapeutic relationship. Moreover, regular review of treatment goals allows for additional, meaningful goals to be formulated as clients feel more comfortable and safe in a trusting therapeutic relationship.

EMPIRICISM

According to Kazantzis et al. (2017), *empiricism* "describes how we help the client to adopt a more 'scientific method' to evaluate his or her experience" (p. 22). When used skillfully, empiricism empowers the client to use their own experience to understand their emotional reactions, design ways to test out their hypotheses regarding explanations for why their experience is occurring or different ways of approaching their experience, and draw new conclusions on the basis of continued observation of their experience. Notice the repeated references to "their experience." Empiricism in CBT empowers the client to apply a systematic, even scientific framework to make sense of their subjective experience, rather than the client relying on the therapist to tell them what to do or how to think. This stance enhances the therapeutic relationship because clients' subjective experiences are accepted and validated, and the therapist is modeling trust in the client's reporting of their experience (oftentimes unlike others in the client's life). It communicates "I believe you" as well as "I believe in you." The application of empiricism to one's own experience is a valuable principle that facilitates many skills that will be useful in years to come, when the client is no longer participating in therapy.

When combined with collaboration (i.e., *collaborative empiricism*), the client and therapist work together as a team to test out their beliefs, rules, and assumptions that have the potential to be exacerbating their emotional distress (Dobson, 2022). In other words, the therapist and client share in the work together (Kazantzis et al., 2017), which further elevates the therapeutic alliance with the shared focus and agreement on the goals and tasks of treatment. More generally, collaborative empiricism enhances the therapeutic relationship because it communicates to clients that they are not alone on their journey to wellness—that someone is very much interested and invested in them. Research has found that combined collaborative empiricism accounts for 12.3% of the variance in outcome after controlling for the strength of the therapeutic alliance and the competency of the therapist (Tee et al., 2017, cited in Kazantzis et al., 2017). This means that empiricism plays a small but unique and important role in outcome, as it cannot be explained by the strength of the therapeutic alliance and therapist competence.

In the previous dialogue with Sarah, she mentioned during the final summary and feedback that she was optimistic about the benefits of keeping a log of successes in her life. This is an example of empiricism because, for CBT homework, Sarah was going to record observations of instances in which she received positive feedback from others, successfully solved a problem, or overcame adversity. All of these observations emerged from her own lived experience and, collectively, they provided evidence that would help evaluate the notion that she is not "good enough." Moreover, the interplay between Sarah and her therapist, in which they adjusted their approach, reflected collaborative empiricism because, together, they took their observations of what did and did not seem to be working in therapy to that point, and they selected another therapeutic intervention. This is an example of the way in which a fundamental CBT principle can be infused in session to address what is happening in the therapeutic relationship and, ultimately, to enhance the therapeutic relationship.

GUIDED DISCOVERY

Guided discovery is the process by which cognitive behavioral therapists use focused questioning or other methods (e.g., behavioral experiments) to help clients consider alternative viewpoints and new solutions to problems. When done in a verbal format, guided discovery relies on Socratic questioning or dialogue, named after the Greek philosopher, Socrates, who encouraged his students to critically evaluate (and even debate) different stances of an argument and draw their own conclusions rather than telling them what to think (cf. Kazantzis, Beck, et al., 2018). Cognitive behavioral therapists adopt a similar stance, in that they ask questions to stimulate the client to think critically about the way they are viewing their lives and to draw their own conclusions. Guided discovery enhances the therapeutic relationship because it shows clients that the therapist is interested in and curious about them. When they ask Socratic questions, cognitive behavioral therapists demonstrate that they are listening carefully to what their clients are saying and are actively engaged in the process of helping clients make sense of their life experiences. At the same time, guided discovery leaves much space for clients to examine all sides of an issue at their own pace and, ultimately, to draw whatever conclusion they see most fit, which enhances their ownership of the course of therapy (Williams et al., 2006) and enhances motivation (Tee & Kazantzis, 2011). Many clients report that they appreciate the guided discovery process because they feel supported as they learn something new and draw conclusions that they can use in their everyday lives.

Guided discovery through Socratic dialogue is not done in a confrontational manner; instead, it is done in a gentle, inquisitive manner that allows the client space to exert their own autonomy (a point elaborated on further in Chapter 5 of this volume). In fact, some perspectives on Socrates' teaching style are that he aggressively pushed students until he caught them with a flaw in their reasoning (Kazantzis et al., 2014)—a style that is certainly inconsistent with that which cognitive behavioral therapists hope to bring to their sessions! Instead, clients are given space to examine different viewpoints and muscle through their implications, with cognitive behavioral therapists interacting in a respectful, reflective manner and asking questions like, "So what do you make of all of this?" (Dobson, 2022; Kazantzis et al., 2014). It should be noted that the term *guided discovery* has the potential to imply that the therapist is guiding the client toward one specific outcome. Perhaps a better term is *facilitated discovery*, in which the therapist provides a foundation for the client to consider multiple possible outcomes (Kazantzis et al., 2017). The term *guided discovery* will continue to be used in this volume due to the decades of scholarship in which it is referenced in this way, but I will be clear that in no way do I want to imply that cognitive behavioral therapists are attempting to "guide" their client toward a conclusion that we, as therapists, have deemed as "correct" or the "right" way to think. When cognitive behavioral therapists enact guided discovery from a relational perspective, they make observations and ask questions that communicate curiosity (e.g., "I'm wondering about . . ."), open-mindedness to various viewpoints (e.g., "What different perspectives could be applied to understanding this issue?"), and belief in the client's agency (e.g., "You know yourself best, and I trust your grasp of the situation").

In fact, one of my recent experiences with a client eloquently illustrates the perils of going "too far" with guided discovery toward a specific conclusion, which had implications for the therapeutic relationship. My client was involved in a long-term romantic relationship with a man who, in my view, was emotionally abusive toward her and whose treatment of her had significant and negative ramifications on her emotional and physical well-being (e.g., not being able to eat or sleep for over a day after he relentlessly berated her for something she had done for self-care, such as getting a haircut). I utilized the strategy of guided discovery with the aim of helping her to see that she was being emotionally abused and that this current situation was unsustainable (gently asking questions to prompt her to consider the value of exiting the relationship). In a poignant session, the client disclosed that she had begun to stop talking about the relationship to me because she knew what I thought of it, but that therapy was the very space she needed to unpack all that was happening in the relationship and his continued maltreatment of her. She stated, more assertively than I had ever heard her state anything, that she was not ready to leave the relationship, that there were also good things about the relationship that she valued and that I was dismissing, and that I was not doing her a service by implementing guided discovery if its purpose was to encourage her to leave the relationship. Although to this day, in my heart of hearts, I believe this relationship adversely affects her mental health, above all I learned an important lesson about guided discovery—it is not the therapist's role to determine or judge what outcome or mindset is best for the client. It is theirs, and theirs alone, to determine. I am grateful to my client for expressing this to me, and we continue to have an enriching therapeutic relationship in which I have learned to be respectful of her choices, even if I would not make them myself or wish them upon others I care about. In response to her assertion, I backed down on guided questioning focused on whether it was in her best interest to remain in the relationship, and I opened up more space for affective expression, support, and validation. Now, we frequently reference this conversation in our sessions to reflect on the openness and care within our relationship (i.e., our real relationship). Importantly, the client now talks much more about this relationship, which has resumed focus within our therapeutic work. She has since concluded, on her own, that it is in her best interest to end the relationship.

The following dialogue illustrates the guided discovery process with Sarah. Although Sarah was able to use her success log to recognize her many areas of strength, she continued to struggle with the idea that Andy had broken up with her because she was not good enough. When she ruminated on the notion of not being good enough, she experienced significant amounts of hopelessness and despair, at times even contemplating nonsuicidal self-injurious behavior to obtain relief from the pain that she was experiencing. Thus, although Sarah responded well to the intervention of recognizing her successes, she continued to move back and forth between feeling mildly optimistic about moving forward with her postbreakup life and experiencing a debilitating sense of worthlessness that continued to cause life interference.

SARAH: I know, intellectually, that I have a lot to offer the world. Even though you wouldn't know it at times, I've really come a long way from where I was as a teenager. But . . . man . . . the waves of worthlessness just come from out of nowhere and overtake me. When that happens, all I can think about is Andy, and how he just dropped me like I was nothing, and how this new girl basically won. I know that's not healthy. But it's what happens. Especially late at night, that's the worst.

THERAPIST: So, it sounds like our focus on your success log does help at times, but the waves of worthlessness are still very concerning. [*This summary statement communicates that the therapist is listening, reinforces at least partial efficacy of a cognitive behavioral intervention, and acknowledges an important focus of continued therapeutic work.*]

SARAH: Totally. It's like grief and loss, and anger and betrayal, and feeling cast aside, like our relationship meant nothing. All rolled up into one. I can't help but think that if I were skinnier, or prettier, or, I don't know, just better, then this wouldn't have happened.

THERAPIST: [seeing the opportunity for guided discovery, and speaking gently] One hypothesis, or theory to explain what happened, is that you are not good enough for him. I'm wondering if there are any other hypotheses? [*This is an example of a question intended to help the client think of other explanations for an upsetting situation.*]

SARAH: Like other reasons why he left me?

THERAPIST: Well sure. From what you described to me about your relationship, there were a lot of layers and complicating factors.

SARAH: [pausing] Yes, I guess there were.

THERAPIST: What might be one that played a contributing role to the downfall of the relationship? [*This is an example of a more specific question intended to follow up on the general question posed by the therapist earlier.*]

SARAH: Well . . . of course he wasn't happy that I was still married. Early in our relationship, he really pushed for me to leave my husband. But, I don't know, I just couldn't do it.

THERAPIST: Interesting. So, he was the one pushing for you to leave your husband. What does that tell you?

SARAH: I know. He was really into me in the beginning. It was like a whirlwind.

THERAPIST: And you didn't ultimately leave your husband, and you had reasons for that. I wonder what he made of that?

SARAH: He was really hurt and sad. One time he even cried and asked me why he wasn't good enough for me.

THERAPIST: [showing especially great interest right here] Isn't that something?

SARAH: Isn't what something?

THERAPIST: That you and I have been grappling with this idea that you weren't good enough for him, but that he expressed the exact same sentiment to you.

SARAH: [looking surprised] Huh.

[*Here, the therapist allows silence and time for Sarah to make sense of this new realization. Silence and time are also important components of guided discovery for clients to evaluate the material that is being covered in session and to draw their own conclusions.*]

SARAH: Well, damn.

THERAPIST: Tell me what sense you are making of our conversation. [*This request allows the client to put words onto the new viewpoints being formulated.*]

SARAH: I wonder if he started to pull away from me for this exact reason . . . because he was not feeling good enough. [*Here, the therapist again leaves silence and time for this viewpoint to resonate.*] Wow, I never thought of it like this.

THERAPIST: [speaking softly and gently] So one hypothesis is that the relationship ended because you weren't good enough for Andy. But there's another hypothesis . . . that perhaps he became discouraged because he started to believe that he wasn't good enough for you.

SARAH: Honestly, as I think about it, I don't think either hypothesis is exactly right.

THERAPIST: That is very interesting. Tell me more about that.

SARAH: You know, it probably wasn't ever a matter of who was or was not good enough. Obviously, it was a very strange situation, with me still being married and having some weird loyalty to my husband. I love Andy, I really do. I even think we are soulmates. We said that on so many occasions; we have so many interests, likes, and dislikes that are exactly the same. But, really, I wasn't fully available. I know that wore on him over time.

THERAPIST: He wanted you all to himself?

SARAH: Yes, totally.

THERAPIST: What does that tell you, that he wanted you all to himself?

SARAH: [sighing] I know he would have married me if I would have wanted that too. I'm sure the whole thing was too much for him to take.

THERAPIST: What an interesting realization you've had here. What are you taking from all of this?

SARAH: Good enough was never the issue. It was really a no-win situation from the get-go. [tearing up] I just . . . I just miss him.

THERAPIST: [speaking gently to communicate empathy] You're allowed to miss him. He was a big part of your life.

It is important to recognize that the process of Socratic questioning in the context of guided discovery is to provide a platform for clients to draw their own conclusions. At times, cognitive behavioral therapists can be over-zealous in their questioning and fire off several questions to "challenge" thoughts that either might be true or are at least experienced as very real by clients and are difficult to subject to empirical scrutiny. This type of questioning, often done in the spirit of a therapist trying to be compliant with the technique of CBT, can backfire and feel invalidating to the client (Kazantzis, Beck, et al., 2018). Thus, it is important to engage in guided discovery in a way that enhances the therapeutic relationship, providing validation and a stance that communicates a desire to understand the client's experience. More is said about this in Chapter 5 on cognitive restructuring.

CUSTOMIZED CASE FORMULATION

Cognitive behavioral therapists hold high respect for individual differences in an array of traits, strengths, preferences, and circumstances that their clients "bring to the table" when they present for treatment. Unless a client has a highly circumscribed condition (e.g., specific phobia, uncomplicated panic disorder) for which a well-validated treatment manual is available, most "real-world" cognitive behavioral therapists rely on the cognitive case formulation of the client's clinical presentation to guide treatment. *Cognitive behavioral case formulation* is the application of cognitive behavioral theory to understand the etiology, maintenance, and exacerbation of a client's mental health problems (Bieling et al., 2021; Kuyken et al., 2006; Persons, 2008). Because every client is characterized by a unique array of cognitive and behavioral traits and features, as well as different past and current life circumstances, every client has a unique cognitive behavioral case formulation. In other words, there are individual differences in the prominent cognitive, behavioral, emotional, and circumstantial traits that are at the heart of understanding clients' clinical presentations. Cognitive behavioral therapists embrace these individual differences from a curious stance, drawing from the available scholarly literature as well as their clinical experience in developing a sophisticated framework from which to understand their clients' experiences and ways of reacting to their environments.

The cognitive behavioral case formulation guides the interventions selected in treatment. The most salient features of the cognitive behavioral case formulation typically serve as the primary targets of treatment. This means that no two courses of conceptualization-based CBT are the same because each client's cognitive behavioral case formulation is unique. Thus, a respect for individual differences is captured in each client's treatment plan because the treatment plan will be tailored to each client's needs and goals.

There exists a vast array of schemes to facilitate cognitive case formulation. Perhaps the most heavily referenced and utilized approach is that taught by faculty and staff at the Beck Institute for Cognitive Behavior Therapy (see J. S. Beck, 2021, p. 53). According to this model, the beliefs that guide the way we operate are shaped by formative life experiences. Many of these key life experiences occur in childhood, but certainly, important life events in adulthood (e.g., military experiences, divorce, sexual assault) shape our beliefs as well. J. S. Beck differentiated between two different levels of beliefs. *Core beliefs* are fundamental beliefs about the self, others, world, and future. Here are some examples: (a) "I am a burden" (i.e., core belief about the self), (b) "Others will take advantage of me" (i.e., core belief about others), (c) "Danger is everywhere" (i.e., core belief about the world), and (d) "Life will not get better" (i.e., core belief about the future). In most clients, negative or unhelpful core beliefs are not perpetually activated; instead, they lay dormant until they are prompted by stressful or aversive life circumstances (Wenzel et al., 2016). *Intermediate beliefs* take the form of rules and assumptions about standards one must reach, expectations for others' behavior, or the way in which life should be. Most intermediate beliefs follow from a person's core beliefs. For example, if a survivor of repeated childhood sexual abuse formed the core belief, "I am not safe," she might also carry intermediate beliefs such as, "If I let down my guard, I will be violated" or "I must be on guard at all times." Finally, *compensatory strategies* are behavioral (and sometimes mental) maneuvers that people make to protect themselves from painful core beliefs. Continuing with the example of the survivor of childhood sexual abuse, she might isolate herself from others, sharing very few personal details, to compensate for the belief of not feeling safe; she might respond aggressively when she perceives (probably very quickly) an attack or a betrayal by others; or, interestingly, she might engage in reckless behavior with the attitude, "Why does it matter? I'm not safe anyway."

Thus, there is an infinite combination of core beliefs, intermediate beliefs, and compensatory strategies that can characterize any one client seen in treatment. The individual differences in such a cognitive behavioral profile are fascinating and vast and, in my opinion, part of the appeal of being a cognitive behavioral therapist is developing such an intricate cognitive behavioral case formulation in collaboration with the client and testing it out against ongoing observations of the client's behavior. Another important feature of such a scheme is that it can help make understandable a client's reaction when they are faced with a particular situation in their life. In other words, the underlying beliefs that a person holds shed light on their cognitive reactions when they are faced with a specific situation (e.g., the meaning the situation holds, the way in which they interpret what is happening in the situation) as well as on their emotional and behavioral reactions. Two people can be faced with the exact same situation but respond to it in very different ways, on the basis of the individual differences in their underlying beliefs and associated compensatory strategies. This framework can be used to understand Sarah's clinical presentation, her reactions to her current life stressors, and the way in which she carried herself in treatment.

> Even at a young age, Sarah was artistic and creative, and she interacted with the world in an "outside of the box" manner. Rather than praising Sarah for her unique insights and problem-solving approaches, her conservative parents often criticized her, gave indications that they were embarrassed by her, and asked her why she could not be more like other girls her age at school or at church. From these messages, she developed core beliefs such as, "I'm an outsider" and "I'm not okay the way I am." When she was in elementary school, she compensated for these beliefs by assuming a quiet, introverted stance and living by rules such as, "If I don't call attention to myself, then no one can criticize me." However, once Sarah began middle school, she became increasingly frustrated by what she perceived as her parents' conservative and judgmental nature. Although she continued to carry the belief of being an outsider, she developed a new compensatory strategy for managing it, such that she flaunted it and almost dared others to call her out on being "weird" or otherwise inappropriate. By nature, Sarah was a polite, kind-hearted, and conscientious girl; but during her middle school and high school years, she rebelled against this disposition and angrily challenged authority and societal norms. She received such a significant amount of negative feedback from many sources—her parents, her teachers, her peers, and law enforcement—that she developed additional and more destructive core beliefs (e.g., "I'm damaged goods" and "I'm not good enough") and ones that cognitive behavioral therapists often see in their most depressed clients ("I'm worthless" and "I'm defective").
>
> In young adulthood, Sarah embraced the core belief of being an outsider. Although she did not flaunt it in the same way she did in high school, she zestfully embraced the behaviors of her community of friends, such as by getting multiple piercings, engaging in marches and protests, and becoming a fixture at local music venues. In contrast, the more serious core beliefs of being "damaged" and "worthless" were not perpetually active, but they were evident in times of interpersonal stress or rejection. At the time Sarah presented for treatment, she was consumed with rumination about the relationship with her boyfriend ending because there was something very wrong with her. As a

result, she reported severe depression and suicidal ideation that was fueled by a sense that she was so flawed that there was no hope for her to have happiness or fulfillment.

In addition to understanding clients' unique histories, life experiences, and ways in which they make sense of their life experiences, as mentioned in Chapter 2, it is essential to consider cultural and environmental forces that shape a client's ways of viewing themselves, others, and the world. In some instances, beliefs that seem distorted or unhelpful to a therapist might make perfect sense and be readily validated by others who share the same culture. Pamela Hays (2008, 2009) has advanced the ADDRESSING framework to enhance therapists' multicultural competence, particularly when using a cognitive behavioral approach. ADDRESSING is an acronym that guides therapists in considering a multitude of cultural influences as they develop their case formulation and propose corresponding therapeutic interventions. The elements of ADDRESSING include the following: Age/generational influences, Developmental disabilities, Disabilities acquired later in life, Religious and spiritual orientation, Ethnic and racial identity, Socioeconomic status, Sexual orientation, Indigenous heritage, National origin, and Gender. Next, we apply this framework to Sarah's case.

Two aspects of the ADDRESSING framework were relevant to Sarah's case formulation. One was her religious/spiritual identity, as she described herself as Wiccan and participated in many Wiccan ceremonies, traditions, and events. Her Wiccan identity often served as a source of strength for her, as it brought her together with likeminded people who formed a close-knit community. Moreover, many Wiccan practices involved unity with nature, which Sarah found soothing and healing. However, her parents were devout Christians, and they viewed her involvement in Wicca as sacrilegious and as signaling that she is a sinner. At one point, her parents disowned her for engaging in Wiccan practices; at the time Sarah started treatment, she was speaking with her parents on a limited basis. On the one hand, Sarah was proud of her involvement with the Wiccan community and felt truly accepted there; on the other hand, her core beliefs of being an outsider and damaged were activated when she experienced her parents as berating her for making this spiritual choice.

In addition, Sarah was female, and she was particularly observant of gender differences in the way in which her male district manager treated her, relative to men who managed other restaurants in the district. Sarah struggled with a lack of assertiveness with her male colleagues, worrying that she would become emotional and would not be taken seriously if she spoke her mind. Sarah compensated for this concern by staying quiet, even taking unwarranted criticism from her district manager. As will be seen in later chapters, Sarah discussed workplace stress stemming from a lack of assertiveness a great deal in sessions with her therapist, prompting the delivery of several cognitive behavioral interventions.

The case formulation is developed collaboratively with the client. That is, the therapist educates the client about key constructs in the case formulation; when the client expresses something that has the potential to be especially relevant to the case formulation, the therapist is transparent about this to the client and obtains feedback from the client as to whether they concur. The therapist is also mindful of their own identity and how it interacts (or has the potential to interact) with the client's cultural background. The case formulation is ever evolving because it is refined over time as the client shares more and more about their subjective experiences, which is another reflection of empiricism. From the formulation, strategic cognitive behavioral intervention strategies are selected to address goals for treatment, again in collaboration with the client by providing the client with the rationale for the intervention and soliciting agreement. Thus, many of the CBT-specific tenets of collaboration, feedback, goal setting, and empiricism are evident in the process of case formulation.

Customized case formulation enhances the therapeutic relationship because it demonstrates to clients that their therapist is making a great effort to truly understand them. In addition, the selection of interventions that directly emerge from the customized case formulation communicates respect for the client's unique characteristics and history, and it shows that the therapist is thoughtfully investing time and effort into molding a treatment package that holds great promise for the client. In the process of gathering information to facilitate cognitive behavioral case formulation, the therapist will see ample opportunities to communicate empathy and positive regard.

CONCLUDING THOUGHTS

As demonstrated in this chapter, there are many fundamental elements of CBT that directly enhance the therapeutic relationship. The six elements described here include collaboration, feedback, goal setting, empiricism, guided discovery, and customized case formulation. They provide a foundation for a strong therapeutic relationship in many ways, including the demonstration that clients' opinions and viewpoints are respected and welcomed, that clients have been heard and are understood, and that the therapist is highly invested in helping clients overcome the issues that brought them to treatment. These features are interrelated; goals emerge from developing the case formulation in a collaborative manner; collaboration is enhanced by soliciting client feedback at every step; and the aims of each session are arrived at through collaboration and client feedback. Moreover, these features of CBT have the potential to enhance clients' investment in the treatment process by creating a welcoming environment, instilling hope that their lives can be different, and providing support and even companionship as they begin to think about and address their life problems in a new way.

As they deliver treatment, cognitive behavioral therapists are acutely aware of the six principles described in this chapter. Thus, their responses to their clients are strategic in that they are reinforcing these elements to both build the therapeutic relationship and provide a scaffolding for change—a hallmark feature of TRF-CBT. This means that cognitive behavioral therapists respond to their clients in an especially intentional manner that is designed to promote these basic principles of CBT. That said, these strategic responses are executed in a way that simultaneously exudes the common factors evident in the delivery of any quality psychotherapy, described in Chapter 2 of this volume. In other words, cognitive behavioral therapists promote collaboration, solicit feedback, set goals, model empiricism, conduct guided discovery, and develop a customized case formulation with the utmost empathy, warmth, genuineness, and positive regard. They allow their humanness to emerge as they are delivering treatment, forming a unique connection with their clients to enhance the real relationship. I believe that the strategic delivery of CBT within the context of one's humanness and genuine connection with the client makes CBT a special and unique experience for both client and therapist.

In Part II of this volume, Chapters 4–9 describe the manner in which cognitive behavioral therapists harness the common and CBT-specific aspects of the therapeutic relationship to establish and cultivate a working relationship and maximize the effectiveness of therapeutic interventions. Part II begins with relationship considerations evident in the very first contacts that a cognitive behavioral therapist has with a new client, beginning with the initial therapy inquiry to the first session.

PART **II** CLINICAL
GUIDANCE FOR
THERAPEUTIC
RELATIONSHIP-
FOCUSED
COGNITIVE
BEHAVIORAL
THERAPY

4

ESTABLISHING THE THERAPEUTIC RELATIONSHIP IN THE FIRST CONTACTS WITH A CLIENT

Although it is tempting to view the therapeutic relationship as commencing at the time of the first scheduled session, in reality it begins with the very first moment that the client is thinking of contacting the therapist, and it continues to develop and take form during the first contacts the potential client has with the therapist before they ever have their first session (cf. Gelso, 2011). This chapter describes ways in which the therapist can be mindful of the developing therapeutic relationship in this preliminary stage of work with a client, setting the stage for a successful course of therapeutic relationship-focused cognitive behavioral therapy (TRF-CBT). Moreover, it considers ways in which the early therapeutic relationship can advance psychoeducation about and optimism for all that CBT has to offer. This chapter also demonstrates the way in which the aims of the initial session, the cultivation of the therapeutic relationship, and the modeling of the CBT approach can be accomplished all at once.

Most clients put a great deal of thought into initiating a course of psychotherapy. It usually takes time for potential clients to recognize that there is a problem for which psychotherapy can be helpful. Then, many potential clients wrestle with a vast array of variables associated with the decision to seek psychotherapy, such as the time and cost involved, how regular sessions will

https://doi.org/10.1037/0000424-005
Therapeutic Relationship-Focused Cognitive Behavioral Therapy, by A. Wenzel

be worked into a busy schedule, and concerns about stigma. When they are contemplating the decision to pursue psychotherapy, potential clients also envision the type of therapist they hope to find. This involves not only the type of psychotherapy that the therapist delivers but also the therapist's style, personality, similarity to the client, competence, and reputation. It is at this juncture that many clients form expectations for the type of therapist with whom they will enter into a relationship.

I happen to be finishing this chapter as the COVID-19 pandemic is becoming endemic, and most people have largely transitioned back to "normal" life. During the pandemic, every therapist I know received an unprecedented number of referrals for services, which probably reflects the tremendous toll the pandemic took on mental health concurrently with many other concerning sociopolitical events. I have heard from many potential clients seeking my services that they made calls to several providers and that I was the only one from whom they received a return call. Imagine how a lack of therapist response would affect a potential client's thoughts and feelings about psychotherapy and psychotherapists in general if they were ambivalent about seeking services in the first place![1]

Thus, from the moment a potential client reaches out, it is important to model responsiveness, respect, care, and concern, all within the context of professional behavior and appropriate boundaries. Such responsiveness models interpersonal effectiveness, which very well might be a target of a specific course of CBT. Moreover, it begins to form a foundation for a healthy therapeutic relationship. Specific therapist behaviors that can help to achieve these aims might include the following:

- Returning a message within a timely manner (e.g., within 1 to 2 business days) upon receipt;

---

[1]Interestingly, in the weeks leading up to submission of this manuscript, I realized that I had a week-old voicemail from a prospective client who I had missed while I was traveling. I immediately returned the call and apologized for the significant delay in responding, stating something like, "It's a big decision to take the step to begin psychotherapy, and you deserve much respect for taking that step. And part of that respect would be a timely return phone call." The client remarked that I was the only therapist who had gotten back to him, so he was just pleased to hear back from me, even after a week-long delay. I expedited the process of working him into my schedule, and I took extra care to develop a strong therapeutic alliance and real relationship (recognizing that I needed to work through my own guilt about taking so long to return his phone call). After the fifth session, the client remarked that he had never remained in therapy for more than a couple of sessions before this experience, that he trusted me to do right by him, and that this trust started the moment that I took ownership over the week-long delay in returning his phone call.

- Supplying reasonable expectations for when the potential client might be able to schedule an appointment;

- Providing at least one referral if the therapist is unable to take on the client due to scheduling or needs that are different than the therapist's expertise;

- Providing thoughtful answers to any client questions about logistics (e.g., payment for sessions) or the therapist's approach;

- If an appointment is set, explaining the new client paperwork that the client will be expected to complete in advance of the appointment;

- If an appointment is set, providing directions to the office or instructions for accessing a session via a telehealth service; and

- If an appointment is set, describing what the client can expect in the first appointment.

The following excerpt describes Sarah's[2] first contacts with her therapist. She made the initial contact by sending an email to the therapist. The email read something like this:

Hello Therapist,

My name is Sarah Carter, and I was referred to you from Dr. Joyce Reynolds. I am experiencing high levels of anxiety. I am diagnosed with bipolar disorder with rapid cycling. I am medicated for the bipolar and also for the anxiety. However, nothing is effective for the anxiety. I cannot sleep. I cannot focus, and I had been having a very difficult time performing at work before I took short-term disability. I am reaching out in hopes that you can be of help. Thank you for your consideration.

Sincerely, Sarah Carter

The therapist received the email in between sessions and quickly wrote something like the following response using her encrypted web-based email service:

Hi Sarah,

Many thanks for your interest in my practice; how kind of Dr. Reynolds to think of me to work with you. I am sorry to hear that you have been going through such a difficult time. I use cognitive behavioral therapy, which is a terrific match for anxiety. Perhaps we can talk on the phone briefly so I can hear a bit more about the situation, and so we can determine if we're a good match to work with one another? I'm available today at 2:30 if you're available to touch base then.

Warmly, Therapist

---

[2]Client identity has been disguised to protect client confidentiality.

Take a moment to reflect on what you notice in this brief correspondence. First, it appears that Sarah received the therapist's name from another provider, which suggests that this provider thinks highly of the therapist. The therapist recognized this and expressed gratitude for Sarah's interest in the practice and for her colleague for referring Sarah to her practice. Not only was this a genuine response on the part of the therapist, but it also created a context for Sarah to feel welcomed into the practice (versus getting the sense that she would be fortunate to be admitted to the practice or she would be another "number" in a long wait-list line). Second, Sarah mentioned that she was going through a difficult time at the moment and seemed eager for help. The therapist recognized this and expressed empathy for Sarah's current circumstances before jumping into logistics. The therapist also ended the email with the valediction, "Warmly," in order to reinforce a warm, inviting stance.

Notice, however, that the therapist did not immediately guarantee Sarah a spot on her caseload. It is good practice to gather additional information through a telephone or in-person consultation before agreeing to enter into a psychotherapy relationship to (a) determine the potential client's level of risk and whether they require a higher level of care; (b) identify the potential client's presenting problems and whether they are within the therapist's expertise; and (c) determine whether the client is in alignment with the logistics of the practice, such as hours of operation, fees, and other policies. Offering the potential client an opportunity for such a consultation communicates interest and responsiveness on the part of the therapist, and it also models appropriate boundaries by communicating that it will be determined whether it will ultimately work out for the potential client and therapist to work with one another.

Sarah and the therapist were able to connect via telephone for a consultation, and together in a collaborative manner, they determined that they would be a good match to work with one another. Sarah scheduled an initial appointment with the therapist for the following week.

DETAILS AFFECTING THE THERAPEUTIC RELATIONSHIP LEADING UP TO THE FIRST APPOINTMENT

Seemingly small details can make an impression on potential clients and affect the establishment of the therapeutic relationship. Applying the cognitive behavioral framework, it is not difficult to imagine that a potential client who feels welcomed by the therapist and is impressed with the therapist's competence and organization might arrive to the first session with a mindset such as, "I'm eager to start working with this therapist, and I anticipate that I will benefit a great deal." This kind of positive mindset would facilitate behavior such as open communication and create the context for a strong therapeutic bond to develop at the outset. In contrast, it is equally not difficult to imagine that a potential client who has a negative reaction to the therapist's initial contact would either choose not to initiate a course of psychotherapy or might arrive to the first session with a mindset such as, "I'm not sure this is going to work out. I don't feel comfortable with this therapist." This kind of negative mindset would facilitate behavior such as stilted communication and create barriers for the development of a strong therapeutic bond.

Potential clients often start with a therapist's website, with a Google search either for therapists in their area or for a specific therapist recommended to them. As might be expected, a website that is organized, easy to navigate, welcoming, and hopeful will instill a different impression than one that is disorganized, difficult to navigate, and sterile. It is helpful to include the therapist's photograph so that potential clients can begin to match a face with the name and credentials. I also include a photograph of the building in which my practice is located so that clients who opt for in-person sessions have a sense of what they are looking for when traveling to their first appointment. In one area of my website, I include links for resources that my clients have found helpful in the past (e.g., *Mind Over Mood* by Greenberger & Padesky, 2016). I have received feedback from many clients that they were grateful for these recommendations and that they consulted one or more of these resources even before contacting me for treatment. Moreover, throughout my website, I include soothing images of nature that I have taken on my various travels over the years as a way to (a) promote a sense of soothing and healing and (b) include a unique piece of myself that I present to the public. My clients give me the feedback that the inclusion of these photographs contributed to the formulation of positive expectations for treatment with me.

Even a therapist's initial paperwork can communicate something about the therapist's style and, thereby, contribute to the therapeutic relationship. For example, in my own practice, I have developed a new client information form inspired by the intake form described by Kuyken et al. (2006). Their form is an eight-page document that asks clients to supply many details about their past and current life as well as their future goals and aspirations. When I first saw the type of information form that Kuyken et al. recommended, I thought it was absolutely fantastic; I also thought many of their ideas would significantly upgrade the quality of my clinical practice because I would have a rich repository of information to begin to develop my case formulation even before I had an initial session with a new client.

However, I experienced an unintended consequence of requiring such an information form. A small subset of clients who begin treatment with me have remarked that the form is off-putting because it is so lengthy. A few clients have even mentioned that they view the form as a bit intrusive because it includes items that, in their minds, inquire about sensitive information that they would not be comfortable sharing with someone with whom they have not yet developed a trusting relationship. Thus, there is potential with these clients for the therapeutic relationship to have started off on the "wrong foot" due to an aversive reaction to the new client paperwork. When these clients mention their reaction to me at the time of the first session, I take care to validate their concerns in order to attend to the therapeutic relationship (and begin repair work if the therapeutic relationship had been compromised). Moreover, I also model the CBT approach by directly addressing their concerns in an interpersonally effective manner. This interpersonal stance does not involve excessive apologizing for the length of and questions on the form; after all, each question included on the form is selected after careful thought on my part, with an eye toward gathering information that would facilitate the development of the case formulation. Instead, I say something like this:

> I really appreciate this feedback, and I assure you that I will consider what you are saying. In fact, you're not the only person who has communicated this to me. I give all of my clients my word that I will carefully review the information supplied and come prepared with a working knowledge of their histories at the time of the first session. I also give all of my clients my word that I will treat this sensitive information with respect and abide by psychologists' code of confidentiality. We will be sure to use the hard work that you put into this form in therapy, as we develop an understanding of the issues on which you want to focus and identify a corresponding treatment plan that has promise.

With this response, I am providing validation, normalization, a sense of being heard, and assurance that clients' hard work will be put to good use, all of which have potential to contribute to a strong therapeutic relationship. Moreover, I am modeling transparency—a hallmark feature of CBT—about what I will do with the information they supply. In describing the way in which I will use the information the client provides, I am also demonstrating a sense of competence to treat the issues bringing them to therapy.

The presentation of the office might also affect clients' perceptions of the therapist, which can, in turn, affect the therapeutic relationship. In fact, the physical surroundings can often be one of the first ways a therapist expresses their "personhood" as they establish a real relationship (Gelso, 2011). For example, I stock my office with many amenities to make clients feel comfortable and welcomed, such as a Keurig coffee machine with a vast array of different coffee, tea, and cocoa cups; a minirefrigerator with bottled water, coconut water, seltzers, and juices; a basket of prepackaged snacks; a magazine rack filled with popular magazines that are interesting to large segments of the population; and a notice indicating the Wi-Fi network name and password. I have had many clients tell me that my magazines are among the "best" that they have ever seen in a doctor's office (oftentimes joking that they are thrilled not to have to page through yet another outdated issue of *Popular Mechanics*). More generally, many clients have commented that they very much appreciate the care that I seem to have taken in making them comfortable, which contributes to a sense of looking forward to coming to my office for sessions and a sense that I genuinely care about their comfort and well-being.

It is also important for the therapist to promote cultural inclusiveness through their choice of photographs on their website and décor in the office. For example, if there are photographs of people, the therapist should ensure that people of color are represented. If there are photographs depicting partner relationships, the therapist should ensure that they are not dominated by cisgender heterosexual couples. Attention to these details will help to counter marginalization.

The first moment in which the therapist and client lay eyes on each other also has the potential to impact the therapeutic relationship. If the therapist appears hurried, aloof, or distracted, the client might form a negative view about the therapist's competence or style. Conversely, if the therapist expresses genuine eagerness to meet the client in person and begin their work together, the client might form a positive view about the therapist's competence or style. When I meet clients for the first time in person, I ask if I can get them something to drink to reinforce an inviting, welcoming atmosphere. I am hopeful that this communicates a sense of respect and genuine care.

At times, clients might express something negative about their journey to the therapist's office, the building in which the office is located, or the directions to connect for the virtual session. The way in which the therapist handles a complaint or criticism can do wonders in setting the tone for the therapeutic relationship. I will never forget my work with an older adult client that could have started off on a very "bad foot." When I introduced myself in my waiting room, he proceeded to tell me that my directions to my office were wrong, that they resulted in him parking in the lot for the building next door to mine, and that this required him to walk much farther than he would have liked in the hot and humid Philadelphia summer weather. Although my directions had worked well for other clients up to that point, I expressed appreciation that the client communicated this to me and assured him that I would review them carefully so that no other new clients were led astray. I also communicated empathy by expressing that I would not be happy if I had to walk in the hot weather from the lot next door. As our therapeutic work together progressed, the client admitted that his attitude likely stemmed from having too much paperwork to complete and wondering whether I would be a "nice" person.

He indicated that he was pleasantly surprised by my personality and style, and we ended up doing fantastic work together in which we often reflected on the strength of the relationship that we had developed (which served as a sound model for his main therapeutic goal, which was to become more open to developing quality relationships in his senior living circumstances to combat his pervasive loneliness).

THE INITIAL SESSION

The initial session is the first "official," often more structured contact that the therapist will have with a client. The therapist and client have either agreed to enter into a therapeutic relationship, or they have agreed to have the first session (or a few sessions) to determine whether they would like to continue to work together. Thus, the first appointment provides more information about what it is like to work with the therapist, relative to a phone call, an exchange of messages, or peripheral experiences like completing the new client paperwork. In this section, I provide some guidance for ways to establish a strong therapeutic relationship in the first CBT session, as well as ways to set up the client for success in CBT. I also provide an excerpt of the initial session between Sarah and her therapist.

It is usually helpful to set expectations for the first session and beyond, in light of research documenting the association between positive outcome expectations and actual outcome in psychotherapy, as referenced in Chapter 2 of this volume. Clients who have not previously participated in psychotherapy can feel a bit unsure and unsettled about the process. Letting them know what to expect can ease their minds. Clients who have participated in one or more previous courses of psychotherapy are likely to be more familiar with the process, but because each course of psychotherapy is so unique, they may have a reaction if the first session of their course of CBT proceeds a bit differently than the previous course of treatment. To set accurate expectations for the first session (and beyond), a cognitive behavioral therapist might say something like this:

> If it's okay with you, I'd like to share a bit about what to expect from this first session and how it's similar to and different than therapy sessions if you choose to proceed. [*The therapist waits to proceed until they get an affirmative response from the new client.*] The first session is devoted to information gathering, so that I can get a more intricate sense of what brings you here, what you hope to work on in therapy, what your current life is like, and key factors from your past that have shaped the person you are today. Together, we will use that information to develop a working model to explain where you are today and the most fruitful

avenues to proceed with in therapy. If you continue to feel that we are a good match to work with one another, we will bridge from the information gathering that is occurring today to treatment planning so we have a clear idea on what we would like to accomplish together in our work and how we will measure progress toward those goals. As we enter into the phase of active treatment, you'll see that therapy is not at all about me asking lots of questions; it is a collaborative endeavor in which you have space to reflect on your experiences, learn more about yourself and ways to create meaningful change, and feel supported and understood.

Some of this communication was inspired by an experience I had in my graduate training, when a new client completed an intake session but did not return. The clinical director called the client for feedback; the client indicated that the intake felt too much like an interview to her, and she did not see promise for the development of a mutually warm and empathetic therapeutic relationship. Because of this experience, I am mindful of the fact that there is no true agenda to be accomplished in any one initial session, other than establishing a connection and obtaining a solid sense of the client's suicide risk to make an appropriate intervention. The most important aim of the first session is to give clients space to share relevant information about themselves, express concerns about stressors in their lives, discuss what they are looking for in their therapeutic work, and feel heard and validated. In some initial sessions, the discussion is heavily focused on diagnosis and symptoms; in other initial sessions, the discussion is heavily focused on current stressors; and in still other sessions, the discussion is heavily focused on the client's history. I find that information not gathered in the first session can be obtained in subsequent sessions to round out the case formulation. In other words, I do not willfully force an agenda in the first session (other than to assess for suicide risk); instead, I follow the client's lead, ask for their expectations and wishes for the first session, and allow discussion to unfold in a way that the client deems most relevant. At times, clients look to me for direction in how to proceed and, in these cases, I let them know that some clients start with their experiences of emotional distress (i.e., diagnosis and symptoms), others start with current stressors in their lives, and still others start with events of historical significance in their lives. When I provide this menu of options, clients readily veer toward the option that feels best to them. Moreover, I have modeled the principles of collaboration, feedback, and guided discovery.

Regardless of the direction the initial appointment takes, I find that the beginnings of the therapeutic relationship are greatly enhanced when the therapist shows evidence that they have read and processed the client's background information in a thoughtful manner. If a client mentions something that they included in the new client paperwork, the therapist might respond with something like, "I noticed that in your paperwork," and pose a thoughtful follow-up question to demonstrate that they had reflected on that piece of information. The therapist can also introduce bits of information included in the new client paperwork without being prompted by the client, which, again, demonstrates that the therapist has invested time and interest in getting to know the client and understanding their background. Many clients spontaneously comment on how much they appreciate this investment from the therapist and that it is different than what they experience from other health care providers.

In light of the fact that the primary focus of the initial session is to form a connection and develop the beginnings of a therapeutic relationship, many trainees ask me what makes an initial CBT session different than an initial session of psychotherapy guided by other theoretical orientations. I believe there are two main CBT-specific features of an initial session, which contribute both to establishing the therapeutic relationship and to advancing the CBT framework that will form the basis of subsequent sessions.

The first CBT-specific feature of an initial session is the posing of questions, and follow-up questions, that demonstrate and reinforce the CBT model and process. I would argue that every question posed should be strategic, in that it should have a purpose in advancing the CBT model and process, nurturing the therapeutic relationship, or both (Wenzel, 2013). The following example illustrates the opposite of what I am suggesting here, or the absence of strategy. In many initial CBT sessions that I have reviewed, I have heard supervisees ask the client where they were in the birth order relative to their siblings. During supervision, when I ask the therapist the rationale for this question, I am typically told something like, "I'm not sure, I just learned this question when I was being trained in graduate school, and I always ask it." If a therapist suspects that knowledge of birth order has the potential to be an important part of the case formulation that is being developed, by all means, they should ask about birth order. They might even go so far as to provide the rationale to the client for asking about birth order, in the spirit of transparency and of developing the case formulation in a collaborative manner (cf. Kuyken et al., 2006). However, if there is no rationale for obtaining a piece of information beyond the vague sense that therapists are "supposed to" ask those questions, therapists run the risk of asking extraneous questions that will detract from the therapeutic relationship because clients view their time as being devoted to superfluous, or even irrelevant, topics.

Second, in addition to asking questions that advance the case formulation, cognitive behavioral therapists are also encouraged to ask questions beginning in the very first session that model the CBT process. The following are some examples:

- "When that occurred, what was running through your mind?"
- "What did that situation mean to you? Or mean about you?"

- "When you had that thought, how did that make you feel?"
- "What do you see as the connection between your thinking and your emotional response in that situation?"
- "How did you respond, behaviorally, in that situation?"
- "How did you cope with the aftermath of that situation?"
- "What steps did you take to solve that problem?"

These questions demonstrate care and interest on the part of the therapist, as they clearly show that the therapist is interested in learning more about the life events that the client is sharing and about the client's internal and behavioral reaction to them. What's more, they are also subtly modeling an important aspect of the theory that underlies CBT—that our thinking, emotions, and behaviors are interrelated and influence one another. Moreover, the therapist will ask these same types of questions when they enact many of CBT's strategic interventions, such as cognitive restructuring and problem solving. This type of questioning provides important socialization into CBT so that clients are primed for it when treatment actually begins.

During these initial visits, most clients provide at least a glimpse into one or more key life events that had a lasting effect on them. Using the language of CBT, it is likely that these key events contributed significantly to shaping the clients' core beliefs about themselves, others, the world, and the future and their strategies to compensate for beliefs that are particularly painful, giving a glimpse into underlying schemas. When a client begins to talk about a key life event, the therapist listens attentively, communicates empathy, and expresses the sentiment that these events may potentially have a great deal of relevance for their cognitive behavioral work. For example, a new client recently described to me an incident from her past that she described as "humiliating," when someone spread awful rumors on social media about her sexual prowess, when, in fact, she was a middle school student with no sexual experience whatsoever. I said something like this to her in the initial session, after she described this incident and her thoughts and feelings about it:

> That experience sounds incredibly difficult, and I'm so sorry to hear you had to go through that. Sometimes, when people experience incidents like this, they develop beliefs about themselves, other people, boys, or friendships that they continue to carry even into adulthood. These are called core beliefs, and they can often explain, in part, the specific reactions we have in any one situation. Do you think this might have been an incident that shaped your beliefs about yourself or relationships? [*Client responds affirmatively.*] In what way?

When the CBT model is illustrated to clients at an opportune time, using a powerful example from their own lives, many clients acquire hope and optimism for treatment because they feel understood (in a relatively speedy manner) and because they begin to see a pathway for change to occur.

At this juncture, let us turn to expanded dialogue between Sarah and her therapist during their initial session. Throughout the dialogue, I illustrate the therapist's mindset and rationale for the questions posed and the stance taken, in the spirit of both developing the therapeutic relationship and in socializing Sarah into the CBT structure, model, and process. I also illustrate some of the therapist's internal reactions to the information that Sarah was presenting, along with the therapist's thought process in managing these reactions to enhance, rather than impede, the development of the therapeutic relationship. This dialogue begins about 10 minutes into the first session, when Sarah is explaining the complicated relationship situation with her (now ex-) boyfriend and her husband.

SARAH: And just like that. He said I needed to get out. [speaking dramatically] Andy had found the love of his life. He had been cheating on me for weeks! And where did that leave me? Out on the street, practically!

THERAPIST: [demonstrating care and empathy] I'm so sorry to hear that you had to endure such an abrupt ending to a valued relationship. [pausing] I noticed on your new client paperwork that you are a homeowner. Am I correct in understanding that you were quickly able to find and purchase a new home after Andy asked you to leave?

SARAH: Well [sighing] . . . I moved back in with my husband.

THERAPIST: [taken aback by this admission because Sarah had indicated her relationship status as "separated" on her paperwork, and the therapist thought that likely meant that she was separated from her boyfriend, although she had previously made a mental note to verify this assumption with Sarah] Oh, when you checked the "separated" box under marital status, you had been referring to your husband?

SARAH: I was actually referring to both of them.

THERAPIST: But now you've gone back to your husband?

SARAH: Living there, yes. Separate bedrooms though. We've always maintained some sort of friendship through this whole thing.

THERAPIST: [finding the details of Sarah's current relationship status to be a bit unexpected, wanting to be sure that she had and could communicate a full understanding of Sarah's situation, and also taking care to communicate a stance of nonjudgment] Let me summarize to make sure I'm right about the details. You met Andy when you were married to your husband, and the two of you developed an intimate relationship in which you moved in together and were together for approximately 2 years? And during this time, you were still married to your husband?

SARAH: Yes, exactly.

THERAPIST: How does your husband feel about your moving back?

SARAH: I don't know. We don't really talk about it. We kind of just picked up where things left off.

THERAPIST: [experiencing a distinctive internal reaction, finding it a bit incredible that Sarah and her husband could resume their previous living and marital arrangements without acknowledging and processing the fact that she had been in a cohabiting relationship with another man, and wanting to be sure that she demonstrated a steadfast stance of nonjudgment and confidence in light of this unexpected information] So you were able to move back into the house that you own with your husband. What is this like for you?

SARAH: I mean, I guess I'm lucky I have somewhere to go, right?

THERAPIST: [keeping her response short so that Sarah had space to elaborate] Yes, for sure.

SARAH: [sensing that the therapist wanted to hear more about what it was like to move back in with her husband] So, I don't know. Carlos kind of does his thing, and I kind of do my thing. Our schedules are pretty different, so we don't even always see each other. It's okay, I guess.

THERAPIST: Is there any tension between the two of you when you find yourselves in the house together?

SARAH: No, not really. I mean, it's really annoying that he leaves his dishes out, and I always have to clean up the kitchen after him. And he's making me sleep in the small bedroom, where there is not enough room for all of my stuff. But I don't say anything.

At this point, the therapist was struck by Sarah's lack of insight into the unusual nature of this situation. The therapist was a seasoned clinician who had heard many stories about infidelity and treated all of them with an open, nonjudgmental stance; the therapist checked herself to ensure that she was not having a judgmental reaction about Sarah's choices, and she determined that she was not. Instead, the therapist was surprised by the fact that Sarah was outraged at Andy for cheating on her, when she had engaged in similar behavior as the transgressor against her husband, and Sarah seemed not to see the parallel between the two situations. The therapist was also shocked that Sarah's husband took her back so easily and that neither one felt a need to talk about Sarah's relationship with Andy.

The therapist felt compelled to ask more questions to pull insight from Sarah, but she realized that this line of questioning was unnecessary at the moment for many reasons: (a) Sarah's lack of insight had already been clearly demonstrated; (b) a motivation for more questioning would have been driven by the therapist's curiosity, rather than a need for gathering additional information to benefit Sarah and the therapeutic process; and (c) an inadvertent consequence of persisting with questioning would be to shame Sarah for being in this situation, which would impair the therapeutic relationship. Thus, the therapist regrouped by reminding herself that Sarah is hurting, that Sarah has put great effort into finding quality psychotherapy and is reaching out for help, and that Sarah has had negative past experiences with the mental health system, which the therapist did not want to perpetuate at all costs. The therapist, then, quickly shifted from a stance of being somewhat incredulous to seeing Sarah's clinical presentation as an interesting opportunity full of potential for them to have an important clinical experience together. The initial session continued as follows:

THERAPIST: In your first email to me, you mentioned anxiety that is problematic in many ways, such that it interferes with your sleep and concentration. Can you tell me more about that?

SARAH: [putting her head in her hands and shaking her head] It's awful. Just awful. I've never felt anything like this before. I've struggled with depression many times, sure. I know what that is. But this anxiety is all new to me, and I just don't know what to do with it.

THERAPIST: What is your anxiety like?

SARAH: It's debilitating. I have a constant sense of dread hanging over my head. It's hard to eat; it's hard to sleep; I can't concentrate. I usually love being at work—when I'm myself, I'm all in—but in the time leading up to when I went on short-term disability, it seemed like I was just counting down the minutes to get out of there. Which is weird, because when I was at home and doing nothing, I was counting down the minutes to go to work.

THERAPIST: [communicating empathic understanding] It sounds like you are a bit lost, and that's much different than the way you usually are, so you're not sure what to do with it.

SARAH: Yes! That's exactly it.

THERAPIST: [taking the opportunity to model the CBT process using the example of Sarah's anxiety at work] Could you take a moment to imagine yourself at work, really bringing yourself back to one of those moments in which you were struggling, feeling anxious, lost, and agitated?

SARAH: Mm-hmm. It was what put me over the edge and made me talk to my district manager about going out on short-term disability.

THERAPIST: What moment at work are you imagining, in particular?

SARAH: It was worst in the middle of the afternoon, when the restaurant was dead, and there wasn't as much to do as there is in the lunch or dinner rush. And my coworker, Sonia. God, she's so annoying. She wouldn't stop jabbering about everything under the sun, and I felt like I was going to jump out of my skin.

THERAPIST: [showing empathy with her tone of voice] That sounds very uncomfortable. Tell me, thinking back to that situation, when traffic was low and Sonia was running your ear off, what was running through your mind at that time? [*Here, the therapist is harnessing the connection that is being forged, via empathy and understanding, to socialize the client into the CBT model and process.*]

SARAH: [pausing] Hmmm. Running through my mind. It felt like my mind was screaming, "I can't stand this anymore!"

THERAPIST: Okay, that you can't stand it. That's really unpleasant. Anything else?

SARAH: [tears forming] That I'm trapped. That I'm trapped in this stupid life, with no one who truly loves me, and all alone! [begins crying in earnest]

THERAPIST: [speaking gently, modeling the cognitive model at the same time] Anyone in the world who believes that they can't stand it, that they are trapped, that no one loves them, and that they are all alone would experience a great deal of anxiety. And probably many other upsetting emotions as well. [*These statements are aimed at deepening the therapeutic connection and communicating understanding by normalizing the client's emotions, done in a way that further reinforces the CBT model and process.*]

SARAH: Oh, yeah definitely, there was sadness. And frustration. And shame . . . oh God, the shame.

THERAPIST: When you have thoughts like that—of being trapped, of no one loving you, of being alone—and emotions like that, like extreme anxiety, sadness, frustration, and especially shame . . . are you able to focus on what you need to focus on? Do the things you need or want to do? [*Here, the therapist is extending the modeling of the CBT process by linking the client's thoughts and emotions to behavior and functioning.*]

SARAH: [shaking her head] No, not at all. [crying some more] That's why I went on short-term disability. Because my anxiety was so bad that I just couldn't function at work.

THERAPIST: What if you were to adopt a somewhat different mindset? Not Pollyanna or a bed of roses, but perhaps a more helpful mindset? [*Here, the therapist is continuing to reinforce the CBT model and process and, at the same time, instilling hope that life can be different.*]

SARAH: I can't even imagine what.

THERAPIST: I'm thinking, for example, of remembering how resilient you are and have been in the past, acknowledging other times in your life that were just excruciating and that you came through on the other side. And remembering those close friends you have. Even though they are not romantic partners, which I know you are very much missing right now, they are people who care and who would not want you to feel alone. If you thought of both of those things, do you think you would feel quite so anxious, sad, frustrated, and ashamed? [*This question offers a concrete glimpse into what one central aspect of CBT—cognitive restructuring—has to offer.*]

SARAH: Maybe not as much. At least a little bit.

THERAPIST: And when you take that little edge off of the anxiety, sadness, frustration, and shame . . . do you think you might be able to focus just a little bit better on work? And other things you'd like to be doing?

SARAH: Probably. I think my functioning, or really lack thereof, goes hand-in-hand with how I feel.

THERAPIST: This, right here, is an example of one aspect of CBT that we can pursue together. Not only can we get an intricate sense of the way in which your thinking, feelings, and behaviors are related, but we can intervene in any one of those areas to affect the other two. And in this example, we illustrated how shifting the thinking part, just a little bit, would have a noticeable effect on your mood and behavior.

SARAH: [brightening up a bit] That's really great. I'm so tired of endlessly exploring my problems, my choices, my relationship with my parents. I'd like to figure out how to manage this and make more permanent changes in my life.

THERAPIST: And it would be a privilege for me to join you on that journey to acquire the tools you need to make that happen.

SARAH: [looking surprised at the heartfelt sentiment, and speaking softly] Thank you. I don't think I've ever had a therapist say that before. They usually take one look at me and run for the hills.

Several points about this initial session dialogue deserve note. Throughout the dialogue, the therapist was mindful of intentionally demonstrating care, concern, empathy, and an open and nonjudgmental stance. As mentioned in Chapter 2 of this volume, these factors are fundamental building blocks of good therapy and a good therapeutic relationship. However, when therapists keep these factors in the forefront of their minds, facilitating the explicit expression of statements consistent with these factors, my clinical experience suggests that the degree to which they are "felt" by clients is enhanced. Second, the therapist made references to the initial email correspondence she had with Sarah, as well as to the new client paperwork that Sarah had completed, to move the questioning forward. This shows that the therapist remembered the specific details of Sarah's case, even though they were still getting acquainted, and has the potential to demonstrate that she values Sarah as a person and truly wants to help her work through the challenges that bring her to therapy.

It is true that the therapist was momentarily taken aback by the unorthodox situation that Sarah was describing. The therapist quickly recognized that she was having this reaction and evaluated whether she was somehow responding negatively to Sarah's choice to have a relationship with another man when she remained married to her husband. The therapist promptly realized that she was not necessarily judgmental of Sarah's behavior, but that she found it perplexing that Sarah did not recognize the parallels between what was happening in her relationship with her boyfriend, Andy, and what was happening in her marital relationship with her husband, Carlos. The therapist also suspected that there was much emotional baggage to "unpack" between Sarah and Carlos now that the relationship with Andy had ended and Sarah had moved back into the house. And yet, Carlos seemed to take her back in without question or any discussion about the way he felt while his wife was living with another man for several years. The avoidance of addressing a broken marriage as demonstrated by both Sarah and her husband in this scenario was profound, in the therapist's estimation. Although the therapist concluded that she was not experiencing countertransference per se, she was indeed experiencing surprise and incredulousness, which still had the potential to be felt (and interpreted negatively) by Sarah. Thus, the therapist quickly reoriented herself by reacknowledging Sarah's pain and what she hoped to extend to Sarah as a helping professional.

Also of note in this dialogue was that the therapist took the opportunity to socialize Sarah into the CBT model and process. Part of the therapist's regrouping after learning more about Sarah's relationship history was to focus on the presenting issue at hand, which Sarah had indicated was debilitating anxiety. The therapist asked for a specific example of a time when Sarah experienced a surge of anxiety and illustrated the interrelations among her thoughts, emotions, and behaviors, as well as the way in which intervening at the level of thoughts would affect the intensity of her anxiety as well as her functioning (i.e., behavior). Not only did this exchange demonstrate a glimpse of what Sarah could expect in CBT, but it also instilled hope and optimism because it showed her a way that therapy would be different from what she had experienced in the past. This was important in light of the fact that Sarah had reported negative experiences with previous courses of therapy.

Finally, take a moment to reflect on the therapist's statement at the end of this dialogue: "And it would be a privilege for me to join you on that journey to acquire the tools you need to make that happen." Sarah was clearly moved by the therapist's expression of teamwork and honor that Sarah had shared some of her life story with her. Such overt statements, when warm, genuine, and authentic, can contribute significantly to establishing and nurturing a strong therapeutic relationship, particularly through the pathway of creating a strong real relationship.

BUILDING A THERAPEUTIC ALLIANCE

As seen in this volume to this point, it is crucial to develop a therapeutic alliance in the early contacts with a client. The therapeutic alliance ensures that the therapist and client are in agreement about the work to be done in therapy, including therapeutic goals; cognitive, emotional, and behavioral targets to be modified; and the way in which goals and psychological modification will be achieved. In addition, the bond that begins to form between the client and therapist—much of which can be cultivated by being mindful of the common factors of psychotherapy, described in Chapter 2 of this volume—can facilitate the work of therapy and, ultimately, successful outcome. As seen in this chapter, even the initial email or telephone correspondence between the therapist and client can begin to cultivate the therapeutic alliance and enhance the client's belief and hopefulness in treatment and in the therapist as the provider.

As discussed in Chapter 2 of this volume, much has been written in the scholarly literature on the nature and predictive capacity of the therapeutic alliance on outcome. However, there is a surprising paucity of scholarship on the factors that contribute to a strong therapeutic alliance (Doran, 2016) and on ways to create a sound therapeutic alliance (cf. Castonguay et al., 2006; Gaines et al., 2021; Horvath, 1994). In one exception, Greenson (1967) wrote, "The analyst contributes to the working alliance by consistent emphasis on understanding and insight, by his continual analysis of resistances, and by his compassionate, empathetic, straightforward, and nonjudgmental attitudes" (p. 46). This statement reflects the balance between strategic therapeutic work within a coherent theoretical framework (in this case, psychoanalysis) as well as the characteristics that would allow this work to unfold in a safe environment for the client (i.e., compassionate, empathetic, straightforward, and nonjudgmental attitudes). Steven Ackerman and Mark Hilsenroth identified several alliance-facilitating therapist characteristics, including being flexible, experienced, honest, respectful, trustworthy, confident, interested, alert, friendly, warm, and open (Ackerman & Hilsenroth, 2003), as well as several alliance-interfering therapist characteristics, including being distracted, self-focused, uninvolved, and disrespectful (Ackerman & Hilsenroth, 2001). In my view, these characteristics are just as important in cultivating the real relationship as they are in building the therapeutic alliance. Moreover, Ackerman and Hilsenroth identified specific therapeutic techniques that therapists can implement to build the therapeutic alliance, including facilitating the expression of affect, collaboratively developing treatment goals, and explicitly affirming the client's past and present experiences. They also identified techniques that impeded the therapeutic alliance, such as overstructuring the session, using self-disclosure or silence in an inappropriate manner, and making superficial interventions. Specifically within the context of CBT, Goldfried et al. (2003) suggested that the thoughtful use of therapist self-disclosure can enhance the bond between the therapist and client.

Paul Crits-Cristoph and his colleagues developed an innovative approach to train therapists to maximize the therapeutic alliance, which they applied to an interpersonally oriented psychodynamic therapy (Luborsky, 1984) and translated into a manualized treatment (supportive-expressive therapy; Crits-Christoph et al., 2010). Agreement on goals was achieved by setting specific treatment goals and reviewing those goals regularly throughout the course of treatment. Agreement on tasks was achieved by socializing the client into the process of therapy and reviewing these tasks throughout the course of treatment to ensure that the client was still in agreement with them. Bond-facilitating techniques were inspired by Orlinsky et al. (1994) and included (a) personal role involvement (i.e., identifying the stage of change that characterized the client and motivating them for change if needed), (b) interactive coordination (i.e., establishing a collaborative relationship, facilitated by therapist empathy and the use of the word "we"), (c) communicative contact (i.e., demonstrating that the client is being heard through accurate reflections), and (d) mutual affirmation (i.e., demonstrating caring, warmth, acceptance, and positive regard). All of these techniques can be implemented in an intentional manner within the context of CBT. Within the framework of contemporarily practiced CBT, and influenced by these sources, I compiled in Exhibit 4.1 suggestions for agreeing on the tasks and goals of therapy, as well as ways to develop a therapeutic bond. Let us now turn back to the case of Sarah to demonstrate the development of a strong therapeutic alliance in the initial phase of treatment.

> As was standard in the therapist's practice, after the initial session that was focused on information gathering, she asked Sarah if she would be willing to complete two tasks before her next session: (a) identify what she hoped to accomplish in their course of CBT and (b) conduct cursory internet research on CBT and return with a list of features that she found attractive and believed would be helpful, as well as any features that she found unattractive or about which she had questions. Sarah readily agreed to take on both tasks. The therapist invited Sarah to elaborate on what she thought would be helpful about these tasks, as she wanted to be sure that Sarah was not simply agreeing to the tasks in order to please the therapist. Sarah responded with, "I've already been looking into CBT a bit, and it's really different than most of the therapy that I've had in the past. I know my thinking can get me into trouble. So getting down on paper some of the thoughts that I've already been having about what will be helpful and what it can apply to in my own life sounds like a good way to start." The therapist assured Sarah that her wishes, preferences, and sense

EXHIBIT 4.1. Strategies for Building a Strong Therapeutic Alliance

Ways to Develop Agreement on the Goals and Tasks of Therapy

- Actively solicit client input about the goals and tasks of therapy.
- Respond in a manner that reinforces the client's input about the goals and tasks of therapy (e.g., "I think you are spot on with that suggestion").
- Prioritize the client's wishes.
- Be sure to ask for feedback from the client when advancing a therapist-driven aspect of the goals and tasks of therapy.
- When providing psychoeducation that is relevant to the goals and tasks of therapy, take time to pause for client questions and input and to check the client's understanding.
- When indicators arise, which signal a lack of agreement on the goals and tasks of therapy, share that observation and invite open and honest discussion to achieve realignment.
- Assure the client that no therapeutic intervention will be pushed on them without their permission, and that declining a particular therapeutic intervention will not jeopardize their status as a client.

Ways to Develop a Therapeutic Bond

- Express genuine delight in taking on the client and in any early therapeutic interactions.
- Express optimism for the therapeutic work that will be done with the client.
- Use nonverbal indicators of warmth and openness, including smiling, an open (versus closed) postural stance, and a soft tone of voice.
- Focus just as much on the relationship and on getting to know the client, if not more, than the "business" of the early sessions of treatment (e.g., paperwork).
- Use self-disclosure judiciously, in a way that demonstrates common ground between the therapist and client (cf. Goldfried et al., 2003).
- Remember small details about the client's life.
- Start the session on time and do not cut the session short in order for the client to develop trust in the therapist and the therapy process.

of what would be most helpful would be valuable and essential information to have as they developed a treatment plan.

When Sarah returned for her subsequent session, she brought in a list of targets for treatment as well as a list of points about CBT that she found to be a good match for her. Sarah's work was used as a catalyst for specific discussion about a customized approach to CBT that could be applied to her clinical presentation and life circumstances. The plan included three main problem areas with which Sarah reported struggling—the issue of immediate concern, the dissolution of her romantic relationship; her difficulties with emotion regulation; and the more distal but daunting issues on the horizon for Sarah, which were decisions she was going to have to make about her future. The therapist took care to provide psychoeducation about each of the treatment strategies in understandable language, and they were only included in the treatment plan if Sarah concurred that she would be open to them and anticipated that they would be helpful. At the end of the treatment planning process, the therapist obtained feedback from Sarah about her experience with it. Sarah remarked that it felt "really, really good" to be a collaborator in the treatment plan, as her experience in the past had been that the goals of treatment were either determined by her parents or by the philosophy of the treatment program in which she was being enrolled.

Throughout these first sessions, the bond between the therapist and Sarah began to solidify. The bond was strengthened when the therapist took seriously Sarah's goals, preferences, and thoughts about the direction of therapy, as Sarah very much appreciated that stance in light of her previous experiences. Less tangibly, the two of them began to enjoy one another as unique individuals. When Sarah presented for each session, there was a change in her appearance—she had changed her hairstyle, gotten another piercing, or was wearing a new outfit that she had sewn from scraps of fabric that she stumbled upon. These appearance changes allowed the therapist to show genuine interest in Sarah's self-expression and artistic ability; Sarah appreciated the therapist's interest because she typically experienced health care professionals as being judgmental about her appearance. These informal discussions helped Sarah to feel accepted and relaxed in her relationship with the therapist, which undoubtedly enhanced their bond as treatment progressed.

Sarah was seen by a therapist in private practice who had autonomy over the practice website, manner of communicating with referrals, new client paperwork, and office space. However, many therapists work in settings (e.g., hospital, corrections) in which they have no control over the impression that clients have of their affiliated organization or of them, or in which clients have little or no information about the setting before the first session. Therapists who work in such settings should keep in mind that they will not have the opportunity to build the therapeutic alliance before the first session. Moreover, it is possible that their client will present in a guarded or skeptical manner because the client is unsure what they are getting into or how they will be received by the therapist. A warm, welcome stance expressing a gentle eagerness to work with the client could help in such a scenario. The therapist could also begin by asking the client how they feel about the setting and the process of scheduling a first appointment so that any client concerns can be heard in an open, nonjudgmental manner. If there are, indeed, concerns or any negative impressions expressed, the therapist can provide validation and solicit client collaboration on how best to ease into the therapy process from that point forward.

CONCLUSION AND FUTURE DIRECTIONS

The seeds for the therapeutic relationship begin long before clients have their initial session with their therapist. The therapist's website, description of their services, interactions on phone calls to answer questions and schedule appointments, and aesthetics of and amenities in the office all contribute to shaping clients' views of their therapist as they begin the initial session. Of course, the degree to which clients feel accepted, heard, validated, and understood in the initial session also carries great meaning as the client and therapist establish their relationship and a therapeutic alliance. Although much work is usually accomplished in the initial session, including the receiving and processing of paperwork, establishing a psychiatric diagnosis, determining the client's presenting problems and goals, and determining suicide risk, cognitive behavioral therapists are strongly encouraged to keep the establishment of a sound, warm, and trusting therapeutic relationship in the forefront of their minds as they proceed.

I firmly believe that the initial session is a great opportunity to model CBT process and structure *simultaneously* as the therapeutic relationship is being cultivated, providing the initial template for a successful course of TRF-CBT. Asking straightforward questions such as "When that happened, what was running through your mind?" or "When you noticed that thought, how were you feeling emotionally?" shows care, interest, and curiosity in the client's experience, and it reinforces the fundamentals of the CBT model—that there are interrelations between our thinking and how we feel. Moreover, it provides a template for the types of questions that will be asked in sessions moving forward, so that clients are socialized into the interactions they can expect to have with their therapist in CBT. The material presented in this chapter is based on clinical experience and the insights of expert clinicians. Thus, it will be important for future research to verify the assumptions posed in this chapter. To summarize, the assumptions are as follows:

1. Clients' expectations for therapy are shaped by impressions formed by a therapist's website, initial contact with the therapist, the therapist's new client paperwork, the therapist's office, and the initial session with a therapist.

2. The strength of the therapeutic relationship is affected by the expectations developed from these initial interactions.

Although there is a rich literature on the way in which client's expectations affect outcome in psychotherapy (cf. Constantino, Vîslă, et al., 2019), there are no studies (to my knowledge) that quantify the ways in which clients' reactions to these specific types of initial contact influence their expectations and then affect the cultivation of aspects of the therapeutic relationship (e.g., the therapeutic alliance, the real relationship). Results from studies designed to isolate the effects of these initial contacts would provide important guidance to therapists as they mindfully begin their work with clients.

In contrast, as discussed in Chapter 2 of this volume, there is a great deal of research indicating that a strong therapeutic alliance established in the early sessions of psychotherapy (and CBT in particular) enhances outcome. Cognitive behavioral therapists can use the strong foundation built from the initial interactions with and impressions formed by clients to hone in on the alliance as they transition to targeted discussion about the goals and tasks of treatment. In other words, cognitive behavioral therapists start with genuine interest in getting to know a new client, and they then focus on the working bond that they are developing to clarify and even build excitement for the work that they are going to do together throughout the course of treatment. In the next several chapters, examples of the collaborative work done in treatment are illustrated, with a focus on continued attention to cultivating and using the therapeutic relationship to achieve treatment goals.

5 COGNITIVE RESTRUCTURING AND THE THERAPEUTIC RELATIONSHIP

Cognitive restructuring is the process by which therapists coach clients to identify, evaluate, and (if necessary) modify unhelpful thinking. Cognitive restructuring is the central strategy used in A. T. Beck's cognitive therapy (A. T. Beck
et al., 1979), and it has remained a staple across most of the broad family of
cognitive behavioral therapies (CBTs) in general. Through cognitive restructuring, clients learn to catch thinking that is associated with life interference
and emotional distress, as well as to adjust it so it is as factual, accurate, and
helpful as possible. When clients practice cognitive restructuring, they often
have the reaction, "Oh, I've never thought about it like that before. There is
some truth to that." As a result, cognitive restructuring often can help clients
to leave the session feeling understood, listened to, and that they obtained
valuable insight. This felt sense strengthens the therapeutic relationship
because clients experience a sense of teamwork, support, encouragement, and
that someone is invested in their lives. This chapter describes specific ways
to implement cognitive restructuring with a simultaneous focus on the therapeutic relationship, supplying tips to enhance the therapeutic relationship
through the use of this intervention strategy, as well as ways in which it can
be a catalyst for repair when there is a potential rupture in the therapeutic
alliance.

https://doi.org/10.1037/0000424-006
Therapeutic Relationship-Focused Cognitive Behavioral Therapy, by A. Wenzel

The primary technique of cognitive restructuring is that of guided discovery. As mentioned in Chapter 3 of this volume, *guided discovery* is a process of focused questioning that allows clients to examine, evaluate, and reshape thoughts associated with excess emotional distress. To facilitate this process, cognitive behavioral therapists use *Socratic questioning* (or *Socratic dialogue*), which stimulates critical thinking about the issue at hand and allows for a person to consider multiple ways of viewing the issue in order to draw a thoughtful conclusion (cf. Kazantzis, Beck, et al., 2018). Active, engaged guided discovery shows that therapists are truly interested in "putting their heads together" with their clients to identify a way to soften their emotional distress, no matter how large or small the problem is. This technique allows therapists to remember small details from their clients' lives that may have relevance to reframing their views of difficult situations. It is often the case that clients are touched when therapists remember these small details, especially those that are communicated in a different session and context but have direct relevance in astute therapist questioning.

Therapists who implement cognitive restructuring are encouraged to do so in a manner that keeps the therapeutic relationship in the forefront of their minds, consistent with the fundamental premise of therapeutic relationship-focused CBT (TRF-CBT). As mentioned in Chapter 3 of this volume, Socratic questioning is designed to be implemented in a curious, sensitive, encouraging manner—not one that clients experience as debating, forcing a viewpoint, or backing them into a corner. Put bluntly, if a therapist feels as if they are in a boxing match with their client, then they are almost surely too heavily focused on proving a point during guided discovery, rather than on using a collaborative, equal, respectful line of questioning that enhances the therapeutic relationship. Consider the differences in the following excerpts.

Excerpt 1: Less Focus on the Therapeutic Relationship

CLIENT: [becoming tearful] I have no friends.

THERAPIST: Oh, come on! You tell me about your friends all the time in session!

CLIENT: [looking down, signaling that she is struggling] Well, I mean, they're not real friends.

THERAPIST: What is the evidence that supports your view that they are not real friends? [*Here, the therapist believes she is asking a standard CBT question that would reflect her grasp of CBT and its procedures.*]

CLIENT: [looking sheepish] I don't know exactly. It just doesn't *feel* like it. I'm not sure they really understand.

THERAPIST: So there doesn't seem to be any evidence that they are not your real friends. What about evidence for the contrary—that they are, indeed, real friends?

CLIENT: [responding timidly] I think you would probably say because I go out with them on a regular basis.

THERAPIST: You bet I would! Don't you think that regular time spent with one another contributes to being a good friend?

CLIENT: Well, yes but . . . there are other things too.

THERAPIST: I agree, good friendship is more than just going out together. How else do you define a good friendship?

CLIENT: [hesitating, as if she is unsure of herself and is feeling as if she is backed into a corner] Um . . . like when they really listen to you and not just brush you off? When you feel like you can share anything with them, without them judging you?

THERAPIST: I agree that those are characteristics of good friendships. Are you saying that those characteristics are absent in your close friendships?

CLIENT: [looking down at her hands in her lap] Well, maybe not all the time. But there are a couple of friends, where it really, really seems like they think I am ridiculous and should just get over whatever is bothering me.

THERAPIST: Ah, but there you go—it looks like you are falling into the all-or-nothing cognitive distortion. [*Here, the therapist is attempting to demonstrate skill in linking the discussion of evidence with another central construct used in CBT—that of the cognitive distortion, in this case, all-or-nothing thinking.*]

CLIENT: [taken aback] I am?

THERAPIST: Yes! At first, you had it in your mind that you have no friends, but when you carefully examined it, it seems like only some of your friends are not treating you the way you'd like to be treated.

CLIENT: [weakly] Oh, okay. I guess my thinking is off on this one.

On the surface, many aspects of this exchange seem somewhat consistent with the premises of CBT. The therapist readily picked up on the client's sentiment that she had no friends, which, on the basis of their previous interactions, was almost assuredly an overstatement that was contributing to the client's emotional distress. The therapist used Socratic questioning to encourage the client to examine the evidence supporting that thought, as well as to identify other aspects of being a good friend that can help her evaluate the status of her friendships. At the end of the exchange, the therapist determined that the client was likely falling into an all-or-nothing thinking pattern, concluding that she had no friends when, in fact, it was likely a couple of friends who were disappointing her.

Despite this exchange having fidelity to one aspect of CBT technique, other parts of this dialogue would likely make some people cringe. For example, when the client became tearful as she stated, "I have no friends," the therapist did not acknowledge the painful affect, nor did she express empathy at how difficult it would be for the client to exist in a state in which she truly believed that she had no friends. Instead, the therapist adopted a bit of a challenging stance to prove her wrong, saying, "Oh, come on! You tell me about your friends all the time in session!" (which could, ironically, be an instance in the therapist's all-or-nothing thinking, when she referenced that the client talked about her friends "all the time"). As the therapist dutifully delivered the CBT technique of examining the evidence for a particular thought, she missed the nonverbal cues that could indicate the client was feeling a bit railroaded, as if the therapist had an agenda of disproving her (at all costs) of the notion that she had no friends. When the therapist and client were examining evidence for the client's statement that she had no friends and were considering the specific characteristics of what makes a good friend, the therapist spoke definitely with expressions like, "You bet I would!" and "I agree that . . ." As you will see as this chapter progresses, in the spirit of collaboration and enhancing the therapeutic relationship, cognitive behavioral therapists take care to refrain from expressing their opinions because the client's opinions and conclusions, in almost all circumstances except when some sort of violence or objective threat is involved, take precedence. Finally, at the end of the dialogue, the therapist proclaimed that the client had fallen into the all-or-nothing thinking distortion, which very well might have provoked a sense of shame and withdrawal in the patient. Thus, at best, expert raters would likely view this example as being a relatively unskilled application of CBT technique; at worst, they likely would view it as lacking in understanding and interpersonal effectiveness on the therapist's part. Moreover, although one could view the therapist's line of questioning as Socratic questioning, the exchange, overall, certainly would not be regarded as a prime example of Socratic dialogue.

In contrast, the following dialogue illustrates how a cognitive behavioral therapist who is more attuned to the therapeutic relationship might handle the same clinical issue. The dialogue begins at the same point, in which the client tearfully expresses her fear that she has no friends.

Excerpt 2: More Focus on the Therapeutic Relationship

CLIENT: [becoming tearful] I have no friends.

THERAPIST: [staying silent for a moment to allow the client to sit with the affect associated with this statement] Tell me more about what goes into your view that you have no friends. [*Here, the therapist hopes to gather more information from a nonjudgmental stance to set the stage for an intervention, rather than solely relying on her recollection of information that she had gathered in previous sessions.*]

CLIENT: [crying harder] It's just that . . . it's just that . . . I had a really bad experience on Saturday night with some friends. That I haven't told anyone.

THERAPIST: [leaning in, looking concerned, and speaking gently] Tell me what happened. [*Here, the therapist recognizes the need to allow the client space to provide detail to develop a sophisticated understanding of the client's troublesome recent experience, rather than pushing to implement a strategic intervention at this very moment.*]

CLIENT: [sniffling] Well, well . . . I was talking to this guy at the bar, while my friends were back in the booth talking to some other guys. [pausing, and crying a little bit] At first, I thought he was really nice, a good guy. I was having a lot of fun talking to him, and I thought, "Finally. Finally. I'm meeting someone nice, someone who is interested in me for me, not for my looks, or my age, or whatever . . ." [pausing again] So I was literally talking to him forever, at least an hour, when he all of a sudden changed, and he started trying to get me to go back to his apartment. [sobbing now]

THERAPIST: [providing empathic understanding] I have a sense of how disappointing this is for you, when you've had such unfortunate experiences with other young men you've started to get to know on a romantic level.

CLIENT: I know, right? Long story short, I told him I wasn't interested, and he literally jammed me up against the bar and started to threaten me, saying he would ruin my reputation if I didn't go home with him.

THERAPIST: [makes a facial expression suggestive that this was an egregious experience]

CLIENT: I got the hell out of there and made my way back to my two friends. But when I got there . . . they were paired up and all into these guys. I tried to grab one of them to tell her what was going on, but she wasn't having it. We went to the bathroom really quick, and she brushed me off, saying I probably imagined it because I can be dramatic like that.

THERAPIST: Oh boy. I can't tell you how sorry I am that that happened. When she said that, tell me what ran through your mind.

CLIENT: That I'm a slut! That no one will ever take me seriously! Doesn't matter if it's people who are my so-called friends, or people who could be my boyfriend, or even a husband. I'm just trash! [begins crying in earnest]

The difference between the two dialogues is immense. The subtle difference in the therapist's response to the client's exclamation that she had no friends led to profoundly different insights, avenues for intervention, and food for therapeutic work. The therapist in the second excerpt asked for more information about the client's view that she had no friends in a way that communicated curiosity and nonjudgment. Unlike the therapist in the first excerpt, the therapist in the second did not immediately jump to challenging that statement, even though she knew very well that the client had referenced a number of close friendships in their previous work.

The therapist's open, nonchallenging, and nonjudgmental stance paved the way for the client to talk about an extremely painful experience that she had over the weekend. Notice that the client did not reference the painful experience at all in the first excerpt. The therapist in the first excerpt was so intent on immediately refuting the client's idea that she had no friends that she did not leave space to learn the important context surrounding the client's exclamation. In contrast, the therapist in the second excerpt indeed created this space, and it opened up four important experiences that would be therapeutically valuable to address: (a) the client's disappointment that a potential romantic interest who seemed to be interested in her turned out to just be interested in sex; (b) the traumatic and humiliating experience of being pushed up against the bar and threatened; (c) the client's despair over her friend labeling her as dramatic when the client had just endured a traumatic and humiliating experience; and (d) the client's profound, self-deprecating beliefs about herself that were activated by this experience. Throughout this exchange, the therapist took the opportunity to express empathy, support, and validation, which would set the stage for continued cognitive restructuring surrounding the meaning that she was associating with this unfortunate situation.

TIPS FOR COGNITIVE RESTRUCTURING THROUGH THE LENS OF THE THERAPEUTIC RELATIONSHIP

It would not feel validating or supportive to any client to leave a session with the sense that their therapist does not believe them or that their therapist believes the problem is "all in their head." When cognitive behavioral therapists are working with nonpsychotic clients, they are alert for the "grain of truth" in their clients' thinking, or the valid reasons underlying the conclusions they are drawing, even if those conclusions are a bit overstated or not entirely supported by evidence. Even when cognitive behavioral therapists are working with psychotic clients, they do not simply dismiss cognitions of a delusional quality (A. T. Beck et al., 2021). In fact, directly challenging the delusions of a psychotic patient usually does not go far, as it shuts down the client, elicits guardedness and mistrust, and dismisses the client's humanness and the values and aspirations they hold. Remember that the ultimate goal of cognitive restructuring is for clients to develop skill in evaluating the accuracy and helpfulness of their thinking and to really own an alternative, more balanced way of thinking, rather than simply being told by the therapist that their thinking is "wrong" or what they should be thinking instead. In this section, I outline seven tips for applying cognitive restructuring in a way that balances the intervention with attention to the therapeutic relationship and can enhance the therapeutic relationship.

Tip 1: Approach Cognitive Restructuring From a Place of Gentle Curiosity

Allow me, at this juncture, to espouse on the notion of "challenging" thoughts. Any avid learner of CBT has undoubtedly come across textbooks and therapy guides that refer to the process of challenging clients' maladaptive thoughts. Indeed, I also took the same stance until I joined the faculty of the University of Pennsylvania in 2004, where I was working with Aaron T. Beck himself. When I joined the faculty, Dr. Beck suggested that he supervise me on a couple of cases so he could get to know my therapeutic style as we developed and adapted cognitive behavioral treatment protocols for suicidal clients with drug dependence. It was an honor to receive supervision from Dr. Beck, and it is not difficult to imagine how proud I was to report on what I thought was skillful cognitive restructuring in which I challenged a client's automatic thoughts. I distinctly remember Dr. Beck's reaction to my description, saying something like,

> You know, Amy, I don't view this process so much as one in which the therapist takes a challenging stance, but one in which the therapist works together collaboratively with the client, almost like codetectives working together on a case, or coscientists working together in a laboratory. (A. T. Beck, personal communication, October 20, 2004)

In other words, my emphasis on challenging was detracting from a fundamental tenet of CBT—that of collaborative empiricism. From that moment on, I referred to the action taken in cognitive restructuring as one of "evaluating with the client," rather than of "challenging the client."

The goal of cognitive restructuring is not for therapists to be so challenging that they get into a debate with the client or the client feels as though they are being "out logic-ed" or backed into a corner. Instead, the idea is for the therapist to approach cognitive restructuring from a gentle, curious perspective, wondering what has gone into the client's thinking and how they drew the conclusions that they did. When cognitive behavioral therapists approach cognitive restructuring in this manner, clients usually feel heard, respected, and a sense of investment on the therapist's part. The gentle, curious approach tends to be much subtler than an overtly challenging approach, which allows clients to feel invested in the conclusions they are drawing from the process and to recognize that they have always had the power within them to step back and reframe unhelpful thinking. Moreover, when paired with overt expressions of validation, empathy, and preservation of client autonomy (e.g., "It makes a lot of sense to me why you'd interpret what was happening in that manner, in light of your past experiences"), the likelihood increases that a client will feel the therapist's positive regard.

Tip 2: Take a Pause and Regroup When Cognitive Restructuring Begins to Feel Like a Debate

Even the most skilled cognitive behavioral therapists experience instances in which they feel like they are trying to convince their clients of something and it is simply not resonating. One telltale sign that this is occurring is when clients repeatedly refute the therapist using statements beginning with, "Yeah but . . ." The moment the therapist perceives that they are debating with their client or even being pulled to convince their client of a different viewpoint, it is probably time to pull back, regroup, and talk about what is happening in order to preserve the therapeutic relationship. The therapist might sense that this is happening because of their own internal reaction, or they might recognize it in their clients with an increased frequency of disagreement, a client's overt expression of sensing that their therapist is trying to change their mind, or behavior indicative of "shutting down" (e.g., aversion of eye contact, single-word responses, defensive posture). We know from research on motivational interviewing and CBT that outcome is poorer when therapists respond to resistance with directiveness rather than with a supportive style (Hara et al., 2022).

Consider the following dialogue between Sarah and her therapist that occurred several months into treatment. Sarah was leaning toward making the decision to divorce her husband once and for all and to move back to the Midwest to restart her life. However, Sarah anticipated that an unbearable, all-out fight would result, which was deterring her from taking action and keeping her stuck in an unfulfilling place in life. Because the therapist had known Sarah for several months and had heard about how both Sarah and her husband handled conflict (i.e., through extreme avoidance), the therapist highly doubted that an unbearable, all-out fight would ensue. As such, the therapist believed Sarah's fortune-telling and catastrophizing about this possibility were prolonging her emotional distress and inaction.

THERAPIST: I hear your concern—that you anticipate that when you finally tell Carlos of your plans, that there will be a major blow-up. [applying the principles of cognitive restructuring] I'm wondering, though, how likely it is that there would be a truly unbearable, substantial blow-out? [*Here, the therapist is applying the standard cognitive restructuring technique of estimating the true likelihood of a bad outcome occurring.*]

SARAH: [showing a bit of annoyance on her face, as if she cannot believe the therapist is questioning her about this] I think there is a pretty high likelihood. I mean, I've never actually left him. I've never told him I am done forever.

THERAPIST: No, that is true you haven't. However, think about your pattern of interactions. How do they typically go, even when there is a problem or an issue in which the two of you do not see eye-to-eye?

SARAH: We typically just avoid it and move on. But that's the point here. We can't avoid it and go on as we usually do because I'm finally saying that I want the divorce and that I'm not even staying here in the area.

THERAPIST: Do you think the fact that this is something new automatically means that there will be a big blowup? [*Here, the therapist applies a slightly different cognitive restructuring technique, inviting the client to consider whether one thing leads to or equals another thing.*]

SARAH: Maybe. Yes. I don't know. Maybe. [putting her head in her hands] It's all just too much to think about.

THERAPIST: [sensing that this process was getting to be a bit much for Sarah, and that the two of them were not "on the same page"] Sarah, I notice that you're a bit further from me right now . . . what is happening for you? [*Here, the therapist is detecting the possibility of a rupture in the therapeutic alliance by the ambivalence with which Sarah was responding, and she steps outside of the cognitive restructuring intervention to address this possibility respectfully and directly.*]

SARAH: [looking up from her hands] I mean, I get what you are doing. You're trying to make me see that there probably won't be the big blowup that I am creating in my mind.

THERAPIST: [smiling] Well, maybe not trying to get you to see something, but at least considering the possibility that a big blowup is not a foregone conclusion. [pausing] Why do you think I was suggesting that we consider this possibility, that a blowup is not a foregone conclusion?

SARAH: I know, I know, because I have a history of avoiding doing things that I know I need to do.

THERAPIST: Yes, I suppose so, only because I'm wondering if, in this instance, your thinking is preventing you from facing an action that ultimately will lead to much life fulfillment for you. [*This statement communicates genuine care that the therapist hopes for Sarah to achieve life fulfillment.*]

SARAH: I get it, and I want that. I really do. It's just . . . it's just . . . [crying]

THERAPIST: It's a loss at the same time. A very real one that perhaps we need to address more fully at your own speed. [*Here, the therapist is*

> *listening and responding to the verbal and nonverbal feedback that Sarah is providing, indicating that she is still not ready to tell her husband that she is leaving him once and for all.*]

SARAH: [looking thankful] Yes, yes, that's it. I know this is what I want, but I also know that it's best to do it at my own pace.

THERAPIST: Then we'll work together to process the loss at your own pace and prepare you so that you feel ready to have this conversation with Carlos, whenever that may be.

SARAH: [looking down, clearly touched] Thank you. That would be great.

Sarah's therapist recognized that tension was developing in their interaction and that, to Sarah, the line of questioning was beginning to feel like an interrogation. The therapist reflected on her ongoing cognitive restructuring work with Sarah and acknowledged her own frustration that while Sarah had demonstrated great skill in restructuring unhelpful thinking across an array of domains, she often became mired in cognitive distortions when it came to speaking her mind to her husband and making decisions about moving on with her life. The therapist is a solution-focused, decisive person who made changes in her own life when she was dissatisfied with something. She realized that she was becoming impatient with Sarah's inaction, which could have been pushing her efforts at cognitive restructuring and detracting from a demonstration of empathic understanding and positive regard. With this recognition, the therapist asked Sarah what was happening right there in the moment between them, and they were able to work through it and repair any rupture in the therapeutic relationship that might have been starting to emerge.

Tip 3: Apply the Principles of Cognitive Restructuring Conversationally

This suggestion arises from my supervision experiences with clinicians training to become certified cognitive behavioral therapists, as I have observed many supervisees ask certain Socratic questions because they believe that they must ask those exact questions to be good cognitive behavioral therapists. Many times, I have observed therapists-in-training hammer the Socratic questions listed in standard CBT texts (e.g., "What is the evidence for that?") over and over, even when the specific question is not especially appropriate for the situation at hand. Cognitive behavioral therapists need not ask any specific question or be limited to the questions listed in CBT texts written by master cognitive behavioral therapists to do effective guided discovery. In fact, the blanket application of those questions is likely to diminish the strength of the therapeutic relationship because it can be experienced by the client as willful, forceful, or abrupt.

Socratic dialogue, in contrast, feels like an engaging conversation with an interested party. Therapists ask questions with curiosity and for clarification, all from a stance of respect for the client's felt experience. Although guided discovery proceeds with a goal of balanced, accurate thinking in mind, it flows naturally, shows open-mindedness and spontaneity, and feels supportive. It is not forced, and it responds to the spontaneous nature of the interaction between the client and therapist (Safran & Segal, 1990). The highest-quality Socratic questioning occurs when the therapist is thoughtful, creative, and intuitive, crafting questions that seem particularly fitting for the situation the client is describing and the client's style. Those questions will never be found in a CBT textbook because they are idiosyncratic to therapy content and the client's personality. They can be based on metaphors, inspirational quotations, verses from a religious text, scenes from a movie or television show, or even memes that float around social media. Take, for example, one of my favorite quotations, "Comparison is the thief of joy" (often attributed to U.S. President Theodore Roosevelt, although there is some controversy around its true source). Throughout their careers, mental health providers will undoubtedly come across numerous clients whose emotional distress is exacerbated by continual comparison to others. When this occurs with one of my clients, I often supply the quotation and see if it resonates with them. If it does, we might develop a question such as, "How is this way of thinking being the thief of my joy?" Many clients report that these customized questions are the ones they find most memorable and helpful as they live their lives. Moreover, when these questions are developed and used in session, clients often have the sense that their therapist truly knows them and has a keen intuition of what will be helpful, which enhances the therapeutic relationship.

Tip 4: Pay Attention to Subtle Ways in Which Cognitive Restructuring Is Coming Across

Attention to tone of voice, pacing of speech, and nonverbal cues during cognitive restructuring can also affect the quality of the therapeutic relationship. When therapists Socratically question with a frown, there is an increased likelihood that clients will feel attacked or will internalize the message that they are doing something wrong. A similar sense might be felt by clients when questions are asked in a rapid-fire manner, allowing little time for them to craft thoughtful responses. I once had a client say something extremely self-deprecating, and she caught it immediately. Although I would like to believe she caught it because of the effective cognitive restructuring work that we had cultivated over the course of many sessions, rather than because of my reaction, she exclaimed, "There it is! There's the CBT glare!" Although we chuckled about this together (and, in fact, it was a repeated source of humor throughout the remainder of our work together), in reality I would not wish for any of my clients to truly believe that I am giving them a "CBT glare." Instead, I aim to communicate attentiveness and curiosity, coupled with warmth and openness.

Interestingly, the increased use of telehealth during the pandemic allowed for mental health providers to observe how they were coming across to their clients, as the default on many platforms is for both parties to see themselves onscreen. For example, I noticed that when I am concentrating intently, I assume quite a fierce look on my face (perhaps my CBT glare?). The use of telehealth platforms allowed me to adjust in real time, observe their effects on the therapeutic connection, and, more generally, on the effectiveness of the intervention I was delivering. This is yet another way that cognitive behavioral therapists conduct themselves as scientist–practitioners, as we adjust our self-presentation on the basis of the "data" that we are observing on camera.

Tip 5: Communicate That You Trust and Respect the Client's Knowledge of Their Personal Situation

When I educate clients about CBT, I talk to them about the tenet of collaboration. I often say something like this:

> I aim to have a 50–50 teamwork type of relationship with my clients. While I have expertise in psychotherapy, and CBT in particular, you are the expert in your own situation, and you will bring important information to our sessions so that we optimize the delivery of CBT. Both of our areas of expertise will come together to achieve a successful outcome.

In other words, cognitive behavioral therapists respect clients' knowledge of their personal situation, and they do not presume what is true or untrue about it or how to think or act in a situation in the client's life that they have not directly observed. Thus, collaboration is essential in implementing a successful cognitive restructuring intervention, and client agency is reinforced.

Clients exist in a vast array of life experiences that are different than our own. Examples include (but are far from limited to) working in a different professional setting (e.g., a client who is an executive in "Corporate America" being treated by a mental health provider in a solo private practice), being of a different race or ethnicity (e.g., a Black client being treated by a White mental health provider in a time of societal racial tension), having different health concerns (e.g., a client with a chronic immunodeficiency being treated by a mental health provider with no chronic medical conditions), and adhering to different religious beliefs (e.g., a client who belongs to the Church of Jesus Christ of Latter-Day Saints and who was taught that sexual practices such as masturbation are sinful, being treated by a mental health provider who is agnostic and who is open to many expressions of sexuality). What has worked as balanced, adaptive thinking and approaches to problem solving in the therapist's world might be very different in the client's world and for the goals that the client hopes to achieve. Recognition of such potential differences can go far in building the client's trust in the therapist. Moreover, clients often appreciate the therapist's explicit statement of this trust in and respect for the client's knowledge of their own situation.

Consider the following dialogue. Here, Sarah had gone back to work after using her short-term disability and was expressing hesitancy in talking to the district manager overseeing her restaurant about an issue bothering her, for fear of retribution. At first, the therapist (who had never worked in the restaurant industry) wondered if this was another instance of fortune-telling and catastrophizing.

THERAPIST: What is the worst thing that could happen if you were to talk with him about your concern?

SARAH: Oh, this guy is really vindictive. If I speak up, he'd see it as disrespecting him, and he could get back at me. Like he could transfer me to a different restaurant an hour away, or to a restaurant in the middle of the city that gets burglarized all the time.

THERAPIST: [wondering if Sarah is catastrophizing] What is the likelihood of such an outcome?

SARAH: I'm not sure it's really likely, but believe me, it has happened many times before. Especially to managers who are female and to managers who are at the higher end of the pay grade. They are constantly looking to replace managers with newbies who don't cost them as much. I can give at least five examples of this happening in the past year and a half, in restaurants in our district.

THERAPIST: [recognizing that these instances serve as evidence to support Sarah's hesitancy] Having never worked in the restaurant industry, I don't have a sense of how much turnover there is among managers, or of the underlying dynamics that make some people at risk for getting replaced or transferred to less desirable locations.

SARAH: No one does, not unless they have experience. Restaurant management is like a secret club.

THERAPIST: Hmm, my gut would have told me to carefully apply interpersonal effectiveness skills to talk to the district manager, predicting that the conversation might be a bit uncomfortable but that, ultimately, two reasonable people could arrive upon a mutually agreeable solution. But it sounds like, perhaps, restaurant management does not operate according to those same rules. [*Here, the therapist is placing the therapeutic relationship and Sarah's personal experience in the restaurant industry above any specific cognitive behavioral intervention.*]

SARAH: No, it really doesn't. You really have to watch your back, even more so as you rise through the ranks. If you anger someone who is higher up than you, it can mean being driven out of your job, even if you had a valid point to bring up.

THERAPIST: I trust your knowledge about the restaurant industry and the things you have observed in other instances with other managers. In light of this type of work environment, I'm eager to hear your perspective on the most effective way to approach this situation. [*Here, the therapist is communicating the message, "I believe you," which communicates positive regard.*]

A mental health provider who "takes the back seat" and allows the client to enlighten them with their knowledge demonstrates openness, respect, and even appropriate deference. This goes a long way in demonstrating to clients that the therapist is willing to acknowledge that they are an authority, which shows humility and could contribute to making clients feel as if the therapeutic environment is safe and nonjudgmental.

Tip 6: Graciously Acknowledge Instances in Which You Made an Incorrect Assumption

In a similar vein as the previous tip, when therapists overtly make incorrect assumptions about a client or their client's situation, they take ownership of it, apologize appropriately, and invite a correction from the client. Consider, in the previous dialogue, if the therapist had said something slightly different than, "Hmm, my gut would have told me to carefully apply interpersonal effectiveness skills to talk to the district manager . . ." Imagine if the therapist had expressed a more pointed assumption, saying something like, "In my experience, going into a situation like this with a balanced mindset and a plan for implementing effective communication skills creates a high likelihood of a positive outcome, or at least one that is acceptable to both parties."

SARAH: Um, I don't know. Maybe.

THERAPIST: I am not hearing a lot of confidence in your voice right now. Tell me your reaction to what I just said.

SARAH: No offense, Doctor, because I think you have really helped me with a lot. But I don't think what's [making her fingers into air quotes] "reasonable" for psychologists necessarily flies in the restaurant world.

THERAPIST: Thank you for sharing that with me. That is really interesting. Tell me more. [*Here the therapist is demonstrating nondefensiveness when Sarah communicates that her assumption is off-base.*]

SARAH: I can give you a million examples of times when reasonable requests are made of people in management and they just aren't having it, and they are out for blood afterward.

THERAPIST: [making one more attempt at cognitive restructuring] Are there any examples to the contrary? Where district managers [DMs] are open to feedback, and they are able to address the concerns of restaurant managers?

SARAH: [responding in a balanced manner] I'm sure not every DM is a jerk, but I do know for sure that mine is. And more often than not, when someone brings a concern or grievance to his attention, they end up being punished for it.

THERAPIST: So, which is more aversive for you—keeping things as they are and dealing with them, or bringing them to the attention of your DM, risking his retribution, but also leaving yourself open to the possibility of change?

SARAH: I have a third option. Not talking to my DM about it, but figuring out a different way of bringing about change. It might take a bit longer, but I can work from the inside rather than from upper management.

THERAPIST: I'm intrigued! Tell me more about how that might work.

In this example, when the therapist continued to push cognitive restructuring, Sarah pushed back. Fortunately, the therapist was open to Sarah's feedback, and she responded nondefensively when Sarah stated explicitly that the therapist's way of approaching the situation was likely inconsistent with what is effective in actuality in a restaurant setting. The openness and curious approach (e.g., "That is really interesting," "I'm intrigued") allowed space for Sarah to think creatively and identify a third option to achieve a "middle ground" that seemed tolerable to her. Moreover, the therapist was able to make use of what she had learned from Sarah in working with other clients who worked in the restaurant industry and were struggling with similar power dynamics. Had the therapist continued to demonstrate a lack of receptiveness to Sarah's feedback, the stage could have been set for a rupture in the therapeutic alliance.

Tip 7: Express Genuine Interest in How the Fruits of Cognitive Restructuring Bore Out Between Sessions

The therapeutic relationship is enhanced when the therapist expresses genuine interest in the client's application of cognitive restructuring in between sessions and the degree to which it softens a negative mood state and allows for more adaptive behavior to be applied. Not only does this expression of interest reinforce the value of CBT homework, but it also communicates that the therapist is truly invested in the client and their collaborative therapeutic work. Demonstrating this interest makes for a warm, engaging review of cognitive restructuring homework. Consider the following example with Sarah, which took place at the beginning of the session after she rated her depression and anxiety levels over the past week:

SARAH: Well, I did it! I started the conversation with Carlos about the divorce.

THERAPIST: You did! This is a big step for you, Sarah.

SARAH: I know! It really needed to happen.

THERAPIST: How did it all unfold?

SARAH: He was talking to me about refinancing the house to get a lower monthly mortgage payment. And he looked at me and said, "That is, if we're going to stay together . . ." I realized that this was the chance to start talking about separating permanently.

THERAPIST: [linking to the cognitive restructuring work they had done in the past in the context of this situation] When we've talked about this in the past, one factor that kept you from discussing this issue in a forthright manner was the anticipation that there would be an awful blowup. How did you overcome that concern in this instance?

SARAH: I remembered what we had talked about in other sessions, that Carlos and I have never really had a big blowup, so the odds were that this time would not be a big blowup either. And, since he brought it up, I figured that he was probably thinking about it as well.

THERAPIST: And? Was there a big blowup? [*The therapist asks this question to facilitate a new learning experience linking Sarah's prediction of a blowup, which she had expressed in the previous session, with the actual outcome.*]

SARAH: No, not at all. It actually ended up being one of the most caring conversations we've had in our relationship. We decided that it is best for us to go our separate ways, but even in spite of everything, it will be done from a place of love and not hostility or bitterness.

THERAPIST: [expressing genuine delight] Oh, Sarah, I can't tell you how happy I am that it is working out in this way. [*Here, the therapist is expressing her genuine happiness for Sarah, enhancing their bond and real relationship.*]

[The therapist and Sarah talk more about the conversation and next steps for permanently splitting.]

THERAPIST: [summarizing, and asking a question to generalize the experience for a healthy mindset in future relationships] You were so hesitant to bring up the possibility of divorce because you expected a big blowup, and once you did so, you realized that a great deal of positive emerged from the conversation, rather than an aversive conflict. What have you learned that you can apply in the future?

SARAH: I definitely admit that the fortune-telling and catastrophizing got the best of me on this one. I need to remember that big conflicts are fewer and further between than they feel. And that sometimes it is best to rip off the Band-Aid and get things on the table so that I'm not in such an uncomfortable limbo for so long.

THERAPIST: Well said, Sarah.

COGNITIVE RESTRUCTURING AS APPLIED TO THERAPEUTIC RELATIONSHIP ISSUES

When issues arise in the therapeutic relationship, it is almost certain that both the client and therapist will have thoughts about the situation, which may or may not be accurate or helpful. Moreover, because we are human, in many instances both clients and therapists attach meaning or significance to the issues based at least partially on the way in which previous experiences have shaped their worldview. Notice that I am using language that gets at the heart of the "C" in CBT—thoughts, meaning, and significance. When issues arise in the therapeutic relationship, it makes logical sense that the cognitive restructuring work already established during the course of therapy can be applied in these instances to facilitate communication, understanding, gentle correction of any misunderstandings, and a corrective learning experience. In this section, I present two common cognitions that clients experience in therapy, which have the potential to cause a rupture in the therapeutic relationship, and illustrate ways to use cognitive restructuring to remedy them.

"I'm Failing in Therapy"

Clients who struggle with depression, insecurity, and low self-worth are often overly critical of themselves in therapy, which increases the likelihood that therapy becomes an aversive experience for them. The underlying meaning associated with this self-criticalness is something like, "I'm failing in therapy," and of even more central relevance to the therapeutic relationship, "I'm failing you." Of course, when a person views themselves as failing, it is logical that they would experience a host of negative emotions, such as sadness, disappointment, guilt, shame, and anxiety. Not surprisingly, when a person views themselves in a negative light and experiences unwelcome emotions, it is logical that they would avoid the experience. In psychotherapy, avoidance translates to being late for sessions, lacking engagement in sessions, missing sessions, being slow to schedule a subsequent session, and avoiding between-session homework. If a client indeed discontinues therapy for these reasons, it would not be surprising if they had a negative view of their experience and would be hesitant to seek therapy in the future. It could also be a source of discouragement that generalizes to other areas of their lives, contributing to a pattern of clients viewing themselves as failing at many things in life.

One relationship-oriented strategy that a therapist can enact across the course of therapy is to reinforce a client's adaptive attitudes and recognize their strengths in a way that could prevent this client reaction in the first place. However, if a client has this reaction, it is important to realize that it provides an opportunity ripe for cognitive restructuring. If a client with this mindset is able to adopt a more flexible cognitive stance (e.g., "Therapy is a process," "I'm learning important things about myself even though I am still struggling"), then there is the potential for the client to view therapy from a more positive stance, facilitating engagement. Moreover, the adoption of a more balanced viewpoint could facilitate self-compassion and generalize to other life experiences outside of therapy. Consider the following dialogue, in which a client was especially hard on herself when she did not complete her homework in between sessions.

CLIENT: I'm sorry! I always do this! I'm totally wasting your time.

THERAPIST: Not a waste of time at all. In fact, this provides an important piece of information. Perhaps it was the case that the between-session work that we developed was, ultimately, not the match that we had hoped it would be.

CLIENT: No, no, it's not anything about you or therapy. It's me. I do this all the time. I think I want to commit to something that helps me to better myself, and I never follow through. [pausing] I'm such a loser.

THERAPIST: I'm wondering if we can take a look at the thoughts that are running through your mind right now, about the therapy homework? [*Here, the therapist adopts a curious stance rather than try to convince the client that she is not a loser.*]

CLIENT: Okay.

THERAPIST: Am I correct that I am hearing you say things like, "Not doing the homework is all my fault" and "I'm a loser"? [*Here, the therapist hopes to demonstrate understanding and listening, as well as to clarify the key thoughts that might be evaluated using conversational cognitive restructuring.*]

CLIENT: [looking forlorn] Yeah, that's it. And also that I'm such a burden on others because I have good intentions, but I oftentimes don't follow through.

THERAPIST: Is that what you think in this case, that you're a burden on me because you did not complete the homework?

CLIENT: Yes, totally. I know how booked you are, how many people need your services. Your time would be so much better spent with someone who actually does their homework.

THERAPIST: If a friend came to you and was extremely down on herself because she perceived that she wasted her therapist's time by not doing homework, what would you say to that friend? [*This standard cognitive restructuring technique is aimed to help clients get distance from their unhelpful thoughts, as they almost assuredly would be kinder to their friend than they are being to themselves.*]

CLIENT: Well . . . I would tell her that the therapist is a professional and probably deals with that all the time. And that therapy is much more than just completing homework assignments.

THERAPIST: How does that apply to this situation?

CLIENT: I know, it's part of the whole process of therapy. [pausing] I just can't help but feel that I've let you down.

THERAPIST: [asking permission to share an honest reaction, which will also serve as evidence for an alternative viewpoint in cognitive restructuring] Is it okay if I share my honest reaction to all of this?

CLIENT: [brightening a little] Yes, go ahead.

THERAPIST: First, I meant what I said when I suggested that not completing homework provides us with important information. We learn as much from times in which homework is completed as we do from times in which it is not completed. [client smiles] And second, what is happening between us, right here and right now, is likely far more important than the homework. We're identifying important beliefs that you have about yourself, and it's giving me a sample of what happens when you get down on yourself. If anything, this experience will move therapy forward tremendously.

CLIENT: Really?

THERAPIST: Absolutely. For example, are there other times in your life when you have the sense that you've failed, wasted someone's time, or let someone down? [*Here, the therapist is generalizing the shared experience in therapy to other situations in the client's life that reflect the pattern of believing that she is a failure or burden.*]

CLIENT: Oh gosh, all the time. Probably three or four times this week alone.

THERAPIST: Then what we're experiencing right now together does have a great deal of relevance for your life.

CLIENT: I never thought about it that way.

THERAPIST: I wonder if we can spend the remainder of the session examining these themes and, together, developing a more helpful way of thinking about yourself when these situations arise, rather than immediately jumping to the idea that you are a loser and have disappointed people.

CLIENT: I think that would be amazing if we can figure this out. Because it seems like I feel like this all the time.

THERAPIST: And when you have the idea that you are a loser and have failed others, what happens? Are you able to accomplish whatever you are trying to accomplish?

CLIENT: God no. I just get discouraged and shut down.

THERAPIST: Do you have the sense that if you were to find an alternative pathway to go down, you'd be able to overcome the tendency to shut down in that way?

CLIENT: That would be really great.

As the session progressed, the client began to understand that there are a variety reasons for homework noncompliance, and many of them ultimately facilitate growth in treatment if they are addressed. By the end of the session, she reported that she believed this notion at a level of 92%. In addition, she was able to craft a statement reflecting a stance of self-compassion, more generally, to apply to homework noncompliance and other situations in her life when she perceives that she has failed or let people down. She left the session with a coping card that read:

> I am a human being who sometimes messes up. But there are lots of times when I do just fine, too. I would have compassion for a friend who does not follow through on occasion, so there is no reason why I cannot have compassion for myself. Tomorrow is a fresh day in which I will try again.

The client readily scheduled another appointment for the following week. Moreover, an important cognitive shift had occurred, all within the context of issues that had the potential to threaten the therapeutic relationship.

"You Are Not Serving Me Well"

The client depicted in the previous example demonstrated internalizing symptoms, such that she directed negative judgments and emotions inward when she did not comply with her therapy homework. Other clients, in contrast, demonstrate externalizing symptoms, such that they express irritability and anger toward their therapist when they are frustrated with an aspect of therapy. Just as there are important cognitions and meanings associated with sadness, disappointment, guilt, and shame about the therapy experience, there are also cognitions associated with frustration and anger about the therapy experience. In many instances, the meaning associated with these cognitions is, "You are not serving me well; you are the problem." Although it is of the utmost importance to demonstrate an open, nondefensive stance when clients express views along these lines, cognitive restructuring can be applied just as readily in these instances as in the previous example.

Consider the following dialogue, in which a client who had been seen for 20 sessions expressed frustration with an exacerbation of symptoms. To this point, she had responded extremely well to a combination of cognitive restructuring, behavioral activation, and acceptance-based strategies. However, at her twenty-first session, the client's mood had deteriorated due to significant work stress; as she was questioning whether therapy had been helpful for her, she began to imply that the therapist was not competent and was not serving her well.

CLIENT: I don't know. I mean, I just think we're missing something here, like we're not getting to the root cause of my depression and anxiety.

THERAPIST: [demonstrating an open, nonjudgmental stance] This is incredibly important feedback. Of course, let's talk more about this. Tell me what makes you say that.

CLIENT: I don't know exactly. But here I am dealing with the same emotions, back to square one. I expected more out of this experience. I don't think it's working. Maybe this isn't the right approach for me. Maybe you're not the right therapist for me.

Here I note that, many times, when clients have complaints about therapy, they have difficulty supplying more detail. Without question, it is understandable for many clients to have frustrations about therapy if, at 20 sessions in, they encounter an exacerbation of symptoms. However, what is often happening is that they are falling into the cognitive distortion of emotional reasoning, such that they are feeling badly, so they conclude that therapy is not "working" or that the therapist is not doing their job. From the standpoint of maintaining and enhancing the therapeutic relationship, of course a therapist would not directly challenge this notion by simply pointing out that the client is thinking about the situation "wrong" or falling prey to a cognitive distortion, or by demanding details to support the client's assertions. However, if therapists can recognize what is happening, then they can distance themselves from their own personalization of the negative feedback and skillfully work from the cognitive behavioral framework to reshape this idea and to re-instill hope and optimism for treatment. The dialogue continues next:

THERAPIST: You have a great deal of expertise and insight into your own life, and it's important to draw on that expertise and insight in order to optimize your therapy experience. Tell me more about finding the root cause. Knowing yourself, how you "tick," how do you think that will help?

CLIENT: Well, I really like to understand myself. You know, understand why I do the things that I do, make the choices I make. I can't help but think that if I knew the root cause, then I could stop these problems from coming up in the first place.

THERAPIST: You do have a strong desire to understand yourself. I've been quite impressed by the depth of your insight into your thought patterns during the time that we've worked together. From my perspective, you've done a terrific job of identifying and reshaping the most powerful and central thoughts associated with your emotional distress, which, up until now, has made a substantial impact on your depression and anxiety. What was different about the events that occurred at work this week? [*Here, the therapist is taking great care not to invalidate the client, even though she has a distinctly different view on the necessity of finding a "root cause."*]

CLIENT: So many things were getting thrown at me at once. Every time I turned around, there was a new fire to put out. And my manager was just horrid this week, insulting and berating us, even threatening our jobs if we didn't complete tasks that we knew were basically impossible . . . [client begins to tear up and whispers] It was just really, really awful. I felt like I was drowning.

THERAPIST: [pausing to allow the client to experience the affect associated with this painful workweek] I'm so sorry to hear all of this. It sounds like an incredibly difficult workweek.

CLIENT: [wiping her eyes, continuing to speak softly] Thank you. It really was.

THERAPIST: To make sure that I am fully understanding what you are saying here, it sounds like this was an incredibly difficult situation in which it was tough to apply what you have learned in therapy so far?

CLIENT: Yes. I was really disappointed with how everything transpired. Nothing is ever as good as it seems. I thought this was going to be my dream job, and look how stressed I am. I thought my new manager was going to be part of the solution, but it turns out that he is even more of the problem than the previous manager. I thought therapy was going to give me some answers, to be able to negotiate life stress better, but it certainly failed me this week. No matter where life takes me, I am always let down. Things are never, never as good as they seem.

THERAPIST: [pausing to let the client's statement resonate] No matter where life takes you, you are always let down. [pausing again] That is a very profound statement. [*Here, the therapist is emphasizing what has the potential to be a core belief—consistent with the client's need to find a root cause—and provides validation of the way that the client is making sense of her difficult week.*]

CLIENT: [eyes brighten, as if something important occurred to her] Yes, I'm always waiting for the other shoe to drop, and when it does, I get extremely angry and let down. Like, "I knew it! Why did I dupe myself into having hope again?" [putting her head in her hands] What's the point of life if a person is continually disappointed?

THERAPIST: [speaking gently and recalling the client's case formulation] This week was incredibly disappointing for you. Work was incredibly stressful, much different than you had expected this job to be. And your manager's treatment of you and your colleagues was unexpected, given the high hopes you had when he replaced the previous manager. [client nods her head] . . . And this is yet another example in a longstanding pattern of life events in which you had high hopes, worked extremely hard to achieve your goals, but yet things did not go as planned. Reinforcing the belief that life lets you down.

CLIENT: [tearful] Yes, exactly. Life lets you down. That is the theme of my life.

THERAPIST: Hmm. We've talked before about core beliefs and the way in which they exert influence on the way we make meaning when we are faced with particular situations in our lives. Do you think we've stumbled upon one? [*Here, the therapist is introducing the notion of core beliefs to respect the client's need to identify the root cause of her clinical presentation, as well as the fact that such beliefs are foundational to the case formulation, as will be seen in greater depth in Chapter 8 of this volume.*]

CLIENT: [nodding her head emphatically] Yes, definitely.

THERAPIST: We started this conversation with your sense that what you have taken thus far from therapy was not helpful this past week, and more generally, it caused you to question whether we are barking up the wrong tree together, or even that you were barking up the wrong tree in working with me. I certainly want to give you the respect of discussing these concerns directly so that you can maximize your experience in therapy. [*These statements directly speak to the rupture in the therapeutic alliance that is threatening to emerge.*]

CLIENT: [pausing in a thoughtful manner] I was really disappointed that I wasn't able to cope more effectively with all of the work stress this week. But I do think I took it really hard, and even blamed therapy a bit, because it was such a reminder of that theme in my life. That I'm always let down.

THERAPIST: [smiling warmly] I get that. Because that idea of life always letting you down has been such a pervasive theme in your life, it's not surprising that this would be the lens through which you view upsetting and disappointing situations in your life.

CLIENT: Yes, that's it exactly. Maybe that is the root cause. My tendency to always expect life to let me down, and when that happens, as it always does, my reaction to it.

THERAPIST: [normalizing the client's experience so that she can practice self-compassion] Honestly, we all have underlying beliefs that are formed from our own unique histories. And these beliefs influence the way in which we all handle stressors that pop up in our lives. Even cognitive behavioral therapists. [*These statements normalize the client's experience and communicate positive regard in light of the client's initial negative feedback for the therapist.*]

CLIENT: [chuckling] That's actually helpful to know!

THERAPIST: I have an idea. What if we were to proceed with a twofold plan? One part of the plan could be to figure out ways to manage high levels of stress and upset in the moment, even in moments in which you are being berated by your manager. And the second part of the plan could be a closer examination of the core belief that life always lets you down, so that we can figure out a way to move toward a slightly softer core belief that, over time, could serve as the filter through which you view stressful situations. [*Here, the therapist is being mindful of the fundamental CBT principle of collaboration.*]

CLIENT: [looking hopeful] I think that plan is right on target.

THERAPIST: [obtaining feedback on what could have been a difficult conversation] How are you feeling about the way in which we have handled this situation between the two of us? [*Here, the therapist also hopes that the promise of working on core beliefs will help to restructure the client's view that therapy is not serving her and that they are not working on the root cause.*]

CLIENT: Truthfully, I didn't think it would go like this. I was ready for this to be our last session. But I think now that I see that the way I was thinking about therapy was a microcosm of the way that I think about a lot of things in my life, that the other shoe has dropped and that I was bound to have been let down. So thank you for bearing with me, for being patient with me as I worked through that.

THERAPIST: Some important realizations have emerged from this session, and it truly is my privilege to have been a part of that.

The therapist employed many relationship-enhancing techniques in this dialogue in order to field the client's concern about therapy in an open, nondefensive manner, working toward the repair of the rupture that had been unfolding. First, she made the overt statement that the client was providing important feedback and that she was willing to talk more about this feedback. In addition, even though the conversation had the potential to be tense and a bit awkward, the therapist took care to give the client credit for her strengths, such as by acknowledging the client's expertise and desire to understand herself and by explicitly stating how impressed she has been with the depth of the client's insight. Moreover, she allowed space during the conversation for the client to experience affect and for the important insights to resonate with the client, taking care not to create a sense of pressure to come to a quick resolution about the possible rupture in the therapeutic relationship. The therapist made overt expressions of empathy (i.e., "I'm so sorry to hear all of this. It sounds like an incredibly difficult work-week"), she made summary statements (i.e., "To make sure that I am fully understanding . . ."), and she made reflections (i.e., "No matter where life takes you, you are always let down"). When she linked the client's concerns to an important aspect of the underlying beliefs comprising a key aspect of the case formulation (i.e., "Reinforcing the belief that life lets you down"), she demonstrated to the client that she, indeed, had picked up on a central core belief, which resonated with the client's need to work on a root cause in therapy. This point cannot be understated, as the therapist took care to acknowledge this belief and link it to previous education on core beliefs to respond to the client's desire to get to a root cause.

In the last segment of the interaction, the therapist used the client's realization about the way in which her core belief was influencing her reaction to therapy as a catalyst for the planning of future work together (core beliefs and their relation to maladaptive schemas are discussed at greater length in Chapter 8 of this volume). The therapist took care to attend to both of the client's original concerns: (a) that she was unable to apply CBT strategies and principles because of the high intensity of chronic stress and overwhelm and stress in the moment and (b) that she had the desire to work on an underlying issue that could account for her style of reactivity. Throughout this segment of the conversation, the therapist took care to show warmth in nonverbal ways (e.g., through smiling) to demonstrate behaviorally that there were no hard feelings about the fact that the client expressed displeasure about therapy, recognizing that handling disagreements with empathy and warmth, rather than directiveness and hostility, is associated with better outcomes (Hara et al., 2022). Moreover, the therapist normalized the client's reaction (i.e., by remarking that everyone has underlying beliefs that influence the way they handle stressors in their own lives) to demonstrate understanding and compassion, as well as to guard against any self-deprecation that would ensue if the client were to get down on herself for being overly critical about therapy. At the end of the conversation, the therapist asked for feedback to ensure that the potential rupture had been repaired, to ensure that the two were "on the same page," and to consolidate the learning that occurred within the therapeutic interaction. It was clear that important cognitive restructuring had occurred in their conversation, in that the client shifted from a view that therapy was not serving her to one in which she realized that she had jumped to that conclusion because of the way she was feeling. In addition, the client also felt respected, heard, and hopeful with the promise of focusing on underlying core beliefs.

CONCLUSION AND FUTURE DIRECTIONS

Cognitive restructuring is perhaps the most essential strategy used in many of the CBTs. Moreover, it is a fundamental strategy for cultivating the therapeutic relationship as well as for clarifying any issues that arise between the therapist and client. Cognitive restructuring contributes to cultivation of the therapeutic relationship in that (a) it allows the therapist to demonstrate genuine curiosity and concern about situations that are associated with emotional upset in clients' lives; and (b) it is often associated with meaningful insights that the client can take from session, which instills hope that therapy will be beneficial and contributes to client satisfaction. Moreover, when there is potential for a rupture in the therapeutic relationship, cognitive restructuring can be essential to clarifying any misconceptions, accurately viewing what is happening in the process of communication, reinforcing client agency, and moving toward reconciliation, which can serve as a corrective learning experience that the client can also apply to other relationships. These experiences can also be growth enhancing for therapists, such that they learn to see that tension and upset within the therapeutic relationship need not be catastrophic and, instead, can be an opportunity for therapeutic growth.

The directions for future research on the association between cognitive restructuring and the strength of the therapeutic relationship are abundant. I propose that, when used skillfully, cognitive restructuring significantly enhances the quality of the therapeutic relationship. Conversely, I would expect that, when used less skillfully, there could be detrimental effects on the therapeutic relationship. Thus, therapist skill level would be expected to moderate the use of cognitive restructuring and the quality of the therapeutic relationship. In addition, it will be important to identify the percentage of variance in CBT outcome accounted for by the interaction of skillful cognitive restructuring and its enhancement of the therapeutic relationship. Moreover, an agenda for future research could be to identify which aspects of the therapeutic relationship are most enhanced (or diminished) by the use of cognitive restructuring (e.g., agreement on the goals and tasks of therapy, the bond, the real relationship) and, conversely, which aspects of the therapeutic relationship (e.g., therapeutic alliance, empathy, positive regard) facilitate the most productive cognitive restructuring. Future research can also isolate the role that cognitive restructuring plays in the repair of ruptures in the therapeutic alliance and in the resolution of transference and countertransference.

Although cognitive restructuring is the focus of this single chapter, in reality this intervention strategy is used in conjunction with the other strategies described in this volume to facilitate cognitive change (even if the primary focus of interest in session is on a client's behavior!). This is especially evident in the next chapter on social problem solving, as many clients present for treatment with dejection and helplessness that stem from their view of their inability to solve problems. In these cases, cognitive restructuring can support the therapeutic relationship-based approach to social problem solving, such that clients develop confidence in their problem-solving ability while enjoying the sense that their therapist shares investment in the solving of their life problems that contribute to emotional distress.

6 SOCIAL PROBLEM SOLVING AND THE THERAPEUTIC RELATIONSHIP

Many clients who present for treatment describe being burdened and overwhelmed by problems that they face in their lives. These clients often hope that therapy will be a forum in which they can work through problems and identify solutions that will begin to ease the strain caused by problems. Some clients are poor problem solvers and can benefit from assistance in developing problem-solving skills; other clients have barriers that impede their ability to enact the effective problem-solving skills they already possess. Thus, there is a focus on life problems in nearly every course of therapy, whether the problem is a mental health disorder, a strained relationship, a major decision that needs to be made, or an obstacle to living a fulfilling life.

Social problem solving is defined as "the process by which individuals attempt to identify, discover, or create adaptive means of coping with a wide variety of stressful problems, both acute and chronic, encouraged in the course of living" (Nezu & Nezu, 2019, p. 14; see also D'Zurilla & Nezu, 2007). Social problem solving is a steadfast strategy that is incorporated into many courses of cognitive behavioral therapy (CBT; e.g., J. S. Beck, 2021). At the same time, social problem solving is the central feature of very specific CBTs

https://doi.org/10.1037/0000424-007
Therapeutic Relationship-Focused Cognitive Behavioral Therapy, by A. Wenzel

that feature a problem-solving focus, such as emotion-centered problem-solving therapy, the latest version of D'Zurilla and Nezu's classic problem-solving therapy (Nezu & Nezu, 2019), and cognitive behavioral treatment for suicide attempts (Salkovskis et al., 1990). The rationale for problem solving being such a central component of CBT is that CBT is known as a problem-focused treatment (D. Dobson & Dobson, 2017), and some conditions treated using CBT are conceptualized, at least in part, as a deficit in problem solving (e.g., suicidal ideation and behavior; Wenzel et al., 2009).

Perhaps the most widely acknowledged approach to problem solving involves the use of steps to help clients acquire skill and confidence in approaching their life problems. At times, many of these stepped approaches make use of clever acronyms to help clients remember the steps in real time when they are called on to solve a problem. One example is ITCH: Identify the problem—Think about possible solutions—Choose a solution to implement—How well does it work? (Muñoz et al., 2000). In this chapter, I use the approach described in the latest volume on problem-solving therapy, now called *emotion-centered problem-solving therapy* (Nezu & Nezu, 2019). This approach incorporates the following steps:

1. *Problem definition*—Describe the specific problem and its components, separate facts from assumptions about the problem, and identify realistic problem-focused and emotion-focused goals.

2. *Generating alternatives*—Brainstorm all possible solutions, without judging or dismissing them.

3. *Decision making*—Examine the advantages and disadvantages of possible solutions, consider the feasibility of possible solutions, and/or consider the personal and social consequences of proposed solutions in order to arrive at one solution or a combination of solutions to implement.

4. *Solution implementation and verification*—Debrief on the implementation of the solution or combination of solutions and consider what was learned in doing so and whether problem-solving efforts need to continue.

I note here that although I focus on the implementation of these problem-solving steps in this chapter, the entire emotion-centered problem-solving therapy treatment package involves many additional strategies. These include skills to overcome cognitive overload (i.e., the tendency to become overwhelmed or shut down when processing a large amount of information), strategies for enhancing motivation for action, and a "stop and slow down" technique to overcome emotion dysregulation associated with problem solving (Nezu & Nezu, 2019, pp. 6–9).

In my experience as a CBT supervisor, this approach to problem-solving coaching is very different than what many therapists implement in actuality when they attempt to deliver a problem-solving intervention. It is easier than we would like to admit to fall into a pattern that goes something like this:

CLIENT: I'm struggling with [insert name of problem].

THERAPIST: I'm sorry to hear that. Have you tried [name of one solution, or perhaps a couple of solutions]?

CLIENT: Gee, no. I didn't think of that. I will do that.

THERAPIST: Sounds great.

[Client and therapist move on to another topic.]

It is true that the client might have experienced the therapist as being helpful in this scenario, which, admittedly, could enhance the therapeutic relationship and the client's satisfaction with therapy. However, I view such an intervention as being problematic for the therapeutic relationship over the long term. As stated many times throughout this book, CBT is not about telling our clients what to do or how to think; if they are struggling with solving a problem in their lives, it is very possible that they lack the skills to go about thinking systematically about a problem and identifying and evaluating potential solutions. If we tell our clients how to solve their problem, we are depriving them of the opportunity to learn how to do so on their own, an important skill that they will be able to apply to future problems they encounter in their lives. Moreover, telling clients how to solve their problems subtly reinforces the notions that they need their therapist to solve their problems for them and that problem solving is beyond their capability. These notions run counter to the basic premises of CBT, which are to respect clients' autonomy and to empower them to acquire cognitive behavioral principles, strategies, and skills so they can function as their own cognitive behavioral therapist and need not rely indefinitely on the services of a professional. In other words, by refraining from making overt suggestions of how to solve clients' problems, cognitive behavioral therapists are enhancing the therapeutic relationship by communicating confidence in clients' ability to acquire and enact these skills.

As we saw in Chapter 5 on cognitive restructuring, problem-solving interventions can be delivered with a lesser or greater focus on the therapeutic relationship. When a problem-solving intervention is delivered with simultaneous foci on strategy and on the therapeutic relationship, consistent with therapeutic relationship-focused CBT (TRF-CBT), therapists demonstrate empathy, compassion, and confidence in the client's ability to solve the problem; respect clients' views of whether a proposed solution is feasible and preferred, as well as clients' ultimate selection of a solution; and show great interest in the client's experience of solving the problem. Moreover, when a client expresses pessimism about the likelihood that a problem will be solved, the therapist does not simply offer hollow platitudes (e.g., "You can do it!"); rather, the therapist allows space for the client to grapple with the problem and experience the weight of the associated emotional experience and communicates that both the therapist and client are partners in the journey to solve the problem. Therapists who implement problem solving also take care to demonstrate much respect and acceptance of clients so self-deprecating beliefs about ineffective problem solving are not reinforced (e.g., a client's belief that they have a fatal defect; Nezu & Nezu, 2019). Moreover, they demonstrate empathy and are open to any signs of resistance to facilitate deep discussion that promotes client agency (cf. Button et al., 2019). The following dialogues illustrate the difference between problem solving with a lesser or greater focus on the therapeutic relationship.

Excerpt 1: Less Focus on the Therapeutic Relationship

CLIENT: [expressed during a Monday CBT session] I just don't know how I'm going to get everything done! I have three deadlines on Thursday, and I haven't even started two of the three assignments.

THERAPIST: It certainly sounds like you have a lot on your plate. What strikes me is that you've had a lot on your plate many times before, and I've even heard you say that you didn't think you'd get everything done. And yet . . .

CLIENT: [looking forlorn, and tone of voice communicating mild irritation] Yes, yes, I know I always get it all done.

THERAPIST: And how is it that you always get it all done? [*Here, the therapist poses this question to ensure that the client can articulate his plan for completing his three assignments.*]

CLIENT: Same thing every time. Work in the library rather than in my dorm room so that I don't get distracted. Pull all-nighters. Wait to do extra things like going to the gym until the assignments are done.

THERAPIST: It sounds to me like you are really prioritizing your schoolwork. I understand that this is a stressful time for you. However, knowing you as I do, I have no doubt that you will persevere and complete your assignments with shining colors.

CLIENT: [shaking his head] That makes one of us. I am completely overwhelmed. Honestly, I think I might just go back to my dorm room and smoke some weed with my roommate.

The problem of focus in this dialogue was how to complete on time the three assignments that were due in 3 days, two of which had not yet been started. The therapist expressed empathy in acknowledging that there was a lot on the client's plate. However, the therapist followed up with the observation that the client had, on many occasions, expressed that he was worried about completing his assignments, and that he had always gotten them done. The therapist meant for this comment to serve as a vote of confidence in favor of the client's ability to successfully complete multiple assignments, as well as a reminder of evidence that the client's previous predictions that he would not complete his assignments had failed to be realized. Unfortunately, this statement did not have the intended effect on the client; rather, the client seemed irritated by this remark and retorted in a mildly sarcastic manner (i.e., "Yes, yes . . ."). The therapist did not follow up on this (possibly) negative reaction to the therapist's previous statement, and instead asked a question to ensure the client had a plan for completing his work over the next few days. Satisfied that the client had an adequate plan, the therapist made an encouraging summary statement (i.e., "It sounds to me like you are really prioritizing your schoolwork"), a statement of empathy (i.e., "I understand that this is a stressful time for you"), and a statement reflecting another vote of confidence (i.e., "However, knowing you as I do, I have no doubt that you will persevere and complete your assignments with shining colors"). Although these statements were meant to provide support, encouragement, and positive regard—all are important statements that can enhance the therapeutic relationship—in this instance, they fell short. I propose the following hypotheses as to why:

1. They dismissed the client's concern and sense of overwhelm, almost communicating that the client was worrying unnecessarily about whether he would complete his assignments.

2. They suggested that the therapist did not pick up on the client's irritation toward her (i.e., a possible rupture in the therapeutic alliance).

3. More generally, they did not match the affect and the intensity of the affect that the client was experiencing in the moment.

By the end of the excerpt, the client was further away from, rather than closer to, enacting a plan of action to complete his assignments. He seemed ready to give up and escape by smoking marijuana, which, of course, would make it that much more difficult to reach the goal of completing his three assignments on time.

In contrast, consider the following excerpt in which there is a relative greater focus on the therapeutic relationship. The dialogue begins in the same manner as the previous excerpt—when the client expresses concern about completing his assignments, and the therapist makes the overly strong statement regarding her confidence in the client's ability to get everything done. However, notice how she shifts to a focus on the therapeutic relationship, and then to collaborative problem solving, when she notices the client's irritation toward her.

Excerpt 2: More Focus on the Therapeutic Relationship

CLIENT: [expressed during a Monday CBT session] I just don't know how I'm going to get everything done! I have three deadlines on Thursday, and I haven't even started two of the three assignments.

THERAPIST: It certainly sounds like you have a lot on your plate. What strikes me is that you've had a lot on your plate many times before, and I've even heard you say that you didn't think you'd get everything done. And yet . . .

CLIENT: [looking forlorn, and tone of voice communicating mild irritation] Yes, yes, I know I always get it all done.

THERAPIST: [noticing the client's irritation, pausing, and regrouping] You know what, I just replayed what I said to you back in my head. If I were sitting in your seat, I would be feeling a bit dismissed. Tell me how you felt when I said that. [*Here, the therapist is shifting to a focus on the therapeutic relationship and any possible rupture that might be emerging.*]

CLIENT: [displaying a sense of exacerbation] Like you don't understand. Don't you think I *know* that I always get it done? But at what price? [putting his head in his hands and becoming tearful] I can't keep this up. It's too much. A first-generation college student at an Ivy League university? Please! What the hell made me think that I could ever cut it here?

[The therapist allows silence for both of them to absorb the magnitude of the client's sentiments and emotional intensity.]

THERAPIST: [speaking softly and gently] It's not easy to be a first-generation college student, is it?

CLIENT: [looking up from his hands and shaking his head] No, no, not at all. Almost everyone else, they went to prep schools where they got used to this kind of pace. These kinds of assignments. The crapload of reading that goes along with each class. They had tutors who helped them get through. Lots of them still do, actually! Tutors that cost an insane amount of money. They learned study skills to manage it all. Me, I didn't have to lift a finger to do well in school in my public high school. I used to think that was a blessing. Now I see it as a curse. Because . . . because . . . I didn't learn what it takes to keep up at a school like this one.

THERAPIST: [continuing to focus first and foremost on the therapeutic relationship] I wonder what it feels like to get those platitudes, those votes of confidence?

CLIENT: Honestly, it doesn't help. It probably hurts. I've been hearing them my whole life. How special I am. How I'm going to go on to do great things. How I'm going to represent my community out there. Blah, blah, blah. What I really need is someone to see through all of that, to see that even I need help sometimes, to understand that I am not Superman.

THERAPIST: That is extremely poignant. And I would like to do my part in that. I am sorry that I was not more astute in meeting that need a moment ago.

CLIENT: I know you mean well, Doc. It's just . . . being here, in this environment. Man, it can really take a toll on you.

THERAPIST: [making a reflection to demonstrate understanding] And you're not Superman.

CLIENT: [immediately picking up on the reflection and appreciating it, smiling] No. No, I am not.

THERAPIST: It sounds like there are two issues here. One is how the heck you are going to complete these three assignments by Thursday. And the other issue, more generally, is how to refine your approach to your classes. [*Here, the therapist is linking the conversation back to problem solving now that it appears that they have averted any rupture in the therapeutic alliance.*]

CLIENT: Yeah, I think that's exactly it. I just need to get through Thursday, and then there will be a lull in my schedule for a couple of weeks. It would be really great to figure out how I can find a low-cost tutor on this ridiculously expensive campus.

THERAPIST: [chuckling in response to client's reference to the "ridiculously expensive campus"] I think this sounds like a solid plan. Regarding the three assignments, tell me what your game plan is for getting these done . . .

This excerpt took a decidedly different turn than the first excerpt. On the basis of the client's irritated reaction to her, the therapist quickly caught on that she said something the client experienced as dismissive and unhelpful. She owned her therapeutic mistake by acknowledging it openly (i.e., "You know what, I just replayed what I said to you back in my head. If I were sitting in your seat, I would be feeling a bit dismissed"). Moreover, rather than leaving it at that and risking that she would continue to misperceive and misconstrue the client's inner experience, she invited him to share his feelings about what she said. Doing so opened the door for the client to elaborate on his reaction to the therapist (that she did not understand) and to identify an issue that was associated with great depth of emotion and meaning—that of being a first-generation college student at an Ivy League university. The therapist allowed space for both of them to sit with this depth of emotion and meaning and made reflections to demonstrate that she was, indeed, acquiring an accurate understanding of his circumstances. In fact, although the focus of the current session remained on problem solving, the insights revealed in this session became the foundation for continued cognitive behavioral work on the client's core beliefs (both positive and negative) and compensatory strategies (e.g., pulling "all-nighters") that were contributing to burnout in school.

In the second half of the session, the therapist and client worked collaboratively from a problem-solving framework to devise an action plan for completing his three assignments. Although the action plan contained some of the elements that the client mentioned in the first excerpt (i.e., working in the library, waiting to pursue optional activities like going to the gym until his work was done), it was much more elaborate in that the client left the session with (a) his assignments prioritized, (b) a realization that he was further along than he had given himself credit for on the two assignments that he had originally viewed as not having been started, and (c) a general structure for breaking up the next two and a half days into chunks to devote to the three assignments. When the therapist asked for feedback at the end of the session, the client expressed that he felt a sense of optimism about his ability to complete the assignments, as well as a renewed sense of commitment to do so (rather than avoiding the assignments and smoking marijuana with his roommate). More importantly, the therapeutic alliance had been significantly enhanced, as both the therapist and client viewed their problem-solving work as meaningful, and they identified two important issues to address in subsequent sessions: (a) the application of problem solving to find a low-cost tutor in his most difficult class and (b) an examination of helpful and unhelpful core beliefs and compensatory strategies that developed from his status of being an extremely intelligent and talented individual who promised to represent his community in a high-pressure environment.

TIPS FOR SOCIAL PROBLEM SOLVING THROUGH THE LENS OF THE THERAPEUTIC RELATIONSHIP

Problem solving is a powerful CBT strategy that enhances the therapeutic relationship because when clients leave the session with a tangible solution to a problem, they perceive that therapy has been productive and helpful and is making an impact on their lives. However, in my training and supervisory experience, therapists have provided the feedback that there are instances in which problem-solving interventions seem a bit rote or bland. One clue that problem solving (or any cognitive behavioral intervention) is being experienced in this way is when clients use words to reference therapy other than "therapy" or "counseling," such as it being a "class" or a "lesson." Although it is true that cognitive behavioral therapists likely provide more psychoeducation and coaching than therapists who practice from many other theoretical orientations, CBT is, first and foremost, a psychotherapy, and the bedrock of psychotherapy is the therapeutic relationship. Thus, if a therapist has the sense that they are lecturing a client or simply providing too much information for it to be absorbed in a meaningful way, I advise them to stop, take a breath, check in with the client's experience, and regroup. All cognitive behavioral interventions, including problem solving, are implemented in a conversational, reciprocal (i.e., back-and-forth) manner. In this section, I outline six tips to simultaneously enhance problem-solving interventions and the therapeutic relationship.

Tip 1: Do Not Rush the Process

As demonstrated earlier in this chapter, it is easy to be lured into the trap of providing a solution to the client's problem, soliciting the client's commitment to enact the solution, and moving on to the next item on the agenda. This is an example of what experts in the motivational interviewing community have aptly referred to as the righting reflex. Remember that the purpose of problem-solving interventions is for clients to acquire and practice problem-solving skills so they can implement problem solving on their own in their own lives without the assistance of a therapist to coach them. In my experience, fully working through the four steps of problem solving mentioned earlier in this chapter (i.e., problem definition, generating alternatives, decision making, and solution implementation and verification) requires a substantial chunk of session time (e.g., 15–20 minutes, although there is no hard-and-fast rule about this). We do not want clients to feel rushed, pressured, or "on the spot" as they work through important life problems, lest the therapeutic relationship become compromised.

One way to pace the problem-solving process and ensure that clients are "on the same page" is to ask for feedback regularly. As mentioned in Chapter 3 of this volume, the solicitation of feedback communicates to clients that their therapist wants to be sure they believe the material being discussed is relevant and helpful, that they fully understand and are digesting the material being discussed, and, if they have any constructive criticism, that their feedback will be taken seriously and heeded as they modify the intervention. Suggested questions for pacing problem-solving interventions through the use of client feedback are as follows:

- What are you learning about problem solving so far?
- Now that we've talked about this a bit, how relevant do you think this approach to problem solving is to your life?
- On the basis of what we are discussing here, how will you approach similar problems that you come across in your life?
- How is the problem-solving approach we're discussing here similar to or different than the ways in which you've approached problems in the past?
- We've covered a lot of material here. Where can I clarify? Or how, more specifically, can I help you to apply it to your personal life circumstances?

When clients provide astute feedback, it is important to embrace it enthusiastically and wholeheartedly to reinforce them for their active participation. Doing so further demonstrates that clients are an essential member of the therapeutic team.

Tip 2: Make It Interesting

My favorite CBT demonstrations are ones in which therapists incorporate their own personalities, humor, anecdotes, and metaphors into conversation to capture clients' attention, as well as ones in which therapists harness clients' personal interests to facilitate an intervention. It is not difficult to imagine that going through a step-by-step process, along with providing definitions and psychoeducation, can be a bit tedious. Thus, it can be helpful to make the problem-solving conversation unique and memorable so that clients can extract tangible pearls of wisdom and insight.

Consider the following problem-solving intervention with Sarah,[1] delivered during a session in which she chose to focus on the problem of chronic lateness by her second-shift employees in her restaurant. Sarah described a scenario in which more than half of the second-shift employees arrived up to a half hour late, which angered the employees who opened the restaurant in the morning and who handled the lunch shift. These first-shift employees had no choice but to stay until the second-shift employees arrived, despite being exhausted at the end of their shifts and having other responsibilities to which they needed to attend. Sarah claimed that, as the manager, she had repeatedly talked to the offenders and even implemented mild disciplinary action. However, she lamented the fact that many people attracted to working in the type of restaurant she managed had a reputation for taking lax approaches to rules established previously by others, and it was so difficult to find people to fill openings that Sarah believed she could not afford to fire any employees. Thus, Sarah described herself as being in a bind, and she had difficulty identifying potential solutions to the problem. This is the point at which her therapist decided to harness her personal interest in and knowledge about the music scene to see whether Sarah could identify creative solutions on the basis of a music metaphor.

THERAPIST: I wonder if we can draw from other related instances of employees not pulling their weight to guide us in approaching this problem.

SARAH: That would be helpful because I'm really not coming up with anything. It seems like no matter what I do, my employees don't listen to what I say. Even if they half-heartedly say that they will be on time at their next shift, more often than not, they don't follow through. It's to the point that I can't get anyone to help me open the restaurant because they just know that they will be stuck there an extra half hour while they are waiting for their replacement to relieve them.

THERAPIST: [demonstrating empathy] That sounds like a difficult position to be in, between a rock and a hard place.

SARAH: Yes! Exactly! It's really stressing me out. I can't even get a day off in peace because I'm constantly getting calls about employees being late for work.

THERAPIST: Sarah, it strikes me that you have a great deal of knowledge about the way teams work. Not just in the restaurant industry

---

[1]Client identity has been disguised to protect client confidentiality.

through your relationships with managers of other restaurants in your district, but also with groups of people in the artistic community or with bands on the music scene.

SARAH: [looking thoughtful] Bands, huh. It's interesting that you say that. One of my favorite bands is going through some turmoil right now due to their lead singer being an . . . well, let's just say he's become totally uncooperative to the point that the band is having to cancel shows.

THERAPIST: Oh my goodness, what happened? [*Here, the therapist is showing genuine interest in Sarah's example, and she also hopes to gather some information to draw parallels with Sarah's current situation at work.*]

SARAH: [rolling her eyes] I think he's gotten such a big ego that he thinks he is better than the band. It's probably our fault, I mean the fans. We all just worship him. But I can tell you that a lot of us are getting really tired of it. I saw them live a few months ago. It didn't seem like the singer was late for that show, but you could totally tell he wasn't into it and that there was a lot of bad blood among the band members. It wasn't the greatest show, that's for sure.

THERAPIST: Huh. How are the lead singer's fellow band members dealing with it?

SARAH: I think they're trying to compromise. I mean, I know they don't want to lose him as their vocalist. He's the face of the band. But it also seems like he wants to venture out on his own as well, like do some collaborations with other people outside of the band, maybe record some of his own solo tracks.

THERAPIST: So, they are trying to solve the problem while keeping the band together, while at the same time accepting that he, perhaps, has a somewhat different personal agenda. Because they know that what is most effective in the long run is retaining him as the lead singer, rather than getting rid of him and finding a new singer?

SARAH: Yes, that's a great way to put it. A lot of bands just fade into oblivion when they go with a new lead singer because the sound is different. So, they're doing what they need to do to stay relevant, I guess.

THERAPIST: Hmm. What parallels do you see with this band and what is happening with your employees?

SARAH: [pausing, and then bursting with laughter] Well, I guess I'd be the one who is the lead singer, and I'm the one who is keeping the band together!

THERAPIST: [joining in the laughter] Ha, so there is one aspect of this example that is the exact opposite of what is happening in the band! You really have been extremely dedicated and responsible in keeping the restaurant operating. [pausing] What can you learn from this example, though, that you can apply to your situation?

SARAH: I get it. The band had to deal with the behavior problem directly, compromising because they knew they weren't going to fire him, but they also wanted to make it work for the rest of the band and definitely not have to deal with worst-case scenarios like canceling a show and having to refund a bunch of money.

THERAPIST: Nicely put! So how can you apply these principles in a tangible way to your situation with your employees?

SARAH: First and foremost, I think I need to do a better job of accepting that this is a problem that I have to deal with. I think I've been resisting even considering the possibility that I have to do something different, like giving them incentives for showing up on time or something, because, in my book, if you're hired to work certain shifts on the job, then you show up on time for those shifts. [sighing] But I know that the world doesn't always operate like that anymore.

With this adjusted mindset of acceptance of the reality of the situation, Sarah was now able to generate a number of potential solutions to address her employees' chronic lateness. These potential solutions included the following:

• Have a restaurant-wide competition for on-time arrivals, complete with a white board to track progress, small rewards for achieving (e.g., an extra 5 minutes of break) certain milestones, and a larger reward for the winner (i.e., the employee who had the most on-time shift starts).

• Periodically take her shift supervisors and associate managers out for drinks and appetizers after closing, as Sarah appreciated that these employees bore the brunt of covering for other employees' lateness.

- Be as flexible as possible with scheduling to maximize the opportunity for employees to take on shifts that were most conducive to their schedules.

- Develop the schedule further in advance so that employees had adequate time to adjust accordingly if they were scheduled for an early shift.

- Remind chronic offenders of the time of their next shift before they leave for the day.

- When conversations involving critical feedback and discipline were necessary, use empathy rather than punitiveness and share her personal experience to connect with the employee.

Throughout the conversation as Sarah was developing potential solutions, she continually referenced the situation with the band and drew additional parallels. When she was asked for feedback at the end of the session, she exclaimed, "Who knew that my therapist would be so down for learning life lessons from a punk band?" Thus, the problem-solving exercise contributed greatly to Sarah's experience within the therapeutic relationship: Not only did she experience relief because she no longer had a sense of helplessness with the problem she was facing, but she was also engaged and had an enjoyable and meaningful time learning from a situation that one of her favorite bands was experiencing.

Tip 3: Evaluate Potential Solutions in Written Format

In a classic psychology experiment, it was determined that the average human being can keep seven (plus or minus two) bits of information in their working memory (G. A. Miller, 1956). When cognitive behavioral therapists work with clients from a problem-solving framework, they are almost always dealing with more than seven bits of information. Even if a client whittles down a list of potential solutions to, say, the top five, and they conduct a straightforward advantages–disadvantages analysis of each potential solution, that still yields 10 bits of information—more than most human beings can hold in working memory. Writing down potential solutions, as well as the components used to evaluate each option (e.g., advantages and disadvantages), helps the process to run more systematically, thoroughly, and smoothly. All of this will give the client confidence in the decision-making process, which has the potential to enhance the therapeutic relationship because clients will perceive that they are getting something valuable from therapy.

Moreover, having a written record of the decision-making process allows clients to reference a model as they apply problem solving, and specifically decision making, in their lives outside of session. This record also serves as a reminder of the active, problem-focused, and (hopefully) helpful nature of CBT. It should be noted here that, at times, clients balk when it is suggested that they write down their therapeutic work on a piece of paper. Or they write it down but quickly lose it. Fortunately, many clients enjoy taking photos and storing them on their mobile phones. So, for example, a therapist could record the decision-making evaluation on a white board in their office, and clients could take a photo to refer to in between sessions as they attempt to select and implement a specific solution to their problem. Some clients even choose to make the photo their temporary background on their mobile phones—a nice reminder of the fruits of the work they have done in therapy. Such easy-access, convenient reminders of therapeutic work have the potential to enhance the therapeutic relationship because they also serve as a reminder of the fact that therapy is making a difference in their lives.

Tip 4: Communicate Trust and Confidence in the Client's Solution

Even after a thorough problem-solving analysis, clients will sometimes choose a solution that seems suboptimal. For example, I once had a client whose faith and participation in religious services were extremely important to her, and she was debating between becoming a member of one of two different congregations. In this case, there were only two potential solutions to consider. Nevertheless, she evaluated numerous factors in the decision-making process, such as the distance from her home, her previous experiences with each congregation, the number of friends and acquaintances in each congregation, the degree to which she resonated with the style of the officiant of each congregation, and so on. After we carefully examined each choice on these many dimensions, it became clear that one choice was associated with decidedly more advantages than the other choice. I was quite shocked that when it came time to choose a congregation, she chose the one with many disadvantages and remarked that it was the direction her heart was telling her to pursue. Although, internally, I was skeptical of the choice, I said something like, "You are the expert on your own needs and preferences, and I have nothing but respect for the choice you made after so thoughtfully considering both options." She later told me in a subsequent session that she was relieved I had that reaction, as she experienced criticism from many family members about making this decision and she appreciated my trust in her. My last session with this client was over 10 years ago, and I receive periodic updates from her. She continues to be a member of this congregation, and she even relocated so that she could maximize her involvement in religious activities.

Therapists are encouraged to reserve judgment about suboptimal solutions, just as we encourage our clients to reserve judgment about potential solutions when they are brainstorming. Cognitive behavioral therapists operate according to the belief that client agency should be supported. In many cases, such as the one just described, therapists are pleasantly surprised at the outcome when clients trust their hearts and enact a solution that does not necessarily follow from logical analysis. These instances demonstrate that even in the most artfully applied steps of problem solving, there is no guarantee that the winner of the decision-making analysis will be the one associated with the most advantages, or even the one that is ultimately the most effective. Like most things in life, problem solving requires some tolerance of risk and uncertainty, and instances in which a client makes a "leap of faith" provide important practice in developing "muscle" for risk and uncertainty in therapists and clients alike.

Of course, if a suboptimal solution toward which a client is veering has the potential to be damaging, then the therapist can gently use Socratic questioning to give space for the client to arrive at this conclusion on their own. Or the therapist can ask permission to consider the likelihood and impact of damaging side effects by implementing that solution, all while demonstrating care, concern, and respect for the client.

Tip 5: Express Genuine Interest in the Outcome of Problem Solving in the Next Session

When a thorough problem-solving intervention is delivered in session, it is often the case that the implementation of the solution in between sessions would serve as the logical homework exercise for the client. Therapists have the opportunity to enhance the therapeutic relationship when they demonstrate keen, genuine interest in the results of problem solving. For example, consider a therapist who says something like, "I was thinking of you on Wednesday when you were going to [implement the solution decided upon in the previous session]. I'm so eager to hear how it went and what you learned from it." Such a statement contributes to the therapeutic relationship because it demonstrates that the client is important to the therapist (i.e., that the therapist was thinking about the client in between sessions regarding something that was important to the client). Moreover, the therapist's use of the word "eager" suggests that they are looking forward to the session and continuing important, productive work together.

Notice that the therapist did not say something like, "I'm eager to hear if the solution worked." I am a strong believer in the notion that problem solving is an important intervention for clients in CBT, regardless of whether their enacted solution achieves its desired effects. In the next section, I discuss ways to deal with clients' negative reactions if problem solving is not particularly effective, in a way that enhances the therapeutic relationship. Here, I will say that refraining from using language that confers real or perceived judgment (e.g., about a solution "working") is preferable for many reasons.

First, in my experience, rarely do enacted solutions "work" 100% of the time. Rather, solutions may be partially successful; they may continue to have potential despite an unexpected obstacle that prevented them from being implemented at that time; or solution implementation may have introduced one or more additional problems to be solved. When a therapist asks a question like, "Did it work?" it has the potential to create an all-or-nothing expectation for the client to have been successful, which could set the stage for shame, embarrassment, or disappointment if the client feels as though they must "come clean" about a less than optimal outcome.

Second, a question like "Did it work?" models an outcome orientation when, in many instances, cognitive behavioral therapists are trying to help clients put more emphasis on process rather than outcome. For example, implementation of a solution could meet with decidedly disappointing results, and yet, that could be essential for a client's growth and development in problem solving. In the process of enacting a disappointing solution, clients may gather additional information that would inform a more refined approach to solving the problem. Alternately, the client may learn something important about themselves, such as the fact that they are more resilient than they had realized or that there is an important area in which they could develop additional skill. Or the client's problem may be difficult to solve at that moment, which may call for distress tolerance, acceptance, and ultimately transcendence—all meaningful principles to incorporate into one's life and desirable outcomes in CBT. Thus, when therapists show genuine curiosity about the outcome of solution implementation, they do so with an eye on the process of what the client is learning and how the client is growing, regardless of the success or failure of the actual problem-solving outcome in the eyes of the client. Such a stance creates a "win–win" situation within the therapeutic relationship and provides a foundation for the client to perceive the exercise as helpful, useful, and growth enhancing under all circumstances.

Tip 6: Use Cognitive and Acceptance Strategies to Manage Negative Emotional Reactions if Problem Solving Does Not Yield Its Intended Effects

Despite therapists de-emphasizing whether problem solving has "worked," many clients, nevertheless, will engage in self-flagellation when they perceive that their solution has "failed." Not only are therapists encouraged to be alert for such reactions when they are debriefing about solution implementation, but they are also encouraged to harness a balance between therapeutic relationship techniques (e.g., empathy, congruence, and positive regard) and broad cognitive behavioral principles such as cognitive restructuring, acceptance, and self-compassion. When clients are critical of themselves for their perception of failing, it can be tremendously therapeutic to have a soft, compassionate, encouraging environment to debrief, learn from the experience, and regroup. This provides an important learning experience in and of itself, as clients learn (a) that they will not be rejected if their efforts did not achieve the desired result; (b) that they are not only accepted as they are, but that important strengths and positive qualities about themselves emerged during the problem-solving process regardless of the outcome; and (c) that they are still worthy of others' confidence and faith in their abilities.

Sarah, for example, decided to enact all six of the solutions she generated when she brainstormed with her therapist. When she returned for the subsequent session, she was excited to share many victories. She had implemented a restaurant-wide competition for on-time arrivals to work, and most employees noticed and accepted the challenge even though it had only been implemented for a few days. Consistent with her new acceptance-based mindset, Sarah was more flexible with scheduling and was sure to schedule the most egregious offenders for shifts in a way that would cause minimal disruption to the restaurant. She pledged to get the schedule out 3 weeks (rather than 2 weeks) in advance so her employees could arrange their own schedules around their shifts accordingly. She organized an after-work social outing with the restaurant's leadership, and she sensed that they seemed to appreciate the sentiment. Moreover, she was taking care to remind employees of their next shift when they left for the day, so their next set of work hours would be fresh in their minds.

Despite these successes, Sarah reported that she had two difficult conversations with repeat offenders, whom she viewed as not receptive to her new campaign. She remarked that these two employees "walked all over" her, which prompted a number of self-deprecating comments and engendered a negative view about her problem-solving and managerial abilities. As Sarah described these interactions, her mood and outlook quickly shifted from excitement and confidence to shame and negativity. Consider the following dialogue:

SARAH: [looking forlorn] I just crumbled when they stood up to me. I started stuttering over my words and did not stand up for myself or for the other employees. I just suck as a manager. Really, I have no business managing that restaurant.

THERAPIST: [leaning forward] Tell me what just happened here, Sarah. [*Here, the therapist refrains from directly challenging the notion*

*that Sarah is an ineffective manager, and instead simply shows
interest in the spirit of maintaining their genuine connection.*]

SARAH: [becoming tearful] You mean as I was telling you what happened
at the restaurant?

THERAPIST: Yes.

SARAH: Overall, I was feeling better about things. But those two guys,
man, they just really get to me. I think I am okay at managing
the reasonable employees, I really do. I've been a server in plenty
of different restaurants throughout my career. So, I do get it, and
I think most people know that I get it. And because they know
that I get it, some of them even want to help me out a little.
[pausing] But when it comes to the tough ones, the ones who
are disrespectful, constantly pointing their finger at others for
why they didn't do their job, rather than taking responsibility
for themselves . . . [shaking her head] I don't know, I just don't
understand it because I've been such a hard worker throughout
my life. I just can't deal with it. But I know, that to be a manager, I
need to deal with people like that. And if I can't, well . . . then . . .
maybe I don't have what it takes to be a manager.

THERAPIST: [speaking warmly] Sarah, I'm actually hearing you say some
important and encouraging things about your managerial abilities. You've been in your employees' shoes before, many times.
You use that experience in an effective way as a manager, and
many employees recognize that. In fact, you've told me some
anecdotes of how you've used that experience in particular situations during the time in which I've known you. Remember how
you pegged that guest who was going to leave without paying
when no one else saw that coming? [Sarah lifts her head, smiles,
and gives a bit of a chuckle] And remember that time when your
assistant manager had just broken up with her partner and was
really having a hard time? [Sarah nods] What happened in that
instance?

SARAH: [sighing] It was actually a really cool moment. When we were
in the break room, she hugged me and thanked me profusely for
having her back. I guess that was a real turning point in our relationship, because before that, I thought I kind of got an attitude
from her and that we didn't work well together. But now, we are
totally in sync. And I think the restaurant runs better because of it.

THERAPIST: [speaking emphatically] Sarah, I have admired you for so many of your managerial abilities that you've described over the course of our work together. However, what is ultimately important is your own opinion of yourself, so that you can thrive and be the person you want to be. [*Here again, the therapist is refraining from telling Sarah what to think about her problem-solving abilities as a manager, while at the same time, overtly expressing positive regard.*]

SARAH: [pausing to reflect] I actually do think I'm a pretty good manager. I'm like a quiet leader. I don't bark orders, and I don't chastise employees, because I know how that feels. And I know lots of people appreciate that. It's just . . . it's just that . . .

THERAPIST: I appreciate that dealing with the difficult, disrespectful employees is never easy, especially when it doesn't seem like there are a lot of other people who can easily step into their position.

SARAH: Exactly.

THERAPIST: How is this for an idea? What if, for homework, you were to work on really giving yourself credit for what is going well from a managerial perspective? And then, we can continue to brainstorm ideas of ways to deal with these two remaining pesky employees? [*Here, the therapist is suggesting an intervention that could facilitate cognitive restructuring of Sarah's view of her managerial abilities, as well as continued problem solving so that they do not abandon the problem-solving thread that is beginning to be woven into sessions.*]

SARAH: [appearing visibly relieved] I really like that idea a lot. I don't give myself enough credit. And look how easy it is for me to get discouraged by two, excuse my language, a--holes, when really, I've made a lot of positive changes even just in the past week, since last week's session.

The therapist in this dialogue could have easily challenged Sarah immediately when she said that she did not have what it takes to be a restaurant manager and that she had no business managing the restaurant (especially after she had just described many problem-solving successes that she implemented in between sessions). However, the therapist recognized that Sarah tended to self-flagellate and that there was a strong possibility she would view such direct challenging as yet another indicator she was doing something "wrong." Instead, the therapist harnessed therapeutic relationship-enhancing techniques to create a warm environment in which Sarah's abilities were respected and even prized. For example, the therapist drew from her previous interactions with Sarah to (gently and sensitively) remind her of some of the victories she has had, such as using her experience to catch an offender and showing compassion for a coworker who was having a hard day at work because of events going on in her personal life. Not only was this intervention meant to remind Sarah of professional accomplishments that deserve praise, but it also showed that the therapist has listened and paid close attention to what Sarah discussed in session, which reinforced the notion of positive regard. When the therapist expressed overt admiration for Sarah's managerial abilities, it communicated that she truly viewed Sarah as an equal within the therapeutic relationship, with special gifts that others can emulate to be successful in life (i.e., prizing the client). By the end of the exchange, Sarah was willing to acknowledge just how much she had achieved in between sessions with her problem-solving implementation, and her tone of voice communicated optimism and hope that something could be done to manage the behavior of (and her emotional reaction toward) her two difficult employees.

SOCIAL PROBLEM SOLVING AS APPLIED TO THERAPEUTIC RELATIONSHIP ISSUES

As with cognitive restructuring, social problem solving can be applied to address issues that arise in the therapeutic relationship. It is hoped that the effective application of problem-solving interventions surrounding the therapeutic relationship will serve as a corrective learning experience that will increase clients' confidence in their ability to solve problems in relationships with individuals in their daily lives. Moreover, it provides an opportunity for the client and therapist, together, to share in the delight of a solution that helps to move treatment forward. The three problems considered in the section are (a) the relatively straightforward, but nevertheless frustrating, problem of scheduling difficulties; (b) the more serious problem of difficulty with homework and its effect on motivation and commitment; and (c) the more serious problem of an intervention that went awry, leading to mistrust in the therapeutic process.

Scheduling Difficulties

If readers' experience with referrals is anything like mine at the time of the writing of this chapter (January 2022), the number of referrals and former clients returning to therapy is absolutely astounding. Providers want to do everything possible to meet the profound mental health needs of people affected by the COVID-19 pandemic and, at the same time, they are increasingly recognizing a need to set some semblance of boundaries and engage in self-care, lest they "burn out." Thus, it behooves all of us to apply the principles of social problem solving to be able to discern guiding principles for taking on new and returning clients, balancing meeting the needs of existing clients and our own well-being.

In my own practice, I identified the following solutions during brainstorming: (a) adding more clinical hours (beyond the 35 clinical hours per week I was already devoting to my clients), (b) turning away new clients, (c) hiring an associate to take on extra referrals, and (d) adopting a flexible model. After applying a decision-making framework, I opted to go with options (c) and (d). I hired an associate who was willing to take on a small caseload to help me field referrals. Then, with the overflow of new referrals and returning clients, I devised the following statement that I shared when I was fielding the inquiry:

> The number of referrals and former clients who have been returning to my practice is nothing short of extraordinary, so my schedule is much tighter than is typical. That being said, the type of therapy that I deliver (cognitive behavioral therapy, or CBT for short) is an active treatment that is often associated with meaningful gains in a relatively short time frame (i.e., a few months). This means that my schedule is always changing, and it often is the case that, when I think my schedule is completely booked, one of my established clients decreases the frequency of their sessions or ends treatment altogether after CBT has been successful.
>
> With this background in mind, the approach I have been taking with new referrals is that they are asked to take whatever slot happens to be available in my schedule. At times, this means waiting for an advance-notice cancellation from someone who had previously held a slot. Fortunately, my caseload is terrific at giving me at least 24 hours' notice of cancellation (usually much more), so people waiting for appointments typically find that, with some patience and flexibility, they are able to be seen. Unfortunately, I will not take a time slot away from an already-established client who is expecting to be seen. However, over time, you will be worked in my caseload, such that you will be one of the already-established clients, and you'll be able to work your way into a regular time slot for therapy that is protected. Once a client is on my caseload, I "have their backs," and I make a commitment to meet their needs, even if we have to be a bit creative in doing so.
>
> It is understandable if this arrangement does not work for your immediate or longer-term needs. I am happy to provide you with referrals for other providers. However, if this sort of arrangement works for you, I'd be happy to talk further to see about getting you on my schedule.

This arrangement is not ideal—what new client in psychotherapy, truly, would want to "fly standby" as they wait for an appointment? In most circumstances, I would not think of conducting my practice in this manner with new clients. However, the circumstances surrounding the need for mental health services during the pandemic were extraordinary. I ultimately found that the transparency and respect demonstrated in this message resonated with clients, and I also received feedback that they appreciated my commitment to my established clients, knowing that they, one day, would be an established client as well. Are there some new referrals who choose to seek services elsewhere? Sure. I applaud that decision, as I truly wish for new clients to make an informed decision and pursue the match that they think would be best for them. However, most clients were grateful to have this opportunity, and within a few weeks, they were worked into regular slots in my schedule. For these clients, I believe that we began our therapeutic journey on a foundation of transparency, respect, and concern for what works best for the client. Moreover, when relevant, I shared with clients the problem-solving process that I went through to arrive at this policy, which modeled the application of this standard CBT strategy.

Difficulty With Homework

Homework is a staple of CBT, as empirical research shows that the more emphasis on homework, the better the outcome in CBT (Kazantzis et al., 2016). When clients enact CBT homework in their daily lives, they practice the skills and principles that they learned in session, which would be expected to be associated with a generalization of the principles and skills learned in treatment. Cognitive behavioral therapists typically take an active stance as they develop homework in a collaborative manner with their clients, asking their clients to articulate their reasons for completing homework in between sessions, the likelihood that they will follow through, how they will remember to do it, and what they expect to learn from it (cf. Wenzel, 2019). Although the completion of homework is ideal in CBT, in reality a common observation among cognitive behavioral therapists is that many clients struggle with it. Difficulties completing homework have the potential to decrease motivation and, ultimately, engagement in treatment, which could, in turn, be a factor in premature dropout or poor outcome. Thus, when a client reports difficulty with homework, it is usually helpful to approach it in a curious manner (rather than in an overly directive manner that would have the potential to shame the client), such that it yields important information to shape future interventions in order to maximize success in CBT.

Moreover, if in retrospect, it becomes clear that the therapist inadvertently contributed to nonoptimal homework development (e.g., the therapist was a bit overzealous in suggesting a substantial exercise), then it is important for the therapist to own that and take an appropriate amount of responsibility to smooth out any "bumps" in the therapeutic relationship.

The following dialogue focuses on a client with obsessive compulsive disorder (OCD) who was considering switching to insight-oriented psychotherapy because, week after week, he was not completing his exposure-based homework. An important part of his case formulation was that he was a highly intelligent individual who was raised in (and continued to benefit from) a family with upper-class socioeconomic status, which afforded him many advantages in life without having to put in a commensurate amount of "blood, sweat, and tears." His therapist truly believed that exposure-based CBT was the optimal match for his pathology (in fact, many cognitive behavioral therapists recognize exposure-based CBT as being so efficacious for a condition like OCD, relative to insight-oriented psychotherapies, that it is unethical to not offer it; Olatunji et al., 2009). Thus, she sincerely hoped that he would continue with CBT, whether with her or another seasoned cognitive behavioral therapist.

The therapist recognized that she did not acknowledge and intervene to address the lack of homework completion early enough in therapy before the client got to this point. In hindsight, she recognized that her lack of timely intervention was probably a clinical mistake in light of the client's background, case formulation, and the way in which he approached his academic and professional work in the past. As she conceptualized the issue from a problem-solving framework, she identified two pieces to be addressed: (a) the client's lack of focus and follow-through in completing homework that they had developed collaboratively in the previous session and (b) her own diligence in addressing homework noncompletion in therapy in a more timely and direct manner before it resulted in negative consequences in the form of discouragement and a lack of motivation and engagement. Although the following dialogue focuses mainly on (a), notice that the therapist takes responsibility for her own piece in the problem described in (b).

CLIENT: I think I'm going to switch psychiatrists. I've had a couple of appointments with this new guy, and I like his approach. I think it's time for something new, as it feels to me like I've exhausted all that I can do with my current psychiatrist.

THERAPIST: It sounds like you've put a lot of thought into this. I will be curious to hear what medication adjustments he might make.

CLIENT: And . . . this guy does a combination of meds and therapy . . . so, um . . . that might affect our work as well.

THERAPIST: [taking care to speak in a warm and nondefensive manner] Ah. Am I right to assume that you are implying that you might switch over to him for psychotherapy as well?

CLIENT: [looking a bit sheepish] Yeah, I think that will likely be the plan.

THERAPIST: [continuing to take great measures to respond in a nondefensive manner] I'm so glad that this is coming up so that we can talk about it further. [asking for permission to continue before asking for feedback so that the client does not feel put on the spot] Is it okay with you if we take a few moments to discuss our therapeutic work and our relationship? We've been working together for some time.

CLIENT: Yes, that's okay with me.

THERAPIST: I'm curious how you've been experiencing our therapeutic work and, in particular, if there's anything with which you are not satisfied?

CLIENT: No, I'm definitely not dissatisfied. I think you are great at what you do. At the same time, you and I both know that I'm not making the most of this, with the homework. It seems like we've fallen into a rut in which I return for session after session with nothing to report. And this new guy, the type of therapy he does is exploratory, really getting into a person's childhood to figure out patterns, you know, why they are the way they are. I think I would really like that.

THERAPIST: Your observation about returning for session after session without completed homework is an interesting and important one. [pausing] You know, I take some ownership, as well, of this piece of our work, as you and I have been in this together since the beginning. It's my professional opinion that exposure-based CBT is the ideal match for OCD, and homework completion is a critical component of success. I could have been more active in recognizing that this was such an obstacle and working with you to brainstorm more creative ways to facilitate your exposure work. [*Here, the therapist is thinking that an insight-oriented psychotherapy would not be the optimal match for the client's clinical presentation, and she is also wondering whether the client's wish to*

> *explore his childhood is a manifestation of avoidance, but she is taking care not to pose these reactions at this time in order to create an open space that would allow the client to express his reservations.*]

CLIENT: Huh. I appreciate you saying that. I've started the leave these sessions feeling more and more discouraged, which just makes me shut down more. So, it was almost like I knew I wasn't going to attempt my homework even before I left the session.

THERAPIST: Oh goodness, I truly am sorry to hear this. [pausing] I certainly respect your decision if you choose to pursue the psychotherapy piece of your treatment with this new psychiatrist, although I will be honest that my professional opinion is that exposure-based CBT is the ideal match for OCD. However, another option is for the two of us to regroup and brainstorm ways to optimize exposure for your personal style and needs.

CLIENT: [appearing to be encouraged] Well, that's an interesting idea. Okay, let's see what we come up with.

The therapist and client spent the rest of the session collaborating on a revised approach to his exposure treatment. They identified several creative exposures that the therapist could supervise over video conferencing while the client had session at home (as the session took place during the COVID-19 pandemic when sessions were held via telehealth). They devised a more inviting way to record his exposures, as he found himself putting off the recording of exposures on the therapist's standard form. They reviewed his original exposure hierarchy; in doing so, the client was reminded of the exposures he indeed undertook and, thereby, the progress that he had made in treatment already. Moreover, in light of the client's history of having few consequences for completing shoddy work, he identified ways to enhance accountability, such as by sending a secure message to his therapist through her client portal each day that he completed exposures and by involving his wife in treatment so that she could encourage him to sequester time for his CBT homework when their lives got busy. The client agreed to try out this new plan. At the time of his next session, he indicated that he completed exposure exercises 3 of the 7 days during the previous week, which was a vast improvement over the amount of time he had been devoting to homework in previous weeks. He noted that he continued to feel a need to explore the option of insight-oriented psychotherapy with his new psychiatrist but that he was feeling better about exposure and, more generally, his work in CBT, and that he understood the value of exposure-based CBT for

OCD no matter what direction he ultimately chose for continued psycho-therapy. Thus, this client's homework noncompliance became an opportunity to enhance outcome, rather than remaining a barrier.

Unsuccessful Behavioral Experiment

A *behavioral experiment* is an experiential approach to cognitive restructuring in which a client attempts to test the accuracy and likelihood of an unhelpful thought that is associated with emotional distress. For example, if a client with social anxiety disorder avoids people because they believe they will be rejected if they attempt to socialize, the behavioral experiment might involve testing out this prediction by asking someone with whom they are friendly out to lunch. Or, if a depressed client believes that an innovative idea will be dismissed by their manager at work, the behavioral experiment might involve testing out this prediction by requesting a meeting with the manager and discussing their thoughts. Behavioral experiments also involve social problem solving because in devising the experiment, the therapist often works with the client to decide on a way to implement the experiment to maximize the likelihood of success and to identify, in advance, ways of coping if the experiment does not turn out as planned. Behavioral experiments often facilitate important learning experiences for clients to realize that what they are expecting from challenging situations is often more aversive than it actually is, that they have the tools to be successful in their endeavors, and that they have the resilience to weather disappointments if the experiment does not work out.

The drawback, of course, with behavioral experiments is that there is always a possibility the experiment will proceed in such a way that reinforces the original unhelpful thought selected for testing in the first place. Although such negative outcomes occur far less frequently than we anticipate, they do occur and they can infuse a sense of mistrust in the therapeutic process.

Consider the following dialogue with a socially anxious client who implemented a behavioral experiment with a woman he was beginning to date. It had been a major feat for this client to begin dating this woman, as his worry about excessive blushing was associated with self-focused attention and preoccupation with temperature regulation that often interfered with effective conversation. The client reported that things were going well with this new romantic interest, but he perceived an "elephant in the room" (i.e., his anxiety) because he believed that he could not fully relax in her presence, thereby creating awkwardness. In this session, the client and therapist considered the utility of sharing an appropriate amount of information about his anxiety to clear the air and create a way for him to feel more relaxed in the woman's presence. Although the client saw many advantages of doing this, he also struggled with the prediction that it would create more awkwardness, not less. The client and his therapist devised a behavioral experiment in which he planned to share a small amount about his anxiety with this new romantic partner to test the notion that it would create additional awkwardness. His therapist was hopeful that, on the basis of things the client had said about this woman in session, that she would be kind, compassionate, and understanding, thereby enhancing their connection.

When the client returned for his next session, he mentioned that the behavioral experiment yielded deleterious effects, much to his therapist's chagrin. He indicated that the woman quickly cut him off as he mentioned his anxiety, indicating that she did not "sign up" for a relationship in which she had to provide support for a mental health problem. The client recounted what, exactly, he said to her, and it appeared to be just what had been practiced in session, which was general and appropriate rather than being indicative of inappropriate oversharing. Thus, it appeared that the client and the therapist greatly overestimated this woman's capacity for empathy and understanding. As a result, the client had a crisis of faith about therapy.

CLIENT: It was so crushing, almost like Dr. Jekyll and Mr. Hyde. I mean, she was so sweet on all of our dates. And as soon as I mentioned anxiety . . . it was like a cloud just came over her. She shut down. And to say what she said, that she didn't sign up for a relationship with someone with mental health problems? I mean, come on! Everyone experiences anxiety! She acted like I'm psychotic or something.

THERAPIST: Oh my goodness, I am incredibly sorry this happened. You did such a thorough job of planning out the experiment and crafting what you were going to say to her. It seemed to strike such a balance between honesty and appropriateness. [*Here, the therapist is mindful of the notion of prizing the client at a time when he did not at all feel prized by this potential romantic partner.*]

CLIENT: I know, I know. [shaking his head] I gotta tell you, though, I can't help but think that I wouldn't be in this position right now if we wouldn't have gone the route of implementing the experiment. Maybe we should have just left well enough alone.

THERAPIST: [speaking warmly and nondefensively] It sounds like there is a part of you that wishes we did not implement the behavioral experiment?

CLIENT: Yes, exactly! Look where I am now! I'm scared s---less of trying to start all over again with someone else! Maybe we should have practiced more ways to manage my anxiety. [sitting back in his seat, looking dejected] God, what did I do? It was going so well!

THERAPIST: I, also, am extremely saddened by this outcome. I know how much you struggle with the fear that others will reject you. And I also know how much you are looking to establish a loving, long-term romantic relationship. [*Here, the therapist hopes to convey empathy and congruence here, attending to their real relationship.*]

CLIENT: Maybe I shouldn't even continue with this. You know, with therapy. I'm not sure how many more times I can put myself out there, just to be shot down royally like this.

THERAPIST: [continuing to demonstrate empathy and nondefensiveness] I understand that you might feel like that; in fact, I might feel the exact same way if I were in your situation. And you are always in the driver's seat with therapy. If it feels as if a break would be best for you, I respect your decision. I wonder, though, if we can discuss this unfortunate incident a bit further so that we can consider it from multiple perspectives and see what can be learned from it?

CLIENT: [speaking in a huffy tone] Well, I guess, since I'm here and paying for the session.

THERAPIST: [proceeding with warmth, especially in light of the client's tone] I appreciate your openness to talking more about this. [demonstrating congruence and genuineness] Frankly, I am experiencing a great deal of disappointment as well. Not only because of the hard work you've put into therapy, culminating in the effort you put into initiating a difficult conversation, but also because another human being whom you valued treated you in an uncompassionate way.

During the remainder of the session, the therapist achieved a balance between cognitive restructuring and acceptance strategies to allow the client to debrief and soften any negative views about himself, his desirability, and his interpersonal abilities that might have emerged from this unfortunate incident. The therapist took care not to push him to assume a more benign view about whether therapy had made things worse for him, as she wanted to demonstrate the utmost respect for his views after he had been disrespected by the woman with whom he was hoping to enter into a relationship. Moreover, although the therapist felt very badly about the way in which the behavioral experiment turned out and was fielding her own negative thinking about ways in which she might have failed her client, she was cognizant of the potential to make the focus of the session about her and her need to rectify his view of therapy. By the close of the session, the client was feeling more centered in light of the incident, and he was nearing a different conclusion about the value of therapy.

CLIENT: I honestly think this says much more about who she is as a person, rather than it being about me and my anxiety. I really liked her, but if I'm honest with myself, there were probably more red flags than I cared to acknowledge. There were times when it seemed like she wanted a rich, good-looking boyfriend to show off to her friends, rather than truly getting to know me. And when I tried to be real with her . . . I don't know, it seemed like she would gloss it over, always bringing the conversation back to talking about other people, or where she wanted to go on vacation.

THERAPIST: [recalling their previous work on recognizing cognitive distortions at work in upsetting situations] I think you are doing a nice job of getting some distance and not personalizing her rejection, even when it seemed so personal at the time.

CLIENT: That's exactly it! In some ways, it was personal—she was saying I don't want you, you're not good enough for me because of your anxiety. But you know what? Maybe she's the one who isn't good enough for me, if she can't handle talking about real feelings, real problems.

THERAPIST: You are a person of great depth, and I would agree that you would do well with someone who also brings great depth to the relationship. At the same time, I understand that this stings, even if you've determined that she was not an optimal match for you. You're still allowed to acknowledge the hurt. [*Here, the therapist is attending to the therapeutic relationship and emotional experiencing, rather than forcing any specific cognitive behavioral strategy.*]

CLIENT: I guess a person doesn't get to experience the good stuff without taking some risks, right?

THERAPIST: [smiling] It is true that relationships can be high risk, high reward. Sometimes that is a tough lesson to learn when a person finds themselves on the risk side rather than on the reward side.

CLIENT: [laughing] Ha ha, isn't that true?

THERAPIST: [speaking warmly] I do hope, when all is said and done, that you can take something valuable from this experience.

CLIENT: I do, I definitely do. I was like really pissed off at everything when this happened—at her, at you, at therapy, at myself for my anxiety. But, honestly, it is probably much better off that I know now that she does not want to deal with my anxiety, rather than first learning that many months down the road when I'm totally in love with her.

THERAPIST: That is a wise observation. So, would you like to schedule another appointment?

CLIENT: Yes, I would. I still need some work if I am going to achieve my goal of getting into a long-term relationship!

In this excerpt, the therapist focused on the therapeutic relationship, first and foremost, when the client experienced an incident that had the potential to be devastating to his self-esteem as a socially anxious man who was trying to "put himself out there" and date. Rather than jumping into any specific CBT intervention, she allowed the client space to experience and verbalize his feelings about the incident itself and about the fact that it occurred when he was implementing a therapeutic intervention. The therapist felt awful that the incident occurred, especially in light of the fact that it resulted from a homework exercise the client was implementing to disprove the idea that discussing his anxiety would introduce awkwardness into the relationship. However, she took care to genuinely express her feelings about what had happened, while, at the same time, focusing on what was important to the client rather than her own agenda to re-instill the client's confidence in treatment so that he would not drop out. Space was made for some cognitive restructuring and acceptance principles to be imbued into the discussion as it ensued; by the end of the session, the client had achieved perspective on the incident and was viewing therapy as a means to continue to work toward his goals.

In this instance, the therapist actually refrained from excessive problem solving. It is not difficult to imagine that the therapist's guilt and disappointment in response to the client's report of the results of the behavioral experiment would facilitate an urge to jump in and "make things better" for the client. Thus, the therapist had to sit with her own distress about the outcome of the experiment, and her own thoughts about what she could have done differently and whether the client would continue therapy with her, to allow space for the client to experience and process his affect, as well as for the bond within the therapeutic relationship to re-emerge. The lesson here for therapists is that there are times when we feel a need to very actively apply problem solving to repair a relationship, and there are other times when perhaps the more fruitful course of action would be to allow the process to unfold naturally, even if it is uncomfortable to do so.

CONCLUSION AND FUTURE DIRECTIONS

Like cognitive restructuring, problem solving is a central strategy that is used at some point during most courses of CBT. When a client implements problem solving in a way that helps advance them toward their treatment goals, it instills confidence in therapy and it reinforces the notion that therapy is valuable. Such attitudes toward therapy feed back into the enhancement of the therapeutic alliance, and they set the stage for a good outcome at the end of treatment. According to the premises of TRF-CBT, the process of problem solving has the potential to enhance the therapeutic relationship because (a) clients develop the sense that their therapist is invested in them solving their life problems, (b) it actively demonstrates the notion of collaboration in the work of therapy, and (c) it allows for therapists to display genuine interest in the events that occur in clients' lives. When a client solves a problem through use of problem-solving tools cultivated in treatment, it allows the client and therapist alike to revel in the success. This shared experience of positive affect contributes to the therapeutic environment being warm, inviting, safe, and supportive.

Problem solving can also be used to repair any potential ruptures in the therapeutic relationship. When the client is having difficulty with one of the therapist's policies, it allows an opportunity for the therapist to demonstrate kindness while maintaining appropriate boundaries, model flexibility (if it is a policy for which some flexibility can be afforded), and help the client identify ways to adapt to the policy. If the client becomes discouraged due to lack of progress in therapy or a CBT homework exercise that they viewed as making a problem worse, then the therapist can apply problem solving in many ways, including the following:

- Revise the treatment plan to identify additional issues to be addressed in therapy that will complement existing aims of treatment to, more fully, help the client reach their ultimate goals.

- Devise creative CBT interventions that capitalize on what is learned by the failed exercise and more precisely attend to the issue that the client hopes to address.

- Provide empathy and understanding about the client's experience with the CBT intervention, and express a commitment to work collaboratively and diligently to support the client through the difficult time in their lives and identify other approaches for addressing the issue.

In many instances, some version of the third approach is sufficient for client satisfaction and trust in the therapeutic relationship. First and foremost, most clients want to be heard, respected, and positively regarded, and attention to these aspects of therapeutic interaction even when a specific intervention has not yielded its desired results is enough. Ironically, implementing the third approach and allowing space for the client to express their feelings and for a natural repair of the relationship to begin can involve the therapist intentionally refraining from implementing excessive problem solving.

There are many directions for future research on the association between problem solving and the strength of the therapeutic relationship. I believe that the skillful, patient, and judicious use of problem solving can enhance the therapeutic relationship and, ultimately, outcome. In contrast, I believe that when problem solving is applied in an overly directive manner, it has the potential to damage the therapeutic relationship because it takes away client autonomy. Moreover, in instances in which there is a potential rupture in the therapeutic alliance, the immediate and direct application of problem solving could exacerbate the rupture because it could come across as forced, as not allowing the client to express their feelings, or as focused more on resolving the therapist's emotional discomfort rather than the client's reaction to the rupture. Thus, it would be expected that not only would therapist skill level moderate the use of problem solving and the quality of the therapeutic relationship, but also that certain problems that arise in the course of therapy might be more amenable to problem solving than others. These sorts of issues can be subjected to empirical scrutiny in process-based psychotherapy research.

It will also be important for future research to identify the ways in which specific aspects of the therapeutic relationship (e.g., agreement on the goals and task of therapy, bond, real relationship) affect the efficacy of problem-solving interventions, and conversely, the ways in which successful or unsuccessful problem-solving interventions affect these aspects of the therapeutic relationship. Specifically, when ruptures in the therapeutic alliance, transference, and countertransference are encountered, it would be beneficial to understand the role that problem solving plays in resolving upset, as well as the way in which problem solving facilitates retention in therapy, continued engagement, and ultimate outcome.

Social problem-solving interventions incorporate a balance between cognitive and behavioral strategies to address life's challenges. In some instances, clients need practice in facing their problems because they have adopted an avoidant coping style; as a result, much anticipatory anxiety has built up surrounding the prospect of addressing these problems head-on. Some of these clients could benefit from exposure, or the systematic contact with a feared stimulus or situation. Exposure often helps these clients acclimate to the anxiety that accompanies problems, learn that they can tolerate the emotional distress associated with these problems, and learn that the "worst-case scenario" associated with these problems is unlikely to occur or is not as bad as once thought. Approaches for using the therapeutic relationship to facilitate exposure in clients who need such practice are described in the next chapter.

7 EXPOSURE AND THE THERAPEUTIC RELATIONSHIP

Exposure, or the systematic contact with feared stimuli and situations, is the premier behavioral intervention for the treatment of anxiety and anxiety-related disorders (including obsessive compulsive disorder [OCD] and post-traumatic stress disorder [PTSD]). Although the efficacy of exposure in the treatment of anxiety-related disorders is unmatched (Hofmann et al., 2012; Kaczkurkin & Foa, 2015; Olatunji et al., 2010), it can be one of the most daunting tasks that anxious clients can imagine taking on because it requires that they intentionally face their worst fears. Moreover, many therapists report hesitation to deliver exposure for fear of premature dropout or even retraumatization (Feeny et al., 2003; Olatunji et al., 2009). Data from large randomized controlled trials evaluating exposure have dispelled these concerns (Foa et al., 2002; Grayson et al., 1982; Hembree et al., 2003). Nevertheless, I contend that a strong and trusting therapeutic relationship is particularly essential as clients with anxiety-related disorders embark on an exposure intervention, as it provides the foundation from which clients develop a willingness to embrace this evidence-based strategy (cf. Björgvinsson et al., 2007;

https://doi.org/10.1037/0000424-008
Therapeutic Relationship-Focused Cognitive Behavioral Therapy, by A. Wenzel

Buchholz & Abramowitz, 2020). Thus, I raise the possibility that adherence to and outcome in exposure-based CBT is maximized when the therapist practices from the framework of therapeutic relationship-focused cognitive behavioral therapy (TRF-CBT).

Exposure often follows a relatively standard trajectory over the course of several sessions. Clients who agree to undertake exposure as part of their CBT treatment plan will first develop a *fear hierarchy*, or an ordered sequence of feared stimuli and situations ranging from those associated with lesser levels of self-reported fear to more severe levels. The idea is that clients will move along the hierarchy, starting with items associated with a moderate level of anxiety and moving toward the more difficult items (although clients can select exposures in random order from the hierarchy as well; cf. Lang & Craske, 2000). Ideally, clients undertake exposure during session, and they practice the same or similar exposures for homework in between sessions (Wenzel, 2013). Although the specific practice of exposure varies, clients usually rate their discomfort as they proceed and assess the degree to which exposure is having its intended effect, such as by providing beginning, peak, and ending discomfort ratings. As they complete a series of exposure trials, clients begin to learn that (a) the dreaded outcome they are expecting is very unlikely to occur; (b) if an aversive outcome indeed occurs, they can handle it, and it is not as bad as they had anticipated; and (c) they can tolerate the anxiety and distress that accompanies contact with a fear stimulus or situation. Point (b) cannot be understated; in my clinical experience, many clients who participate in exposure come to realize that their anticipation of how bad it will be to have contact with a feared stimulus or situation is much worse than how bad the actual encounter is. Clients who report this realization often have a very positive view about their experience in therapy, as before embarking on exposure, they could not have dreamed that they would have gotten to the point at which they feel this way.

As with the other cognitive behavioral strategies described in this volume, exposure can be conducted with the highest level of integrity along with a simultaneous focus on the therapeutic relationship. The following excerpts contrast the conduct of exposure with a lesser or greater focus on the therapeutic relationship. In these examples, the therapist is working with a client who practiced interoceptive exposures to address his fear and avoidance of the sensation of dizziness. In between sessions, he worked on spinning in a chair at home for increasingly long periods of time, and then he moved to spinning in a chair at work (where he was even more fearful of negative consequences if he felt dizzy). Here, the therapist is reviewing the client's homework with him.

Excerpt 1: Less Focus on the Therapeutic Relationship

THERAPIST: Let's take a look at what you've done here for exposure homework.

CLIENT: Sure. Here is my Exposure Recording Form [where the client maintained a record of the exposures that he completed and the corresponding anxiety ratings that he assigned].

[The therapist saw that the client's initial spinning exposures were associated with discomfort ratings of 8 out of 10, and his latter spinning exposures dropped to discomfort ratings of a 0 out of 10.]

THERAPIST: It looks like you worked really hard this past week, and that your discomfort ratings dropped, the more exposures you completed.

CLIENT: Yes, I was pleasantly surprised. I didn't think this process would work as completely as it did.

THERAPIST: I'm pleased that this has been so helpful. Tell me what, then, you learned from these experiences that you will take with you moving forward.

CLIENT: I learned that it wasn't as bad as I was making it out to be. It even became kind of fun after a while.

THERAPIST: This is great news. Should we plan another round of exposures?

CLIENT: I'm not sure what is left to do. This is really what I came in for, and it was a success. I'm pretty good as is.

THERAPIST: I can think of a couple of directions to take. One is to continue the spinning exposures to reinforce the gains you made, perhaps even generalizing the spinning to other environments to promote generalizability. The second direction links back to something we discussed when you first came to treatment— your discomfort surrounding the potential for embarrassment and social judgment. I realize that you had indicated that you were really only interested in pursuing the interoceptive exposures that targeted physiological sensations of dizziness. But now that you have had some success, I wonder if you might reconsider?

CLIENT: Honestly, you've really helped me a lot for what I came in for. At this point, I don't think I need a lot more. Maybe we can schedule again after some time passes, like in a month, and we can see how I am doing with the dizziness?

The therapist in this excerpt did her due diligence as a cognitive behavioral therapist. She reviewed the client's homework, expressed encouragement, and asked a question that allowed the client to consolidate the learning that he achieved. When the therapist tried to continue their exposure work, the client expressed satisfaction with what he had achieved and implied that he had met the major treatment goal that brought him into therapy. By all indications, this is a treatment success.

Consider, however, what happened when the therapist put a bit more emphasis on nonspecific counseling skills to utilize the power of the therapeutic relationship to a greater degree. The following dialogue begins in the same manner as in the previous excerpt.

Excerpt 2: More Focus on the Therapeutic Relationship

THERAPIST: Let's take a look at what you've done here for exposure homework.

CLIENT: Sure. Here is my Exposure Recording Form [where the client maintained a record of the exposures that he completed and the corresponding anxiety ratings that assigned].

THERAPIST: [expressing enthusiasm and smiling widely] Oh my goodness. I'm not sure that I've seen a response like this before! You started with initial and peak discomfort ratings of 8 out of 10, they dropped a bit on the next two exposures, and then they plummeted to zeros out of 10. Tell me more about your experience with these exercises.

CLIENT: [feeling encouraged by the therapist's enthusiasm] It was the most interesting thing. At first, I was surprised by my high discomfort ratings. As you know, I had been skeptical that these exposures would approximate the anxiety that I get in panicky situations . . . and boy, did they! But I kept at it, and it made me think about being a little kid at the playground, spinning on the merry-go-round. When I looked at in that way, all of the anxiety went away. It was whimsical, rather than scary.

THERAPIST: Whimsical, huh? That is a fantastic example of a mindset shift that resulted from your exposure work.

CLIENT: It was quite uncanny. I started to actually look forward to doing the exposures each day. Can you believe that? [laughing]

THERAPIST: [sharing in the laughter] I'll take it! That is one great exposure success story. [sharing her own reflection, to demonstrate partnership and genuineness] You know, when we were developing your fear hierarchy together, I was really hoping that these interoceptive exposure exercises—particularly the spinning on the chair—would be just the match for you to have a different experience with the sensation of dizziness. I'm just delighted that it worked out in this manner—it has made my day! [pausing] Tell me what, then, you learned from these experiences that you will take with you moving forward.

CLIENT: This is going to help a lot the next time I am having to speak in front of my colleagues. Sometimes I get a wave of dizziness when I see a bunch of eyes on me, waiting for me to make a statement that will lead the team. Now I know that I don't have to be so scared of the dizziness. It really isn't that bad, and it doesn't last very long. And, if I can approach it with a different mindset, like, "Oh, this feels kind of fun," rather than, "Oh, this is the absolute worst because it means I'm going to have a panic attack in front of all these people," then I should be able to get through anything, no matter how many people I am speaking to.

THERAPIST: That is quite profound, really. [making a reflection] You've learned three things—that it does not feel as bad as you had anticipated, that it is transient, and that shifting your mindset can help you get through it. I commend you on your hard work and your thoughtfulness in taking away key pearls of wisdom that you can bank on in the future. [*Here, the therapist is prizing the client, expressing admiration for the work that he has put into exposures.*]

CLIENT: Absolutely!

THERAPIST: Should we plan another round of exposures?

CLIENT: I definitely think I should practice the spinning some more to make sure I maintain my gains.

THERAPIST: I agree wholeheartedly with that. Perhaps we can even consider other places to practice spinning so that we can enhance the generalizability of the new learning that you've achieved.

CLIENT: I think that is wise. I started at home and then did it in my office . . . [starting to have some fun with exposure] maybe I can bring my office chair into the conference room at work to try it there.

THERAPIST: That is a fantastic idea! Any other places you can think of, where it has relevance because you've experienced dizziness in the past?

CLIENT: I generally don't like feeling dizzy when I'm in public, where others can see me. So, maybe in an office supply store, where the employees and other customers would be in the vicinity?

[The therapist and client worked collaboratively to plan the specific elements of the exposures, such as when he would embark on them, how long they would last, and so on.]

THERAPIST: Is it okay with you if I also bring up another area for exposure, outside of the dizziness? [*This question is asked to obtain permission from the client to move in a new direction, reinforcing collaboration and value of client feedback.*]

CLIENT: Yes, that is fine. [smiling] I have a feeling that I know what you are going to propose.

THERAPIST: [returning the smile] Yes . . . now that you've had success with the interoceptive exposures focused on dizziness, I wonder how you feel now about considering some of the exposures for potential embarrassment.

CLIENT: [taking a deep breath] It's really interesting that you're bringing this up because I've been thinking about this as well. When you first introduced the idea of exposure to me, I was on board with some of the physiological exposures because that was what I had hoped to reduce when I started therapy. Then you, very astutely, raised the possibility that I have an underlying fear of being embarrassed. You probably remember that I was less on board with addressing that in therapy.

THERAPIST: [smiling and nodding her head] I remember.

CLIENT: I think I've had a change of heart, at least somewhat. If I'm honest with myself, I just didn't want to hear it because then I knew that I would have to do something about it. And I wasn't ready for that. I came in with a very specific agenda for treatment, and that was about all I wanted to do. But now, after seeing how effective exposure was for my dizziness . . . it makes me think that softening the edge of my aversion to being embarrassed, of people looking at me in a way that seems like they think something's wrong with me . . . maybe that actually *would* be something that would be good for me to work through.

THERAPIST: You just had to be ready for it in your own time. Especially after you got a feel for the way in which exposure worked and a glimpse of how powerful it can be.

CLIENT: [breathing a sigh of relief] Yes, exactly. Thank you for understanding that. I wasn't trying to be difficult, or like question your judgment or anything. I needed to work up to it, and I appreciate that you gave me the space to do that.

THERAPIST: And when you think about it, some of these new spinning exposures for dizziness . . . they actually do target the fear of embarrassment a bit because they will be conducted in places where others could possibly be present.

CLIENT: That's what I was thinking! Killing two birds with one stone!

THERAPIST: Yes, definitely. I will be very interested to see how your exposures this week speak to that target of anxiety. In the meantime, in our remaining time here in session today, shall we brainstorm some ideas to target the fear of embarrassment that we might include on a hierarchy geared toward that issue?

CLIENT: Let's go for it.

Notice how much more information the client contributed about his experience in the second excerpt. The therapist, both verbally and nonverbally, demonstrated great interest in his experience and pleasure in the outcome, which encouraged the client to reflect in a more complete way than he did in the previous excerpt. The therapist then provided her own reflection in the spirit of partnership (i.e., collaboration) and genuineness. Not only did her genuine reflection cultivate the real relationship, but it also enhanced the therapeutic alliance because it reinforced the goals and tasks of therapy. Also notice that the therapist asked the same question about learning in each excerpt: "Tell me what, then, you learned from these experiences that you will take with you moving forward." In the second excerpt, the client expressed much more than a generic, "I learned it was not so bad" type of statement. In fact, he put words to a mindset shift that he will apply in future instances that have, historically, been associated with a sense of dizziness that was threatening to him.

Perhaps the most striking differences in these excerpts are in the latter part of the dialogue when the therapist asks the client about scheduling additional exposures. In the first excerpt, the client indicated that he did not necessarily see a need to do so, and that he was satisfied with what he had achieved, even after the therapist explained her rationale. In contrast, the same client was much more open to additional exposure work in the second excerpt. Not only was he willing to commit to additional spinning exposures in different environments to promote generalizability, but he was also more open than he had been earlier in the course of therapy to participating in exposures that targeted a fear of embarrassment. In fact, when the therapist had originally suggested exposures targeted toward this fear, the client was quite insistent that they focus only on interceptive exposures that evoked the physiological sensations that he dreaded. However, between the success of his interoceptive exposure work and the genuine collaboration and partnership that was evident in the second excerpt, the client developed a sense of comfort, confidence, and commitment to embarking on exposures that very likely were more centrally related to his case formulation than the interoceptive exposures. The take-home point here for readers is that the therapeutic relationship can serve as a foundation that opens a door for clients to consider and commit to exposure exercises that they otherwise might continue to avoid.

TIPS FOR EXPOSURE THROUGH THE LENS OF THE THERAPEUTIC RELATIONSHIP

Despite the power of exposure, at times therapists bring a guarded or even negative mindset toward the delivery of exposure because they worry about the drawbacks of exposure described previously, even if there are little data in support of them. This mindset has the potential to create a self-fulfilling prophesy, such that the therapist does not fully commit to the delivery of exposure, the client senses hesitation, and then the client does not fully commit to the execution of exposure (cf. Zayfert et al., 2005). Instances in which the therapist indeed encounters client avoidance or resistance can be conceptualized as an opportunity to enter into the client's world and solidify a partnership in the work of therapy, rather than as a barrier to good outcome. In this section, I describe eight tips for using the therapeutic relationship to facilitate exposure for clients with anxiety-related disorders, which I hope will increase therapists' comfort with and confidence in the procedure.

Tip 1: Deliver Psychoeducation About Exposure in a Manner That Strengthens the Therapeutic Relationship

The term *psychoeducation* has been referenced in passing on many occasions to this point in the volume. The provision of psychoeducation occurs when the therapist educates the client about principles of behavior change, the rationale and procedures associated with a therapeutic strategy, or the theory underlying the intervention and its proposed mechanisms of change. Most cognitive behavioral therapists feel quite strongly about the provision of psychoeducation because they operate from a standpoint of transparency, and they hope that their clients will acquire knowledge that they will be able to mold to their own lives, eventually without the help of a therapist. Many clients participating in CBT report that they appreciate the psychoeducation that they receive and find it empowering. Nevertheless, I encourage cognitive behavioral therapists to be mindful of therapist skills for enhancing the therapeutic relationship (e.g., empathy, positive regard) when they are delivering psychoeducation to guard against instances in which clients might feel overwhelmed with too much information or "lectured at."

I believe this is especially true for the provision of psychoeducation in anticipation of a course of exposure. Some clients with anxiety-related disorders balk at the notion of exposure, indicating that they cannot imagine why one would want to engage in exercises that put them in a position in which they would face their worst fears. Thus, it is important to provide a rationale that is compelling and easily grasped. For example, it is common to hear exposure experts liken one proposed mechanism for exposure—habituation—to immersing oneself in a swimming pool that is first uncovered in the spring. At that time of year, the water is very cold; but if one stays in the pool long enough, the water no longer feels as cold. The temperature of the water has not changed in that short period of time; rather, the person's physiological homeostasis has adapted.

In my experience, many clients find this explanation to be quite intriguing and, ultimately, motivating as they make a commitment to exposure. However, it is important for cognitive behavioral therapists who deliver exposure to stay abreast of the contemporary literature on this intervention, as Dr. Michelle Craske's impressive analysis of the literature suggests that habituation does not necessarily always occur when clients with anxiety-related disorders undergo exposure (Craske et al., 2008, 2014). Moreover, a focus on the fear reduction that accompanies habituation could inadvertently reinforce false beliefs that anxiety is shameful, dangerous, and intolerable (Abramowitz et al., 2019; Jacoby & Abramowitz, 2016). Thus, it is important not to instill the expectation that habituation absolutely will occur if clients undertake exposure, as they could lose confidence in the therapist and in the therapeutic process if it does not. Fortunately, Craske et al.'s (2008) critical analysis suggests that outcome in exposure-based CBT can be successful even without the experience of habituation because new learning occurs, such as the new learning that anxiety is tolerable (through *inhibitory learning*, or the forming of new, safety-based associations between the feared stimulus and perceived threat; cf. Abramowitz et al., 2019). In my experience, when presented with confidence and enthusiasm, clients come away from this psychoeducation with the notion that exposure is a win-win proposition—either they achieve a state of habituation and feel less anxiety, or they learn through experience that their anxiety is tolerable. In both scenarios, the end result is an increase in quality of life because clients are able to more readily engage in the things in life that they find valuable and meaningful. Thus, knowing the research literature, and being able to describe it in a compelling way, can be used to a great advantage in CBT.

It is also my experience that clients are very interested in a detailed description of the process of exposure. Although the research in this realm is limited, there is some indication that agreement on the goals and tasks of therapy (one part of the therapeutic alliance) is particularly predictive of outcome in exposure therapy (Buchholz & Abramowitz, 2020). Thus, it is important to present and discuss psychoeducation in a manner that is engaging, collaborative, and that builds the therapeutic alliance. Most clients want to know that they will not be forced to participate in any exposures for which they do not feel ready. It is true that clients who express such concerns are manifesting subtle forms of avoidance (e.g., they are very willing to undertake exposure exercises for mildly to moderately threatening stimuli and situations, but they reserve the right to stop before they undertake the most threatening exposure exercises). However, it is equally as true that cognitive behavioral therapists respect clients' autonomy above all in almost every circumstance (unless there is an imminent threat of violence). I say something like this to my clients who are considering exposure:

> You are in the driver's seat with this course of exposure. The idea behind our plan is that we work together, carefully and systematically, in a planful way. This is likely different than the haphazard way in which you might have had exposure experiences in the past. I will never force or insist that you engage in any one exposure. After all, as we know with any therapeutic intervention, clients obtain the greatest gains when the motivation and commitment come from within, rather than being forced on them by another person. That being said, there very well might be some instances in which I notice subtle maneuvers to avoid certain fears as we go through exposure. Is it okay with you if I gently point those out as we work together? [obtain client's permission] I appreciate that you granted me this permission to make such observations. One thing I do not want to do is to inadvertently reinforce your anxiety by being complicit in the avoidance of certain fears—that would be contrary to my pledge to you to deliver high-quality exposure-based CBT in a way that is based on principles of human behavior and the research data.

As cognitive behavioral therapists provide psychoeducation, they often find that it can be helpful to share success stories of former clients who recovered from their anxiety-related disorder through exposure (removing any identifying information, of course). In addition to success stories, I often share a story of someone who, after careful consideration, decided not to undergo exposure and who instead chose to live with her anxiety disorder. I find that this story reinforces my claim of respecting clients' autonomy, preferences, and personal wishes.

Tip 2: Use Motivational Interviewing for Ambivalent Clients

Motivational interviewing is a clinical approach in which therapists converse with a client in such a way that allows the client to "dig deep" and to find and articulate reasons for engaging in therapy, rather than being told how to think about therapy (Arkowitz et al., 2015; W. R. Miller & Rollnick, 2013). The origins of motivational interviewing lie in the addiction treatment literature, grounded in the observations of its developers (William Miller and Stephen Rollnick) that the confrontational approach used in treating people with alcohol and drug use disorders back in the 1980s was ineffective, such that it was associated with high rates of relapse and premature dropout from treatment. Instead, Miller and Rollnick reasoned that respecting clients' autonomy and reasons for changing or not changing was paramount in providing an environment in which clients could move from a precontemplative or contemplative stage of change to a preparation or an action stage of change (cf. Prochaska & DiClemente, 1982; Prochaska & Norcross, 2011). To achieve this aim, therapists who use motivational interviewing rely on a client-centered stance of making reflections to demonstrate understanding of the client's position, particularly in a manner that reinforces clients' *change talk*, or expressions of reasons why participating in therapy and making changes would reduce unwanted negative consequences and have the potential to bring about positive consequences in their lives. Change talk is in contrast to *sustain talk* (sometimes called *counter-change talk*), or clients' expression of reasons why moving forward with therapy might be undesirable or why they are benefiting from staying as they are.

A full description of motivational interviewing is outside the scope of this text. However, motivational interviewing is relevant here because it has been applied successfully with clients with anxiety-related disorders who demonstrate ambivalence about treatment as they consider participating in a trial of exposure-based CBT, even despite having presented for treatment of their own volition (Van Horn et al., 2021; Westra, 2012; Westra & Aviram, 2015). Indicators of ambivalence about and resistance toward exposure include (but are not limited to) being late to sessions, cancelling or missing sessions, not completing homework, presenting to session with a "crisis" that seemingly requires immediate attention, and/or introducing irrelevant or trivial items for the session agenda, all of which have implications for the therapeutic alliance. The application of motivational interviewing prior to the commencement of a course of CBT has been associated with increased treatment engagement (e.g., higher reports of readiness to change, increased treatment attendance; R. T. Murphy et al., 2009), increased homework completion (Westra et al., 2009), and, in some instances, better outcome after treatment (e.g., Westra et al., 2016). Moreover, the adoption of a motivational interviewing mindset during the course of therapy, when the therapist detects ambivalence or resistance, can help to overcome a therapeutic impasse.

Thus, inclusion of a section on motivational interviewing in a chapter on therapeutic relationship considerations in the use of exposure is relevant for several reasons. First, motivational interviewing is a client-centered approach that emphasizes the use of many of the therapist skills described in Chapter 2 of this volume to cultivate the therapeutic relationship. Second, it is a gentle approach that allows the therapeutic experience to unfold at its own pace, rather than forcing any particular agenda or intervention. Such a natural pace has the potential to provide a sense of welcoming and controllability for the client, which will help them to move on their own to a position in which they embrace exposure rather than have the sense that it is being imposed on them. Third, the hallmark feature of motivational interviewing is its reliance on reflective listening, and reflections usually communicate to clients that they have been heard and understood. Finally, the use of motivational interviewing communicates an understanding that even clients who initiate psychotherapy of their own accord have some ambivalence and trepidation about change and all that working toward change would involve. Thus, therapists who use motivational interviewing in these instances recognize the subtle nuances of motivation for change and use the therapeutic relationship to ensure that the client is ready for the action stage of therapy.

The following dialogue provides an example of motivational interviewing with a 22-year-old college student who presented for exposure-based CBT to address a debilitating vomit phobia. The primary features of her clinical presentation were (a) avoidance of parties and bars (i.e., common social outlets for college students); (b) drinking a maximum of a half glass of wine on any one occasion; (c) consistent questioning of her partner, friends, and family members if they felt sick, to the point that many of these close others became frustrated by the questioning; and (d) (perhaps most indicative of the great extent of life interference posed by this phobia) avoidance of most foods for fear of choking while eating or some sort of contamination that would result in vomiting. In the following dialogue, the therapist had just educated the client about the aims, process, and anticipated results from exposure. When the client expresses ambivalence about moving forward, the therapist uses reflections guided by the principles of motivational interviewing to demonstrate understanding and compassion for reasons that were keeping her from embracing therapy, as well as to reinforce instances in which she expressed reasons to move forward with therapy. In this dialogue, the reader will see examples of (a) simple reflection (i.e., repeating back what the client has said, adding little extra, to demonstrate that the client has been heard and to reinforce the message that the client is communicating); (b) amplified reflection (i.e., repeating back what the client has said in an exaggerated manner, which often prompts the client to turn to the other side of an argument); (c) open-ended questions asking for elaboration to reinforce change talk; (d) summarizing; and (e) decisional balance, or the weighing of factors that go into the decision to change or not to change.

CLIENT: Oh my gosh, this seems so daunting. I can't even imagine how to start with all of this. I can see myself having panic attack after panic attack.

THERAPIST: You see yourself experiencing a great deal of anxiety if you were to participate in a course of exposure. [*This statement is a simple reflection of the client's sustain talk to demonstrate that the therapist has heard the client.*]

CLIENT: Yes, for sure. I don't know if I have it in me.

THERAPIST: You might not be ready for this therapy yet. [*This statement is an amplified reflection, taking the client's statement one step further to open up room for the client to back down on her statement and move toward change.*]

CLIENT: Well, I'm not sure that I mean it like that. I put a lot of thought into seeking out CBT because I read about how well it works for anxiety disorders. And I've been in therapy for a lot of my life from middle school, and nothing helped with this problem. Some therapists taught me some breathing techniques, but those techniques don't help when you do everything that you can do to avoid being in a situation in the first place.

THERAPIST: What, in particular, did you read that you found to be a good match for you? [*Here, the therapist asks for more detail because she detects a hint of change talk, and she hypothesizes that the client would become more invested in such change talk through elaboration.*]

CLIENT: Well, I did like that it could be gradual. I had nightmares of being made to stick a finger down my throat at my first session! I also read something somewhere that said that most people find that the anticipation of the exposure is usually a lot worse than the actual exposure. That one really stuck with me because I find that's the case with me as well. Like, I get worried about getting car sick, so sometimes I dread going on long car rides. But then I get in the car and go, and I'm fine. I barely feel nauseous. So, it was a lot of time spent worrying about it for nothing.

THERAPIST: You read some things that you liked and that resonated with you. [*Here, the therapist is making another simple reflection, this time to reinforce the change talk.*] [Client nods] What does that suggest for the work that we could do together with exposure? [*The therapist poses this question in order to extend the client's change talk and look forward to the future.*]

CLIENT: I hate to admit it, but I think it's exactly what I need. I'm scared to death of facing my fears. But at the same, I can't keep living like this anymore.

THERAPIST: Tell me more about that, not being able to live like this anymore. What have been the effects of your fear of throwing up? [*Here, the therapist is reinforcing the client's change talk by asking a question about the consequences of living her life as is.*]

CLIENT: Oh my gosh, so, so many! The only time my boyfriend and I fight is when I badger him about being sick. I ask him over and over and over again. And over! When he tells me he is fine, I don't believe him. And my family [becoming tearful] . . . they've missed out on so many things because of me. I can't fly because I'm afraid of motion sickness. And of being trapped on a plane with someone else who has motion sickness. So we never go on any real vacations, not the kinds that they want to go on. I feel so badly, I know my mom, my dad, my sisters . . . everyone would like to go somewhere more exotic than the same old beach where we rent a house every summer.

THERAPIST: How would you envision your life if this anxiety were not as much of a problem for you? [*Here, the therapist is asking for elaboration on change talk in a different way by asking the client to consider the benefits of undergoing treatment for anxiety.*]

CLIENT: [leaning back and closing her eyes for a moment] I honestly think it would be blissful. So much bliss. I'm not sure I've fully described the way in which I completely run my life around the anxiety. And I can see it in other people's eyes, too, like my boyfriend's and my roommates'. How they are afraid of saying things that will get me all worked up and ruin everyone's night. [becoming tearful] I would just love to see the people I'm closest to being 100% comfortable around me, just able to be spontaneous as they tell me what they are thinking and feeling, how their days have gone, what they want to do that night or for spring break or whatever. Totally free of walking on eggshells and being in fear of saying something that will upset me.

THERAPIST: You've identified a number of ways that anxiety has impacted your life, and you've also painted a portrait of the freedom that you would experience if you were to overcome the debilitating aspects of your anxiety. What do you see, then, as the advantages and disadvantages of moving forward with CBT? [*Here, the therapist is making a reflection on what the client has said in the form of a summary, and she moves toward a decisional balance to evaluate whether the client would fall on the side of opting toward change through CBT.*]

The client went on to list many reasons to move forward with CBT and only one reason not to move forward—her fear that her anxiety would become so all-consuming that she would be disabled to the point of not functioning, and that she would be unable to "come back" from such a state. At the conclusion of the discussion, she expressed cautious optimism about CBT and, at the same time, continued ambivalence about taking on the most difficult of exposures. In response, her therapist utilized the fundamental tenets of CBT described earlier in this chapter—collaboration and respect for clients' autonomy—and provided assurance that the client would have the opportunity to provide consent before embarking on any specific exposure. With that assurance, the client visibly relaxed and moved toward developing her fear hierarchy with her therapist.

Tip 3: Model Flexibility

Many clients make great gains very quickly using exposure, such as the client depicted earlier in this chapter who reported near total relief from his anxiety associated with dizziness when he engaged in interoceptive exposure. Such success stories can generate a great deal of enthusiasm in cognitive behavioral therapists, as well as an eagerness to offer their clients all that exposure-based CBT has to offer. However, at times, clients arrive for a session and are not in the best mindset for exposure, for reasons such as feeling physically ill, experiencing an unusual amount of life stress, or having just had an unsettling experience in the time before session. These types of contextual factors render it so that clients are less "ready" for exposure than what is usual. It is not difficult to imagine that such a scenario could create a mismatch between what the enthusiastic cognitive behavioral therapist hopes to address and accomplish in session and where the client is at in the moment.

Such instances can create a fine line for cognitive behavioral therapists to walk. On the one hand, it is important not to abandon exposure based solely on how a client is feeling and reinforce subtle (or not so subtle) expressions of avoidance. On the other hand, it is important to demonstrate flexibility and allow clients a bit of grace as well. When the therapist adopts an attitude of, "We're all human, and it's part of being human to have occasional 'off' days," the therapeutic relationship is enhanced because clients feel compassion and understanding. Moreover, the modeling of flexibility in session serves as an important learning experience so that clients recognize the need to have flexibility in their own lives, to recognize they will have occasional "off" days, to have self-compassion on those days, and to recognize that an occasional "off" day does not have to signify being back at "square one." The demonstration of flexibility when a client is not feeling up to exposure can also allow for a celebration of what the client is able to accomplish in session, even if it is not of the same magnitude as they accomplish in many other sessions. This experience has the potential to be more powerful and lasting than yet another experience in which a client quickly ascends the fear hierarchy in a more straightforward manner.

Tip 4: Be Sure to Conduct Exposures Together in Session

In my previous writings (Wenzel, 2013, 2019), I have strongly recommended that cognitive behavioral therapists be sure to practice exposure in session and not just rely on therapy homework outside of session for clients to get in their exposure practice. In other words, it is important for the therapist to facilitate the engagement of exposure in session, not just talk about facilitation of exposure outside of session. For example, if a client has a fear of elevators, the client and the therapist could ride in an elevator in the therapist's building during session, and the client could do so in various buildings for homework in between sessions. If the therapist does not have access to an elevator in their building, they can approach exposure in a creative manner by conducting an imaginal exposure exercise or by simulating a similar felt sense (e.g., the sense of feeling trapped) during session. The rationale for this suggestion is three-fold, including (a) to ensure that the client gets practice with exposure; (b) to provide an opportunity for a success experience; and (c) to observe the client during exposure to determine whether any additional intervention is necessary (e.g., whether the client subtly avoids the experience of anxiety during an exposure, such as by distracting themselves from a full focus on the task at hand). All of this increases the likelihood that clients will have productive experiences with exposure when they implement their therapy homework in between sessions.

I contend here that conducting exposures during session also enhances the therapeutic relationship. In-session exposures are a way for therapists to communicate a "we're in this together" attitude. It is an opportunity for therapists to provide gentle and compassionate encouragement (though, it is important that the therapist refrain from being too effusive with praise so that they do not inadvertently provide reassurance [see Tip 5 next] or create a scenario in which clients are completing exposures more for their therapist's approval than for their own personal reasons). If the client struggles with exposure, the therapist can demonstrate a tolerance for any negative affect associated with that struggle, as well as positive regard for the client even in spite of a difficult moment in therapy.

Tip 5: Refrain From Providing Reassurance

Most of us became mental health care providers because we truly care about the well-being of others, and we have a great deal of compassion for people who are in distress. Part of this disposition means that if someone in distress comes to us for support, we (naturally) want to provide them some sort of reassurance that all will be okay. Unfortunately, reassurance seeking is behavior that clients rely on to neutralize the distress associated with the object of their anxiety, much like a compulsion or ritual. When a person, particularly a mental health provider who is deemed an expert, communicates reassurance, it deprives the client of the opportunity to fully experience the anxiety that ultimately will be honed by the exposure exercise, and it (inadvertently) teaches the client that they do not have the capacity to accurately assess the experience on their own. In extreme cases, clients who do not engage in exposure without their therapist's reassurance acquire the learning that they cannot face contact with a feared stimulus or situation on their own, without the support of another person or an expert like a therapist.

Many therapists feel guilty when their clients ask for reassurance and they do not give into them. They worry that they are not being supportive, kind, and understanding; in other words, they worry that they are compromising the therapeutic relationship. It is important for therapists to remember that these thoughts can be examined and reshaped using cognitive restructuring, just as we ask our clients to do. In fact, in every instance in which I have had a supervisee (i.e., a cognitive behavioral therapist-in-training) worry that their behavior has compromised or will compromise the therapeutic relationship, I have encouraged them to check out this assumption with their client. In every instance, their client responded with something like, "I totally understand what you are saying; in fact, I tend to ask for reassurance, and I know it hasn't been helpful in the past. I want you to do whatever is necessary to help me overcome my anxiety disorder."

To take the extra step to preserve the therapeutic relationship, therapists can certainly educate their clients at the outset that part of their job is to refrain from providing excessive reassurance in order to maximize the benefits of exposure. The following is a sample script that a therapist can use to address the issue of provision of reassurance:

> During the course of any one exposure exercise, you'll find that it is human nature to look to me for reassurance. It could be reassurance that "everything is okay," it could be reassurance that you are doing it correctly, or it could be reassurance that your anxiety is "normal" and like the anxiety of others who have similar problems and have gone through exposure. The thing about reassurance is that, while it feels nice to receive in the moment, it actually makes the anxiety worse in the long run. This is because reassurance neutralizes the anxiety, not allowing you to receive the full benefit of the exposure because you inadvertently teach yourself that there is something that is truly dangerous and should be avoided, whether that is object of the exposure or the experience of anxiety itself. You might find yourself asking for reassurance without fully realizing that you are doing it. If this happens, I will not provide reassurance. Please know that this has nothing to do with me, as a human being not wanting to give you reassurance; in fact, I care a great deal about you and do not wish to impose any extra distress on you. However, because I've seen the way in which anxiety becomes further entrenched when reassurance is given, I would actually be hurting you if I provided it to you. I'm curious what you think of all of this.

When the rationale for the lack of reassurance provision is provided in this manner, clients usually appreciate the therapist's reasoning and foresight that this issue may arise. Moreover, they feel supported because of the therapist's overt comments that they care for the client and do not want to do anything that will hurt them, even when the thing that will hurt them (i.e., reassurance) feels good and helpful in the moment.

Tip 6: Make a Special Effort to Commend the Client's Bravery and Strength

Carl Rogers' (1957) notion of "prizing" the client allows the therapeutic relationship to serve as a catalyst toward successful outcome in exposure interventions. I will often say something like this:

I truly commend you for the hard work that you took on today with these exposures. I realize how daunting it is to face some of your worst fears—fears that you have had for much of your life. It takes a lot of strength and bravery to do what you are doing, and I admire that.

Of course, therapists want to be sure that clients are not complying with exposure simply to obtain their praise. However, in my experience, many anxious clients view themselves as weak and vulnerable, and hearing a statement expressing genuine admiration for their strength and bravery can go far in healing and in recovery from a mental health disorder. In fact, it can facilitate a shift in clients' view of themselves from being weak and vulnerable to having the resilience to overcome adversity.

Tip 7: Point Out Avoidance in a Gentle Manner

Clients with anxiety-related disorders can be extremely logical and articulate in arguing why an exposure is not relevant or not something that would be wise to undertake. Take, for example, a client with contamination fears. If one follows the guidelines published by the U.S. Centers for Disease Control and Prevention regarding handwashing, safeguards against asbestos, handling of raw chicken, and so on, the recommended behaviors can, at times, begin to look very similar to what we observe in clients with OCD. Thus, the suggestion to do something that is different (and presumably less "safe") than guidelines published or espoused by authorities can be confusing and daunting to clients who are about to embark on exposure.

One "golden rule" of exposure is that cognitive behavioral therapists should not suggest exposure exercises that result in anything more than everyday levels of risk (Abramowitz et al., 2019). However, the definition of an everyday level of risk is crucial for both therapists and clients to understand—it is the type of mild harm that people might inadvertently experience while living their daily lives. Take the example of not washing one's hands after using the restroom. When faced with this prospect, most people in Western society would grimace and view executing this as undesirable, especially when we have recently lived through the COVID-19 pandemic. And yet, on occasion, people do not wash their hands after using a restroom (e.g., if a sink is out of order). Moreover, in some cultures, it is not customary to wash one's hands after using the restroom. Thus, on the basis of our definition, refraining from washing one's hands after using the restroom would be considered a permissible exposure because it is consistent with occasional experiences that we have when we live our lives. It is important to educate clients at the outset of therapy about this definition.

Despite being mindful of this definition, there will be times in which clients, invariably, balk at doing an exposure because it does not make sense to them on the basis of tightly held rules about the way people "should" live their lives or the way that things "should" go. Examples of reasons for not doing exposure include the following:

- "I wouldn't ever do that in real life, so this just feels too artificial."
- "Most people I know wouldn't do something like this."
- "What you are suggesting requires that I go out of my way to do something, and I would choose the most efficient way."
- "This requires too much setup, and I don't have time for it in my everyday life."
- "This is completely different than the way I was raised."

When clients express these sorts of reservations, it can be helpful to concur that there is some truth in their observations. Nevertheless, it is also important for clients to know that these reservations are often indicative of subtle avoidance behavior. I let clients know that I would be doing them a disservice if I did not gently point out a subtle avoidance behavior when it arises as we are planning exposures.

Note the word "gentle" in the title of this section. The idea is not at all that the therapist is trying to out-logic clients, back them into a corner, or guilt them into doing an exposure. In fact, many clients do not recognize that their rationalizations are indicative of avoidance behaviors, and they find it fascinating how quickly and frequently avoidance manifests itself in their everyday lives. Thus, cognitive behavioral therapists are encouraged to point out subtle manifestations of avoidance behavior in a compassionate, supportive way, in which it is clear that the therapist is genuinely helping the client to meet their goals. Oftentimes, it becomes a source of humor in therapy that allows the therapist and client to share a laugh. Sometimes, I will begin by saying, "Don't shoot the messenger, but I'm wondering if you are noticing anything about what you just expressed?" Or, before we begin a series of exposures, I let clients know in advance that if I detect avoidance, I will point it out in order to be serving them to the best of my professional ability. Over time, clients begin to catch themselves when their first inclination is to avoid an exposure, and they proactively apply the principles they have learned in treatment to identify what is happening and to overcome it. Such instances are truly gratifying moments for therapists, and ones that facilitate a sense of genuine positive regard for the client and all of their accomplishments.

Tip 8: Manage Your Own Fear-Based Thinking

As mentioned earlier, therapists are encouraged to apply cognitive restructuring surrounding predictions that the therapeutic relationship will be compromised if they do not provide reassurance. More generally, many therapist concerns about exposure therapy have been identified, and any one of these concerns can thwart a therapist's commitment to exposure, their decision to inform clients that exposure is an option for treatment, and/or their delivery of exposure in a thorough, systematic manner (Olatunji et al., 2009). When a therapist begins to doubt whether exposure will be helpful (versus harmful) or to fixate on imagined catastrophic outcomes, they will not introduce or deliver the intervention with confidence. It follows that when a therapist does not deliver an intervention with confidence, there is an increased likelihood that the client will express hesitation and demonstrate a lack of commitment or engagement.

Thus, therapists who deliver exposure are encouraged to be astutely aware of any reservations they might have when they are considering exposure for a particular client. Then, they are encouraged to apply the principles of cognitive restructuring to manage their own thinking. From a factual perspective, they can consult the empirical literature to identify rates of people who have adverse outcomes after participating in exposure. They can also conduct themselves as scientist–practitioners and collect careful observational data about the degree to which exposure is achieving its intended results with the individual client. In the majority of instances, therapists will see that their fears are unfounded and they will be able to deliver the intervention with increasing confidence, which could, in turn, enhance the degree to which the client invests in the therapeutic relationship and in the course of treatment.

EXPOSURE AS APPLIED TO THERAPEUTIC RELATIONSHIP ISSUES

Unlike cognitive restructuring and social problem solving, a therapist will likely not actively select exposure as a therapeutic intervention to address or resolve an issue within the therapeutic relationship. Nevertheless, if a therapeutic relationship issue must be addressed with a client who reports anxiety associated with interpersonal strife or anxiety associated with affective experiencing, then the above-board resolution of that issue may, in retrospect, be considered an important exposure experience for the client. For example, consider a conflict-averse client who experiences shame associated with missing a scheduled therapy appointment without providing ample notice. When this client contacts the therapist to reschedule and attends a subsequent session, the therapist can commend the client's courage for doing something difficult for them and use the exposure framework to learn from the experience. The therapist could even help the client apply this new learning to other interpersonal situations that they are avoiding. Although this "exposure" was not necessarily planned in advance, it nevertheless can have great therapeutic value. The therapeutic relationship can, however, be used as an agent for planned exposures that do not necessarily involve a rupture in the relationship. Next, I describe two ways in which this can occur.

Social Interaction Anxiety

Social anxiety disorder is an extremely prevalent mental health problem (Kessler et al., 2005), and many clients in psychotherapy report problems with social anxiety even if they do not carry an "official" diagnosis. Thus, the very act of interaction with a therapist can serve as a form of exposure. The therapeutic relationship can provide fertile ground for exposure, depending on the social interaction fears that are most relevant to the client's case formulation (cf. Buchholz & Abramowitz, 2020; Goldfried & Davila, 2005). Ways that the therapeutic relationship can be used for exposure include the following:

- practicing small talk
- sharing personal information about oneself
- asking for information about a topic of interest
- making a request
- saying "no" to a request
- expressing dissatisfaction

One advantage of using the therapeutic relationship for exposure in this manner is that the therapist can respond strategically on the basis of the aspects of interaction that the client needs to practice, or on the basis of the variables that are associated with increasing levels of anxiety. For example, suppose a therapist uses the therapeutic relationship as grounds to give the client experience in making small talk. In the first exposure, the therapist could respond in a way that makes the interaction run smoothly and that is focused on topics of conversation that are relatively easy for the client. As the therapist and client continue to conduct exposures in session, the therapist could play increasingly difficult (and more anxiety-provoking) roles, such as contributing very little to the conversation (resulting in awkward pauses or the client having to be active in directing the conversation), introducing topics about which the client has very little knowledge, and/or communicating a sense of impatience or hostility. The advantage of conducting such exposures in session is that the therapist is able to respond in a way that would be therapeutic and that would facilitate a learning experience in the client, as opposed to an in vivo exposure conducted in the client's life, where the person with whom the client is interacting is a "wild card" and could respond in any number of ways.

Fear of Vulnerability and Closeness

One of the great joys of the therapeutic relationship is the unique sense of closeness that can develop between the therapist and the client (Mearns & Cooper, 2018). As has been demonstrated to this point in the book, clients who experience closeness in the therapeutic relationship often report (a) looking forward to having sessions with their therapist; (b) feeling heard and understood by their therapist; (c) having the sense that their therapist knows them extremely well and remembers important details from their lives; and (d) having confidence that their therapist likes them, respects them, cares about them, and has their best interests at heart. Such a close therapeutic relationship can serve as an important corrective learning experience that generalizes to other close relationships in the client's life. For some clients, however, the fear of entering into a close therapeutic relationship is daunting. They may be characterized by a history of difficult, failed, and even traumatic close relationships, rendering them guarded and wary of sharing vulnerability. Entering into a therapeutic relationship is a huge step for such clients, and the therapist has a pivotal opportunity to enhance client autonomy, agency, confidence, and comfort with themselves and in their interactions with close others (Khattra et al., 2017; Macaulay et al., 2017).

The process of therapy, then, can serve as an exposure to vulnerability, interpersonal closeness, and emotional experiencing. When framed specifically as an exposure, clients can develop a hierarchy of increasingly difficult topics to share, and they can move through them as the course of therapy unfolds. Throughout the process, the therapist can assess for any predictions the client makes about negative consequences of sharing; as the client shares, they can evaluate whether these predictions were realized and the benefits that emerged from sharing. Consider the following dialogue with a female client, who described a history of rejection by others. As therapy progressed, she began to share a number of these rejections, and she was working up to sharing a previous experience that was associated with great shame. At the 22nd session of treatment, she chose to describe this situation with her therapist, and for the first time, she allowed herself to cry in the therapist's presence. In the following dialogue, the therapist and client discuss her experience with sharing this level of vulnerability with the therapist:

CLIENT: [sniffing, wiping her eyes, averting eye contact, and speaking softly] Oh boy, that was a lot. Once I got started, it was hard to stop.

THERAPIST: Why do you think that was?

CLIENT: Probably because I have kept this bottled up for so long. Shame is an incredible burden to carry alone.

THERAPIST: [speaking softly and genuinely, with a tone demonstrating that she has great reverence for the client] Yes. Yes, it is.

CLIENT: I've wanted to get that off of my back for a long time. I just didn't know who I could trust it with.

THERAPIST: [smiling warmly] I remember when the two of us first met 6 months ago. You weren't sure at all about therapy, about sharing personal details about yourself.

CLIENT: To be honest, it sounded awful. I knew I needed it. But it was excruciating for me.

THERAPIST: And that's why we worked up to what we discussed today, slowly and systematically. You needed to get used to opening up and sharing about yourself, especially details that you have held close to your heart for so long.

CLIENT: [sinking back into her chair] I'm really glad you framed it as practice, and that we first started with topics that weren't as difficult for me. If you would have pushed me to get into what we just talked about, like when we were first getting to know each other, I would have bolted. I never would have come back.

THERAPIST: I suspected that would be the case. It's truly important for me when I work with clients to go at their own pace and let them open up as they feel ready to do so. [pausing] What have you learned, then, from this gradual experience of opening up and sharing vulnerability?

CLIENT: [pausing to think a moment] I always get afraid that people will use it against me. I know, logically, that a therapist would never use it against me. But it was nice to live that out first-hand.

THERAPIST: Most definitely. How will this experience affect the likelihood that you will open up and share with others outside of therapy?

CLIENT: I'm never going to be one of those people who is an open book, who dumps their lives on other people. But I do understand that my close relationships can only go so far if I don't let them in. And I'm ready for closer relationships. My life can't continue to be all about my work and my cat. I'd like to have the kind of friendships in which I am comfortable enough with someone to call them out of the blue to spend a Saturday night together. Maybe even go on a girls' weekend, or spend a holiday together. To have these kinds of relationships . . . I have to be close to someone. And being close involves a two-way street of sharing.

The client had five more sessions before ending treatment. She provided her therapist with feedback about qualities of the relationship that enabled her to share vulnerability, including being a good listener, being nonjudgmental, providing empathy, allowing the conversation to unfold naturally (versus pushing the client), and remembering important details. These qualities were particularly important to the client because she knew that what she was saying was being respected and heard by the therapist, and she did not feel like she needed to repeat herself to bring the therapist "up to speed." When the client returned for a "booster" session 4 months later, she indicated that she was beginning to cultivate a close relationship with a friend from work, and they even spent the Independence Day holiday with her friend's family at their lake house. Moreover, her therapist was pleasantly surprised to learn that the client had been on a few dates with a man that she very much liked. Although the potential romantic relationship was clearly in the early stages, the client expressed much less trepidation about developing a sense of romantic closeness than she had reported when she initiated treatment. The client stated that her experience in therapy, framed as gradual exposure to sharing personal information and vulnerability, paved the way to take reasonable interpersonal risks in the spirit of cultivating closeness with others.

CONCLUSION AND FUTURE DIRECTIONS

Countless clients with anxiety-related disorders have been helped by exposure. Comments I have received from clients about their experience with exposure-based CBT include "truly amazing" and "transformative." Clients who wholly embrace exposure usually see great gains quite quickly, which reinforces their sense of confidence in therapy and in the therapist, contributes to satisfaction, and instills much hope that their lives can be free of debilitating anxiety. Not surprisingly, these outcomes enhance the therapeutic relationship, instilling motivation to continue taking on new exposure-based challenges as treatment progresses. Moreover, when clients have such a positive view of their therapy experience, it stands to reason that they would not hesitate to return if they noticed indicators of relapse.

Of course, some clients find exposure to be a daunting prospect, as it involves facing their worst fears that have been associated with highly ingrained patterns of avoidance. It stands to reason that despite reporting much motivation for treatment, such clients would demonstrate ambivalence about moving forward with systematic exposure. I contend that a therapeutic relationship characterized by support, encouragement, respect, and positive regard can serve as a catalyst in the client's ultimate decision to embark on a course of exposure. Therapists who deliver exposure-based CBT must be careful not to inadvertently provide reinforcement or serve as a safety figure on which clients rely to implement their exposures. At the same time, a warm therapist who communicates an inspirational "You've got this" type of message, combined with genuine delight when the client accomplishes a meaningful exposure, can go a long way in shaping a positive experience for the client.

At times, interactions within the therapeutic relationship itself can serve as stimuli for exposure. It is not difficult to imagine that socially anxious clients could achieve exposure-related benefits by conversing with a therapist. Moreover, conversations can be strategically set up to target specific social interaction fears of clients, such as expressing an opinion or making a request. If the client and therapist face a potential rupture in the therapeutic alliance, discussing it in a collaborative, respectful manner could provide a fantastic opportunity for exposure in clients who struggle with assertiveness and who typically refrain from speaking up, for fear of a "confrontation." On another note, other clients have fears of emotional experiencing and emotional expression, and conversations about different topics can serve as exposure that could result in generalization of learning to discuss these topics with other important individuals in their lives.

Of course, it will be important for future research to examine the association between aspects of the therapeutic relationship and outcome in exposure-based CBT. For example, we know that the strength of the agreement on the goals and tasks of therapy (i.e., two of the three key components of the therapeutic alliance) correlates positively with engagement and outcome in exposure-based CBT (Buchholz & Abramowitz, 2020); can this be replicated and quantified? It will also be important to verify whether some of the intangible aspects of the therapeutic relationship referenced in this section, such as the bond between the therapist and client, mediate the relation between agreement on the goals and tasks of therapy and engagement and outcome in exposure-based CBT. More generally, it would be a major contribution to the literature to investigate the central premise of this chapter—whether a strong therapeutic relationship is a prerequisite for engagement in exposure-based CBT in all clients, or in a subset of clients (e.g., those who report substantial ambivalence about embarking on a course of exposure), and it would be most helpful to know which particular therapeutic relationship-enhancing behaviors of therapists (e.g., the provision of empathy, respect, and/or encouragement) predict the magnitude of outcome, as well as the speed at which clients complete exposure-based CBT. Perhaps a research agenda of this nature could start with qualitative research by soliciting clients' perspectives of aspects of the therapeutic relationship that they view as being pivotal in their experience with exposure-based therapy.

All of the cognitive behavioral strategies described in the book to this point—cognitive restructuring, social problem solving, and exposure—focus on problematic thoughts, behaviors, and reactions to life issues in the here-and-now, or that clients are facing in their daily lives at the same time that they are participating in CBT. However, cognitive behavioral therapists will undoubtedly encounter clients who have a history of adversity and trauma, which shaped the way in which they view themselves, others, and the world around them. As a result, they may have developed distinctive—and often maladaptive—response patterns to protect themselves from further adversity or trauma. These long-standing beliefs and behavioral patterns often provide a rich context for the presenting problems that bring clients to treatment. In the next chapter, these long-standing beliefs and behavioral patterns are considered, and the key role that the therapeutic relationship plays in promoting healing will be illustrated.

8 SCHEMA MODIFICATION AND THE THERAPEUTIC RELATIONSHIP

The cognitive behavioral therapy (CBT) model outlines multiple layers of problematic psychological factors that contribute to the understanding of the development, maintenance, and exacerbation of pathology. Because of its focus on the here and now, many cognitive behavioral therapists work with their clients to address the cognitive, emotional, and behavioral issues that are currently causing difficulty in their lives. That is, these cognitive behavioral therapists help their clients identify and, if necessary, modify unhelpful thinking that arises in particular situations that clients encounter in their lives during the course of treatment (often in the form of cognitive restructuring, described in Chapter 5 of this volume). They help their clients to manage aversive and life-interfering emotional reactions to these challenging circumstances. And, they help their clients to recognize self-defeating behaviors that they are enacting to prevent or navigate these difficulties (often in the form of social problem solving or exposure, described in Chapters 6 and 7 of this volume, respectively). Countless clients focus nearly exclusively on their here-and-now cognitive, emotional, and behavioral reactions during the course of CBT, and they emerge from therapy as a treatment success.

https://doi.org/10.1037/0000424-009
Therapeutic Relationship-Focused Cognitive Behavioral Therapy, by A. Wenzel
Copyright © 2025 by the American Psychological Association. All rights reserved.

However, this heavy focus on the here and now is, perhaps, not the ideal match for all clients. Many clients present for treatment with long-standing difficulties rooted in their past, which have exerted profound effects on their psyche and functioning. They might endorse a history of trauma, insecure attachment with parental figures, a history of unrelenting social rejection or bullying, an unstable childhood environment, and/or a host of other historical variables that shape the very essence of who they are and how they respond to the world. Although these clients have the intellectual capacity to learn the tried-and-true principles, strategies, techniques, and tools offered in CBT, they can struggle with feeling the benefits emotionally, or with believing that the acquisition of these skills and principles can make a meaningful difference in their lives. For several decades now, it has been recognized clinically that these clients respond well to the additional focus on schema modification. This chapter describes the core components of schema modification, the key role that the therapeutic relationship can play in facilitating schema modification, clinical guidance for delivering schema modification strategies through the lens of the therapeutic relationship, and cognitive behavioral approaches for repairing ruptures in the therapeutic relationship when a maladaptive schema has been activated in the course of the work of therapy.

A *schema* is a hypothetical cognitive structure that influences the way in which people process, make sense of, and find meaning in information that is formed from previous experiences with others and situations. It is a cognitive representation of individuals' past experiences with other people, situations, and themselves, which helps them understand events that are happening in similar realms that they encounter in life (Goldfried, 2003). The schema construct has been influential across many fields of psychology. Within developmental psychology, it explains how children acquire knowledge and begin to make sense of their worlds (Piaget, 1952). Within cognitive psychology, it captures the rules by which and the speed at which people categorize information and then later retrieve content from memory (Brewer, 2000). Within social psychology, it accounts for the way that people form impressions of others and their social and interactional world, such as the way in which we form impressions of others, develop stereotypes, and even promote prejudice and racism (Pennington, 2000). Within clinical psychology, it explains the core beliefs that people with mental health disorders carry with them and the way in which they process information that reinforces those beliefs. Thus, clinical psychologists view schemas as reflecting pathology-relevant content and process—content reflective of the core beliefs that people have formed about themselves, others, the world (cf. A. T. Beck et al., 1987), and the future, and preferential processing of information that reinforces those beliefs. I have referenced core beliefs in many sections of this volume to this point, especially when illustrating the underlying meaning of thoughts that are subjected to cognitive restructuring. In this chapter, I focus on the core beliefs that form the basis for maladaptive schemas that are the subject of some of CBT's deepest and most meaningful work.

Take, as an example, Sarah,[1] whom we have been following throughout this volume. Sarah reported a long history of perceived rejection, beginning with her experience of rejection by her parents. She absorbed parental rejection in a number of ways, such as when her parents criticized her appearance and interests and made snarky comments about the friends with whom she was spending time. This sense of rejection was further reinforced when Sarah was hospitalized and then sent to live with her best friend's family because her parents believed that she was incapable of fitting into their family's culture and household rules. In fits of frustration, her parents would often exclaim, "Something is wrong with you!" which contributed to a related core belief that Sarah internalized (i.e., defectiveness).

These beliefs about rejection and defectiveness followed Sarah in her relationships from adolescence and beyond. She was quick to interpret benign behavior of others as a sign of rejection unless she was extremely secure in the relationship (e.g., if an acquaintance did not respond to a text message right away, Sarah assumed that she was bothering them and that they did not want to hear from her). If a guest dismissed her at the restaurant, she assumed that they viewed her as being unworthy of their attention. If she noticed other people staring at her (as they often did because of her colorful appearance), she assumed that they were making fun of her rather than admiring her courageous expression. Thus, not only did these beliefs facilitate the specific, and usually self-deprecating, way Sarah interpreted situations that she encountered in her daily life, but they also influenced the direction in which she deposed her attention. That is, she would zero in on perceived signs of rejection, while at the same time, dismissing indicators of warmth, acceptance, and good will. When she experienced an actual rejection (i.e., her boyfriend leaving her abruptly to begin a relationship with another woman), she quickly reached a place of emotional crisis because her most painful schema was reinforced.

Fortunately, a specific approach within the general CBT family to work with these fundamental core beliefs and the interpersonal consequences of these beliefs has been in existence for many decades. *Schema therapy* was developed by the renowned Dr. Jeffrey E. Young, a former trainee of Dr. Aaron T. Beck's (Young et al., 2003). Dr. Young's schema therapy is an approach in which clients with comorbid mental health problems, personality disorders,

---

[1]Client identity has been disguised to protect client confidentiality.

and/or extensive histories of trauma and discord are understood according to their dominant schemas. This approach addresses long-standing beliefs and self-defeating behavioral patterns that stem from damaging experiences that take place earlier in life. Many of these beliefs and behavioral patterns are associated with interpersonal problems, which could also manifest in the therapeutic relationship and thus make it an ideal place to nurture a new way of being and responding.

Dr. Young and colleagues (2003) identified 18 early maladaptive schemas (i.e., schemas with roots that were established at a young age and that manifest and are reinforced throughout a person's life) that stem from previous experiences and influence the way in which people make meaning of their life situations. These schemas include the following:

1. *Abandonment/instability*—the view that others are unavailable or unreliable in their provision of support

2. *Mistrust/abuse*—the assumption that others will be hurtful or will mistreat them

3. *Emotional deprivation*—the assumption that others will not meet expected needs of nurturance, empathy, and/or protection

4. *Defectiveness/shame*—the view that one is defective, unwanted, inferior, and would be deemed unworthy if others were to detect this in them

5. *Social isolation/alienation*—the view that one is different from others and separate from a community

6. *Dependence/incompetence*—the view that one is helpless and unable to execute the responsibilities of life without the help of others

7. *Vulnerability to harm or illness*—the view that one cannot prevent an imminent catastrophe

8. *Enmeshment/underdeveloped self*—the assumption that one cannot achieve normal development without the overinvolvement of others

9. *Failure*—the view that one has failed in areas of achievement

10. *Entitlement/grandiosity*—the belief that one is better than others, and therefore, is entitled to special privileges or suspension of rules

11. *Insufficient self-control/self-discipline*—difficulty applying self-control over one's behavior and emotions, and the belief that one cannot tolerate aversiveness

12. *Subjugation*—an overemphasis on relinquishing one's needs, preferences, or emotions to avoid anger, conflict, retaliation, or abandonment

13. *Self-sacrifice*—an overemphasis on meeting the needs of others at the expense of one's own needs in order to avoid guilt or rejection

14. *Approval-seeking/recognition-seeking*—an overemphasis on gaining recognition from others at the expense of sharing one's true self in order to elevate one's status

15. *Negativity/pessimism*—the assumption that things will go wrong, along with a minimization of the positives or things that are going right

16. *Emotional inhibition*—the view that one should inhibit spontaneous action or emotion for fear of disapproval, shame, or losing control

17. *Unrelenting standards/hypercriticalness*—the view that one must meet excessively high standards in order to avoid criticism

18. *Punitiveness*—the view that people should be punished for making mistakes

Schema therapists work with their clients to educate them about schemas, notice when their personal schemas are activated, and apply an array of traditional and schema-focused strategies and techniques to modify the schema itself as well as the typical cognitive, emotional, and behavioral reactions that arise when these schemas are activated.

As can be seen from this list, nearly all of the early maladaptive schemas involve a relational component. This means that the activation of these schemas can exert their effects within the therapeutic relationship, and what is happening within the relationship can serve as fodder for clients to develop a rich understanding of the way in which their schemas are activated and affect their relationships. Examples of ways in which each of these schemas can be activated and affect the therapeutic relationship are as follows:

1. *Abandonment/instability*—This schema could be activated when the therapist is away for a period of time, such as a vacation or a maternity leave. It could also be activated in more subtle ways, such as the therapist returning a phone call after a longer period of time than the client had hoped.

2. *Mistrust/abuse*—This schema could be activated when a therapist provides gentle feedback to the client that the client does not want to hear, interpreting the feedback as harsh or rejecting and, thereby, hurtful.

3. *Emotional deprivation*—The activation of this schema could be "tricky" for a therapist who is trying to meet a client's needs and simultaneously maintain appropriate professional boundaries. Consider the following example: A client is moving to a new apartment complex and wants an emotional support animal. The client asks the therapist to write a note to the complex management team requesting permission for the emotional

support animal. The client then perceives that their therapist is not protecting them when the therapist gently refuses to write such a note.

4. *Defectiveness/shame*—This schema could be activated when a client regrets sharing their inner-most thoughts and fears with a therapist, worrying that the therapist will now view them as defective or unworthy because of the repugnance of these private thoughts.

5. *Social isolation/alienation*—This schema could be activated when a client believes that their therapist does not understand them.

6. *Dependence/incompetence*—This schema could be activated when the client is having difficulty implementing CBT skills for homework in between sessions.

7. *Vulnerability to harm or illness*—This schema is likely to be less related to the therapeutic relationship itself than many of the other schemas, but it is common in clients with anxiety disorders and can lead to difficulties in the therapeutic relationship if the client feels invalidated by the therapist or perceives that therapy is not helpful.

8. *Enmeshment/underdeveloped self*—This schema could be activated when a client has the expectation that the therapist will solve all of their problems for them.

9. *Failure*—This schema could be activated when a client is not achieving the expected aims of CBT, thereby souring their view of the therapy experience.

10. *Entitlement/grandiosity*—This schema could be activated when the client expects basic rules of therapy not to apply to them, such as payment for a session canceled with less than 24 hours' notice.

11. *Insufficient self-control/self-discipline*—This schema's activation is evident when a client has an outburst in session, particularly toward the therapist when another early maladaptive schema is activated.

12. *Subjugation*—This schema's activation is evident when the client relies on the therapist to direct the session (e.g., when the client has nothing for the agenda and responds to the therapist with a statement like, "I'll let you take the lead").

13. *Self-sacrifice*—This schema's activation is evident when the client attempts to go out of their way to accommodate the therapist (e.g., "It's okay with me if you want to switch my appointment time with someone who needs it more at the last minute. I'm not doing anything important").

14. *Approval-seeking/recognition-seeking*—This schema's activation is evident when the client asks the therapist for validation that they are doing "better" than the therapist's other clients.

15. *Negativity/pessimism*—This schema's activation is evident when the client dismisses the therapist's insights and suggestions, often displaying a "yeah, but" posture.

16. *Emotional inhibition*—This schema's activation is evident when a client deflects discussion about their private thoughts and fears. The client in Chapter 7 of this volume who underwent exposure to the sharing of personal information and the experience of vulnerability would likely have been characterized by this schema.

17. *Unrelenting standards/hypercriticalness*—This schema's activation would be evident when the client puts themselves down for their view that they did not complete their CBT homework well, when in reality their homework was thorough and contributed to significant gains made in treatment.

18. *Punitiveness*—This schema's activation would be evident when the client overtly criticizes the therapist for not making "progress" in therapy or for having "unreasonable" rules or boundaries.

In addition to the rich way in which most of the schema therapy content areas can manifest in the therapeutic relationship, schema therapy also incorporates two constructs that cut across a focus on any specific schema, cultivating the therapeutic relationship in general. Both strategies are woven into the fabric of the entire course of treatment—and are entirely consistent with the central premises of therapeutic relationship-focused CBT (TRF-CBT). First, *empathic confrontation* involves the balance between demonstrating empathy when clients' maladaptive schemas are activated and helping them to see that the resulting ways in which they are interpreting and coping with events in their lives are unhelpful. Empathic confrontation involves the provision of honest feedback to the client, lest the therapist might be inadvertently reinforcing an unhelpful pattern of interacting with the world. However, it is done in a way that is sensitive, respectful, and understanding of what it might feel like to receive such feedback. When I implement this principle with my clients, in my mind I conceptualize it as *empathic sharing*, as the typical person often carries unhelpful connotations of the word "confrontation." When I implement empathic sharing, I often ask the client for permission to share honest feedback and, if relevant, I note that their pattern of responding makes sense in light of the schema that is activated, even if, ultimately, their response is self-defeating.

Limited reparenting refers to instances in which the therapist, appropriately, gives clients something essential that they did not receive from their parents during childhood, meeting their core emotional needs. The word "limited" is included because it would clearly be inappropriate for a therapist to function fully as a parent; yet, the therapeutic relationship could serve as a platform for the client to have a corrective learning experience that would repair some of the damaging effects of invalidation, rejection, and abuse by parents and that would provide a secure base from which the client can explore other ways of being (cf. Safran & Segal, 1990). For example, when clients' negative schemas are activated and they act out as a result, the therapist might respond in a validating manner that does not feel like punishment, serving as a very different experience than the client endured during childhood. It is crucial that therapists recognize the activation of maladaptive schemas, understand the core emotional need that was not met by the client's parents, and gently meet that corresponding need to facilitate the corrective learning experience. For example, a client with an abandonment schema might lack a sense of secure attachment to others; when the therapist recognizes that this has been activated, the therapist can then provide comfort, soothing, and a sense of acceptance (Gülüm & Soygüt, 2022).

Schema therapy incorporates therapeutic relationship-enhancing techniques into its very definition. Nevertheless, as with any of the CBT strategies described in this volume, clinicians can work on schema modification with more focus or less focus on the therapeutic relationship. Consider the following two excerpts, which were conducted with a client with a defectiveness/shame schema. In my clinical experience, I view this as a particularly heart-wrenching schema with which to work, as it is often associated with profound beliefs of worthlessness and of being a burden to others. In these excerpts, consider the therapist's style in working with the client's defectiveness/shame schema. Note that the client has already completed an inventory to identify his maladaptive schemas in a previous session, with defectiveness/shame coming out on top (therapists who wish to administer such an inventory to their clients can contact the Schema Therapy Institute [https://www.schematherapy.org/]).

Excerpt 1: Less Focus on the Therapeutic Relationship

CLIENT: I don't know what is wrong with me. I'm a successful guy, a CEO of my own company that I started from scratch. I have business associates who respect me across the globe, and I've won so many awards. Why is it that I'm 52 years old and still not married, without a family?

THERAPIST: You certainly have achieved so much. This is the one area of struggle for you. [*Here, the therapist chooses to make a reflection to demonstrate empathy.*]

CLIENT: It sure is. I mean, I'm clearly doing something wrong. All of these relationships, they start out great in the beginning, and over time, they just don't work out.

THERAPIST: [recalling the schema inventory completed by the client in the previous session] What schema do you think is being activated here?

CLIENT: Defectiveness/shame for sure. It really does feel like something is wrong with me. I think I really need to take a closer look at what I am doing in these relationships so that I can detect some patterns and correct them.

THERAPIST: I think that is a fantastic idea. Should we start with your most recent relationship, the one that just ended?

On the surface, this dialogue achieves several aims of schema therapy-based CBT. The therapist linked what the client was saying to the beginnings of their schema work done in the previous session (i.e., the completion of the inventory). Moreover, when the client mentioned examining patterns within his relationships, the therapist was wholly on board, as the examination and modifications of patterns of behavior is a hallmark of schema therapy. Notice, however, that something seems to be "missing" in this dialogue. The client has clearly identified a painful schema in the context of talking about an important aspect of his life that remains unfulfilled. And yet, there is no visible affect. As a successful CEO of his own startup company, the client has exceptional intellectual and problem-solving skills. However, these strengths also translate to a tendency to "intellectualize" about the issues that bring him to therapy, limiting the opportunity for the shared experiencing of affect with his therapist that very well might be an agent of change. In the second excerpt, his therapist harnesses the power of therapeutic relationship-enhancing techniques to elicit affect and work collaboratively together within that affect.

Excerpt 2: More Focus on the Therapeutic Relationship

CLIENT: I don't know what is wrong with me. I'm a successful guy, a CEO of my own company that I started from scratch. I have business associates who respect me across the globe, and I've won so many awards. Why is it that I'm 52 years old and still not married, without a family?

THERAPIST: You certainly have achieved so much. This is the one area of struggle for you. [*Here, the therapist chooses to make a reflection to demonstrate empathy.*]

CLIENT: It sure is. I mean, I'm clearly doing something wrong. All of these relationships, they start out great in the beginning, and over time, they just don't work out.

THERAPIST: [recalling the schema inventory completed by the client in the previous session] What schema do you think is being activated here?

CLIENT: Defectiveness/shame for sure. It really does feel like something is wrong with me. I think I really need to take a closer look at what I am doing in these relationships so that I can detect some patterns and correct them.

THERAPIST: [pausing and speaking from the heart] Defectiveness/shame. What a painful notion that is, viewing oneself as defective. And what a painful emotion shame can be. [*Here, the therapist attempts to share in the painful affect in a genuine manner.*]

CLIENT: [looking rattled] Nobody understands how difficult it is to live in my skin.

THERAPIST: [speaking gently] Tell me what you mean by that.

CLIENT: [voice is shaking] I have to make all of these decisions every day. Decisions that affect the lives of the hundreds of people that I employ. Decisions that affect the lives of my clients. And of the people who use the product we've developed. It seems like there is so much riding on everything I do. And you know what? I do it! And I do it well! [pausing, becoming tearful] That's why it makes it all the more difficult to understand how I can be so successful in one area of my life, and how I can be such a failure in another area of my life. I truly, truly believe that I am defective interpersonally. My only friends are my colleagues, and even then, sometimes it feels like I have to buy their adoration. Every romantic relationship I have turns horribly volatile. And there, I get used too, because I feel like I have to buy back their affection. [pausing again] At the end of the day, after all of the stress I experience on a daily basis, I just want to come home to a partner who loves me for who I am. Not for the money. Not for the status. Not for the jewelry or expensive clothes or whatever. I just want to have what it seems like everybody else has, and I don't seem to have what it takes to do that.

THERAPIST: I hadn't fully appreciated, until now, just how deep the sense of defectiveness/shame runs for you, interpersonally.

CLIENT: This is the last frontier, Doctor. We've tackled my depression, we've tackled my unhealthy drinking, and we've even tackled my suicidal thoughts. But this . . . throughout it all . . . this *thing*, this defectiveness/shame when it comes to my relationships . . . this, in some ways, underlies it all.

THERAPIST: Well, it would truly be my pleasure to work with you to soften the effects of this schema, and ultimately reshape it. [*The therapist makes this statement as a reflection of the real relationship in order to join together in an authentic manner to address a pivotal issue.*]

CLIENT: You're the only person I would trust with that level of vulnerability.

Notice that one sentence made by the therapist propelled this dialogue in a different direction, immediately following the client's observation that his defectiveness/shame schema was activated and his suggestion that he examine patterns in his relationship. Instead of replying with, "I think that is a fantastic idea. Should we start with your most recent relationship, the one that just ended?" the therapist made a simple statement about how painful defectiveness and shame can be. This response created space for the client to experience the affect associated with his schema and open up a bit about his lived experience. Ultimately, as in the first dialogue, they agreed to work together on this schema, but in the latter instance, this agreement was made from a more profound place of empathy, congruence, and mutual positive regard.

TIPS FOR SCHEMA MODIFICATION THROUGH THE LENS OF THE THERAPEUTIC RELATIONSHIP

Schema modification work can be some of the most profound work that is done in CBT, in part because it inherently weaves in a focus on the therapeutic relationship through therapist–client interactions that take place in session. In this section, I provide some suggestions for schema therapy-based work with clients from a framework of TRF-CBT.

Tip 1: Attend Closely to the Client's Affect

As demonstrated in the previous excerpts, affect plays a central role in schema therapy work. It tends to be the case that the most painful schemas are associated with significant affect; clinical experience suggests that the most substantial schema modification occurs when this affect is elicited, and clients experience the corresponding shift in affect as they achieve the aims of schema modification. Moreover, the expression of affect can help both the therapist and client identify when a maladaptive schema is activated. The most common affective expression that signals the activation of a painful schema is tearfulness. However, more subtle affective indicators could point to the activation of a maladaptive schema, including the following:

- averting eye contact
- frowning
- shaking
- fidgeting
- wringing of hands
- playing with hair
- inappropriately laughing
- changing the subject
- closing one's posture (e.g., crossing one's arms, bending the legs and bringing one's feet up on their chair)

When therapists notice one of these or other indicators of affect, they can stop and gently ask what is happening for the client in that moment. They can also educate their clients that the presence of such affective indicators can mean that a maladaptive schema has been activated, which can help clients to acquire skill in recognizing this on their own.

In general, the experience of intense affect within the therapy session is powerful for the therapeutic relationship. It requires vulnerability on the part of the client, and the therapeutic relationship will be enhanced when the therapist treats that vulnerability with the utmost empathy and respect. Moreover, it allows an opportunity for congruence between the therapist and client when the therapist is touched by the client's affective expression.

Tip 2: Normalize Schema Activation

As clients begin to get a sense of the reach that maladaptive schemas can have in their lives, they sometimes feel secondary guilt and shame when they recognize that their schemas are active and causing damage. Common reactions to the activation of maladaptive schemas include the following:

- "I'm weak for allowing this to come to the surface."
- "I haven't worked hard enough to manage the effects of my schema."
- "That my schemas keep being activated means that I'm truly damaged and will never improve."

- "Other people shouldn't have to deal with the effects of my schema activation."

It is important for clients to know that all people are characterized by a combination of positive (or healthier) and negative (or less healthy) schemas. According to basic cognitive theory (see Wenzel et al., 2016), during times of relative calm, the positive, healthier schemas predominate. However, in times of stress the negative, less healthy schemas are activated and exert their influence. Although it is true that many people for whom schema therapy is appropriate are characterized by the chronic activation of the negative, less healthy schemas, nevertheless, the presence of negative schemas can be normalized with the observation that almost everyone has had life experiences that contribute to the development of negative views of themselves or others. Another form of normalization that clients often find helpful is the understanding that the way they are feeling makes perfect sense, in light of the schema that is activated that is, in large part, determining what aspects of the situation they attend to and the way they are interpreting those aspects. Clients often come away from such a discussion of normalization with a sentiment such as, "Okay, I'm not crazy. The way I am feeling makes sense because of the schema that formed from very real, and difficult, early experiences."

Normalization of schema activation enhances the therapeutic relationship because it allows an opportunity for the client to experience the therapist as understanding and nonjudgmental. When a maladaptive schema is activated, the therapist has the opportunity to remain present with the client's affective expression, as aversive or as difficult to endure as it might be. This sends the message to the client that the therapist will not abandon them, even when a maladaptive schema is at work and when the client is exuding strong affect. It also allows the client to conclude that they can be at their "worst" in the presence of their therapist, and the therapist will nevertheless accept them and treat them with respect.

Tip 3: Recognize That Schema Modification Takes Time

Schema modification often occurs some time after therapy has commenced, after clients have acquired many of the fundamental CBT principles and tools relating to cognitive restructuring, behavioral activation, exposure, and/or problem solving. Part of the reason is that having this foundation in CBT can help clients apply the principles in a sophisticated way to their maladaptive schemas. Another reason is that schemas are typically very ingrained in clients, sometimes to the point that they take the contents of their maladaptive schemas as facts rather than as filters through which they view the world that can be altered with quality CBT. This means that schemas are not usually shifted noticeably with the application of any one CBT strategy on only one occasion. Instead, the benefits of these CBT strategies accumulate over time, and the schema shifts very gradually through continued attention given to schema modification.

This point is being made here so that the therapist and client both understand that schema modification takes time. It is not difficult to imagine a client becoming frustrated in an instance in which they exhibit a very skillful application of a CBT strategy, only to experience their maladaptive schema being activated the very next time that they are faced with stress or adversity. Such an experience could easily form the basis for a rupture in the therapeutic alliance if the client were to conclude that therapy has not been helpful or that the therapist has lacked competence in helping them to achieve lasting change. By knowing that schema modification takes time, the client and therapist, together, can celebrate small victories in modulating the effects of a maladaptive schema; when more substantial schema modification has occurred, that victory will be that much sweeter. In some instances, appreciable schema modification does not occur—and this does not necessarily mean that therapy is unsuccessful. From a standpoint consistent with that advanced by the developers of acceptance and commitment therapy (S. C. Hayes et al., 1999, 2012), therapy is just as much of a success if clients recognize the activation of a schema, accept that it is influencing cognition and need not be taken as truth, and continue to live their lives in a thoughtful prosocial way consistent with their values.

Tip 4: Recognize the Reactions That Stem From Your Own History

Schema modification work is challenging for clients and therapists alike. Clients who engage in schema modification typically face painful experiences from their past and painful beliefs that they might have a difficult time articulating to themselves, let alone others. Many clients who work with their therapist on schema modification disclose that they have never before shared these thoughts with another human being. It is not difficult to imagine that there will be some instances in which a client pulls back out of a sense of shame or embarrassment, even after a seemingly powerful and productive session. For example, they might cancel or even fail to report for the next session, even after they expressed that they were looking forward to continued schema modification. They might steer the conversation toward "safer," more mundane topics. They might even demonstrate hostility toward the therapist for inviting vulnerability in the first place.

Because therapists are human beings, they are likely to have their own maladaptive schemas as well. When a client responds to them in a (seemingly) negative manner, the situation could be ripe for the therapist to interpret the client's behavior in a manner that reinforces their own schema, which could, in turn, influence the therapist's reaction to the client and create countertransference. For example, a therapist with a defectiveness/shame schema could interpret the client's behavior as a personal rejection. From that stance of personal rejection, the therapist might not reach out to reschedule the client who cancels a session for fear of continued rejection, when reaching out would have been what the client needed to reinforce the therapist's care, concern, and competence. A therapist with a failure or unrelenting standards/hypercriticalness schema could interpret the client's behavior as signaling that they are no good as a therapist. This stance could facilitate a response in which the therapist overcompensates by forcing along the process of schema modification to achieve success at all costs. A therapist with a punitiveness schema could assume a blaming stance for the client's stalled progress in schema modification, which would likely negatively affect the therapeutic relationship in subtle ways that could shut down the client's sense of security in continued schema modification work with the therapist. In fact, research shows that therapist perceptions of a power struggle with the client, sense of helplessness and that they should be doing more, and feelings of guilt, frustration, and being drained are associated with client resistance, perhaps through the mechanism of reducing the competency of treatment delivered (Westra et al., 2012).

It is important for therapists to pay close attention to the reactions they are having to their clients (Kohlenberg & Tsai, 1991; Safran & Segal, 1990). An indicator of a reaction to a client might be emotional in nature (e.g., a sense of dread in anticipation of the next session with a client), physiological in nature (e.g., chest and throat tightening in anticipation of the next session with a client), or behavioral in nature (e.g., ending the session a few minutes early). Exhibit 8.1 displays questions that therapists can ask themselves as they notice these indicators to determine whether they are having a reaction to their client that (a) might serve as "grist for the mill" in therapy that would ultimately help the client reach their treatment goals, (b) could be indicative of a therapeutic alliance rupture, and/or (c) might signal a countertransference reaction. Many of these questions were specified by Tsai et al. (2010) and Leahy (2012).

EXHIBIT 8.1. Questions to Facilitate Reflection on Therapist Reactions to Clients

- In what ways is the client having a negative impact on you, and why might that be?
- Do you find your attention wandering in session, and why might this be?
- In what ways are you frustrated with the client?
- Does your client avoid answering questions or respond to your questions in a way that is not straightforward?
- Does your client exhibit behavior that is unreasonable, and if so, what impact does that have on you?
- Do you have concerns about your client making on-time payment for services?
- Does your client respond to your warmth and humor, and if not, how does that make you feel?
- Does the client remind you of anyone in your past or current life, and if so, how is that affecting your work with them?
- Does your client do or say things that are particularly aversive for you in light of your past experiences?
- Does your client seem to "push your buttons," and if so, in what way?
- Is there anything you are avoiding discussing with the client and if so, why?
- Is there anything about your client's pathology that you have overlooked, and what made you do so? (Leahy, 2012)
- Are there some types of clients who bore you? (Leahy, 2012)

It is vitally important for therapists to keep client reactions to schema therapy work in perspective and to recognize when their own schemas are activated and affecting the way in which they are reacting to their clients. It is only natural that some client behaviors will be challenging to process and handle because they bring up past issues that were particularly upsetting or hurtful to the therapist. However, it is the therapist's responsibility to do the required work to ensure that it does not affect the therapeutic relationship with the client. More generally, if a therapist notices repeated occasions in which their own maladaptive schema is activated in the context of clinical work with their clients, then it would behoove them to embark on their own schema modification work. Avenues for adjusting the way in which schemas affect clinical work include the following:

- seeking schema-based CBT with a trained cognitive behavioral therapist

- seeking supervision with a trained cognitive behavioral therapist

- actively using CBT principles and strategies to address schema-related thoughts, emotions, and behaviors

- reviewing the client's session documentation and engaging in honest reflection about one's reactions to the client and the way in which their schemas are affecting therapeutic interactions

SCHEMA MODIFICATION AS APPLIED TO THERAPEUTIC RELATIONSHIP ISSUES

As mentioned previously, nearly all of Young's early maladaptive schemas have a relational component, and interpersonal relationships are a central feature of many of them. In this section, I illustrate ways to work with a subset of six of Young et al.'s (2003) early maladaptive schemas, ending with an illustration of the defectiveness/shame schema with Sarah, the case we have been following throughout this volume.

Activation of the Abandonment/Instability Schema

As mentioned earlier, people who endorse the abandonment/instability schema believe that others on whom they thought they could depend will not be there in times of need or will abandon them altogether. One of four types of compensatory behavioral patterns within the therapeutic relationship typically emerges in clients with this schema. Some clients with an abandonment/instability schema will be especially "clingy," checking in with their therapist frequently on (often) trivial matters with the underlying goal of obtaining reassurance that the therapist is still there for them. Other clients with this schema come across in a demanding manner, almost as if they are taking control of the therapeutic relationship as insurance that the therapist will be there when they need them. Still other clients with this schema take on a guarded stance, as if they are waiting for the therapist to "abandon" them so that they can say something like "I knew it!" when their beliefs, in their minds, have been validated. Finally, other clients with an abandonment/instability schema can approach therapy in an apathetic manner, almost as if they have an attitude like, "Why bother investing in therapy? My therapist will invariably show me that she won't really be there for me when I need her."

Fortunately, many of the tenets and practices of good therapy, and good CBT in particular, go a long way in modeling behavior that can help to reshape this schema. Good therapists get back to their clients in a timely and a consistent manner when their clients reach out to them. When an unexpected client need arises, good therapists make reasonable accommodations to schedule a session sooner than they might have otherwise. Moreover, good therapists are clear about the boundaries of their practices so that clients have clear expectations about the types of issues for which it is appropriate to reach out to a therapist, as well as the timeliness with which they can expect a response. For example, in my practice, I (unlike some other providers) have a no-texting policy so that I do not inadvertently create the expectation in clients that I will respond in a relatively immediate manner or engage in ongoing messaging, as often occurs in casual texting.

Despite modeling of responsiveness consistent with well-articulated and agreed-upon boundaries, clients with an abandonment/instability schema are at an increased likelihood for reacting to a scenario in which they perceive that the therapist was unavailable when they were needed. Many CBT strategies can be used to address a potential rupture in the alliance that could follow from such an event. For example, cognitive restructuring could be used to reframe the idea that the therapist does not care for them. It could also be applied as the therapist and client revisit the expectations that the client has for the therapist to ensure that those expectations are consistent with the agreement that they made at the beginning of their professional work together. Social problem solving could be used to continue to reinforce professional boundaries, as well as to devise a plan for negotiating another delicate situation should one arise. Breathing and self-soothing strategies could be used to work through difficult moments before the client says something to the therapist that they do not really mean. Acceptance-based strategies could help the client cultivate a spirit of acceptance over the professional nature of the therapeutic relationship, boundaries and all. All the while, as the therapist uses these strategies with a client with an abandonment/instability schema, they could inquire as to what the client is learning from the therapeutic relationship and consider ways in which this learning would apply to other relationships. In this way, the experience can be used to soften and provide alternatives to the abandonment/instability schema.

Activation of the Mistrust/Abuse Schema

As mentioned previously in this chapter, clients with a mistrust/abuse schema believe that others will mistreat or harm them. These clients often present for treatment as guarded and even hostile as a means of self-protection from injury. It can be difficult to form a therapeutic relationship with these clients because it is challenging for them to express vulnerability and to believe that their therapist has their best interests at heart. Not surprisingly, then, it can be difficult for therapists to muster and express genuine warmth toward these clients because these clients tend to provide the therapist less positive reinforcement than many other types of clients. Thus, therapists who work with clients characterized by a mistrust/abuse schema may find themselves in a precarious position in which their own maladaptive schemas are activated, as they often perceive that their clients are not having a good experience in therapy (which could be associated with the activation of a failure or defectiveness/shame schema).

Trust takes time to develop in all relationships, and the therapeutic relationship is no different. If anything, it can be diagnostic when a client immediately places full trust in a therapist before truly taking the time to learn what the therapist has to offer and about the therapist's style. Nevertheless, trust usually develops more slowly with clients characterized by a mistrust/abuse schema than with clients who are not characterized by this schema.

Many of the same practices described in the previous section on the abandonment/instability schema apply to work with the mistrust/abuse schema. Examples include getting back to clients in a timely manner, making reasonable accommodations for clients in need, and communicating and modeling clear boundaries. Whereas the curative message for clients with an abandonment/instability schema is that of consistency (i.e., "I will show you that I will follow through on my word no matter what we are working with in session"), the curative message for clients with a mistrust/abuse schema is that of having their best interests in mind (i.e., "I am going to treat you with respect and not intentionally harm you"). As therapeutic work unfolds, it is hoped that the client with a mistrust/abuse schema will develop the view of the therapist as a kind, compassionate individual who can be trusted to treat them with courtesy, respect, and care. This can be a powerful experience for a person who does not believe that they have people with these characteristics in their lives to provide support.

I encourage therapists who work with clients characterized by a mistrust/abuse schema to pay special attention to the therapeutic relationship-building strategies described in countless texts on psychotherapy and in Chapter 2 of this volume. Warmth, empathy, and positive regard likely will not be readily accepted by a client with a mistrust/abuse schema at first, but the consistent demonstration of these qualities over time can build good will and create an environment in which the client can relax enough to absorb the benefits that can be had from a genuine relationship characterized by mutual respect and kindness. When a client has a mistrust/abuse schema, forming and maintaining a genuine relationship with someone who does not harm them can serve as a pivotal life experience that can pave the way for the development of closer and healthier relationships outside of the therapy office.

As with all the early maladaptive schemas, clients with a mistrust/abuse schema are prone to interpreting events that occur in their lives through the filter of that schema. It is not difficult to imagine, for example, that a therapist's honest feedback that is inconsistent with what a client wants to hear would be interpreted as the therapist causing harm to the client. Above all, it is essential for therapists to refrain from justifying their behavior and overtly trying to convince a client to interpret their behavior in a benign manner. Rather, when the therapist demonstrates the ability to sit with the client's anger and disappointment, the therapist enters into the client's emotional space, experiences it with them as a partnership, and, importantly, demonstrates that they will not punish the client for having and expressing negative feelings.

Activation of the Emotional Deprivation Schema

Clients who are characterized by an emotional deprivation schema expect that others will not provide nurturance, warmth, and support. It is not difficult to surmise that many people who become mental health providers do so, in part, because they naturally provide a great deal of nurturance, warmth, and support to others in their lives. Thus, a sound therapeutic relationship has the potential to be an ideal corrective learning experience because these clients can get practice in experiencing and responding appropriately to such gestures. Such an experience has the potential to combat all-or-nothing perceptions that "no one cares" or that they are undeserving of warmth, care, and concern from others.

However, imagine what would happen if a client with an emotional deprivation schema perceives that their therapist is not meeting their need for nurturance. Such a scenario would be ripe for transference to occur, as these clients could be experiencing the therapist in the same type of way in which they experienced others (e.g., parents) as withholding affection, and their response to the therapist could be similar. Take, for example, an instance in which a therapist must enact a boundary by communicating that the session must end at the prescribed time despite the fact that the client was late and did not get a full 45- or 50-minute session. When the emotional deprivation schema is activated, it could facilitate an interpretation of the therapist as being cold, harsh, and/or "too clinical"—all of which could affect the therapeutic relationship moving forward.

When therapists practice in a way that is well within their professional right with a client characterized by an emotional deprivation schema, they are encouraged to identify the meaning associated with events that are experienced negatively by the client. If the meaning is influenced by the filter of the emotional deprivation schema, the therapist can use cognitive restructuring to examine it more closely. This occurs in the following dialogue, in which a client had a negative reaction to a therapist when she indicated that she would not read the client's lengthy email exchanges with her husband, with whom the client was in a volatile relationship, outside of session. Until the time at which this dialogue took place, the client had made many remarks about the bond she felt with the therapist and the ways in which she experienced the therapist as "having her back."

CLIENT: I'm assuming that you read through those emails I sent you, where I had pasted in all of the back-and-forth between my husband and me.

THERAPIST: Ah yes, this is something I wanted to add to our agenda.

[The client and therapist decide to discuss this issue first, before diving into the contents of the client's email exchanges with her husband.]

THERAPIST: [taking care to speak in a warm, inviting tone, despite setting a boundary] I want to remind you of my policy that I do not process lengthy emails in between sessions. I'm more than happy to talk about exchanges like this one in session, and in fact, I encourage it because it is something significant that occurred in your life in between sessions.

CLIENT: [quickly assuming a hurt expression, the smile disappearing from her face] Oh . . . but we always have so much to talk about in session, I thought this would save some time so that you have some level of familiarity with what was going on between us in the time since we last met.

THERAPIST: I understand where you are coming from. I appreciate that the tension and conflict with your husband is front and center in your life, and I think we've done some good work to sort through it all as you are debating between various courses of action with your marriage. Is it okay with you if I share the rationale behind this policy? [*The therapist asks permission to share the rationale, rather than launching immediately into it, in order to (a) reinforce a sense of collaboration and (b) refrain from "lecturing" in a manner that might be interpreted as defensiveness and "turn off" the client.*]

CLIENT: Well, yeah. I mean, I guess so.

THERAPIST: [leaning forward and speaking with a warm tone of voice] My ultimate goal, for all of you, is to be as helpful as possible. Unfortunately, when I receive lengthy correspondence to read in between sessions, especially in the form of heated email or text exchanges, I have a hard time processing it all and grasping the nuances. I've found that it is more helpful in session to discuss the main points, and importantly, what it all means to you.

CLIENT: Well, okay, but . . . this is really it. He's threatening divorce now. I'm really all alone here to make these decisions, and I don't have anyone else to turn to. I can't text or call my friends because the phone plan is in his name, and he will see that I am reaching out to them. He hates them. He knows that they support me and think badly of him . . .

THERAPIST: [taking the opportunity to gently interrupt the client's spiral] You said something powerful there. "I'm all alone here." The fact that I'm asking you to wait and describe email exchanges with your husband, rather than agreeing to read them in advance . . . do those boundaries exacerbate the notion of being all alone? [*The therapist asks this question to begin to consider the link to the emotional deprivation schema.*]

CLIENT: [becoming tearful] Yes, they absolutely do. You don't understand how lonely it is to be in my household. There is stone cold silence between my husband and I almost all the time—no kindness. No laughter. No care. And then if he does speak to me—it's just a bunch of insults and digs.

THERAPIST: [making a facial expression that demonstrates empathy] Yes, that certainly seems to be the case right now in your home. And it can be excruciating. [pausing] I'm wondering if something happened between us, just now, that was close to what you experience at home? [*The therapist asks this question to use the therapeutic relationship as a vehicle toward reshaping the emotional deprivation schema.*]

CLIENT: [looking surprised with insight] Yeah, I think it just did. I mean, we've always worked so well together, you and I, and it's been so easygoing. I know you care about me, so I thought that, of course, you'd want to see the email exchanges. And, I don't know, it just seems a bit harsh that you won't read them before our session.

THERAPIST: Does it feel to you as if that boundary is taking away from the feel of our relationship to this point?

CLIENT: [again, looking surprised with insight] It does, a little. [averting eye contact] It's just been so different in here. My family growing up, I know they care about me, but with their ethnic heritage, they don't show a lot of emotion, so there was not a lot of warm fuzzies. And I think I'm a person who needs warm fuzzies. My husband, I can never count on him for warm fuzzies, let alone basic human decency. I get it from my friends, but I have to be careful how much I talk to them because my husband thinks that all we do is bash him behind his back. So that leaves the sessions that we have here.

THERAPIST: And up to this point, here in session with me, you have experienced the warmth and kindness that you feel have been missing from your life? [*This question further reinforces the link between the possible rupture in the therapeutic relationship and the emotional deprivation schema.*]

CLIENT: Yeah, I have. I can't tell you how nice it's been.

THERAPIST: And now?

CLIENT: Less so. [pausing]

THERAPIST: I appreciate your honesty. [pausing] I'm wondering if you have been operating under the assumption that others will not provide warmth and nurturance. And, you experienced a bit of that in here over the course of our sessions, but when I didn't read the emails, it brought you right back to that place of not expecting such positivity from those you trust the most.

CLIENT: That's exactly what happened. I'm so beaten down by my husband. And, like I said, my family. [sighing] My family is there for me, I know they are, but in more of a stoic type of way, rather than an emotional sort of way.

THERAPIST: What can you conclude from all of this, that has just happened in here between us, today? [*The therapist asks this question to consolidate meaningful learning from this experience in the therapeutic relationship to have relevance to her emotional deprivation schema.*]

CLIENT: [chuckling] I guess I have some issues!

THERAPIST: Well, to be fair, we all have "issues." What I'm wondering is if something was easily activated in you, and it was easy to draw conclusions based on whatever that was, which was activated?

CLIENT: No, absolutely, I think that is right on target. I've gone without emotional support for so long, it's pretty much how I experience the world, how I expect it to be. Therapy is different. It's been so nice, actually, to have someone really listen to me, to really show that they care, to really want to hear what I am feeling.

THERAPIST: What does this experience with me, right here today, show you?

CLIENT: [sighing] That it is really easy for me to go down the road of concluding that just because a person draws a boundary with me, it does not mean that they aren't trying to help me or that they don't care. I'm so starved for emotional connection that it's really easy to set myself up for disappointment if it feels like I am not getting it. But I have to see that I really am still getting it.

THERAPIST: That's an important insight. And to be fair, I think the current state of your marriage, which is so filled with tension and conflict, makes the situation ripe for you to feel as if you're not getting emotional needs met in other contexts. But, that's part of the goal of our work together—to find ways to get your emotional needs met, to view others' provision of emotional support, or lack thereof, in a balanced manner, and to be able to meet some of your own emotional needs.

CLIENT: That is exactly what I'm hoping to get out of our therapy experience together.

The client's expression of "I'm really all alone here" was a pivotal point in this dialogue. It reflected significant vulnerability that she was experiencing within the context of her current life situation. This statement could have been indicative of a number of maladaptive schemas, including the abandonment/instability schema and the social isolation/alienation schema. The therapist linked this statement to an emotional deprivation schema on the basis of what she had known about the client to this point in the course of therapy. The client actually had a supportive, involved family-of-origin (albeit one in which it was uncommon to show much emotion), as well as friends who were interested and who provided camaraderie. The therapist knew that the client was struggling with the accumulation of years of coldness and emotional abuse by her husband, which had solidified her emotional deprivation schema. This schema was perpetually activated due to ongoing tension and conflict in the marriage, so it created a ripe context for the client to interpret the therapist as withholding emotional support. Fortunately, the therapist was inviting and nondefensive as she examined this notion with the client, and the client was able to use this experience to develop a keen awareness of just how powerfully her emotional deprivation schema operated in her life.

Activation of the Subjugation Schema

Clients with a subjugation schema operate according to the belief that the needs and opinions of others are more important than their own needs and opinions. Cognitions associated with a subjugation schema include the following: (a) "My needs and opinions are silly or insubstantial," (b) "I would be inconveniencing others if I communicate my needs and opinions," (c) "Others might get offended if I express my needs and opinions," (d) "I might be rejected if I express my needs and opinions," and (e) "I don't deserve to have needs and opinions." As a result, clients characterized by a subjugation schema usually defer to others to make decisions and refrain from speaking up if there is something about the needs and opinions of others that makes them uncomfortable or that does not sit right with them.

Many therapists find the experience of working with clients characterized by a subjugation schema to be pleasing, as they present as low maintenance. The profile of a client with a subjugation schema is one of a client who faithfully keeps their appointment, is ready to begin the session on time, pays for their session at the time the session is held without hassle, completes their between-session therapy homework, and does not make excessive demands on the therapist. Such clients can be a welcomed break from many other clients who have many needs that must be attended to in between sessions.

However, we, as therapists, must be alert to the possibility that we are inadvertently reinforcing these clients' subjugation schema with subtle complicity. Clients characterized by a subjugation schema can also pull therapists into an excessive caretaking role, which does not help these clients to develop assertiveness in expressing their own needs and opinions (versus waiting for others to meet or express needs and opinions for them). Consider the following dialogue:

THERAPIST: For when would you like to schedule our next session?

CLIENT: Um, it would be great if we could meet again next week. But I know that you are in such high demand, so it's really okay if we have to wait.

THERAPIST: It looks like I only have two openings next week. One on Tuesday at 10:30, and the other on Thursday at 3:30.

CLIENT: Well, I know you have a lot of high school students who probably could really use the 3:30 time. So I'll take the 10:30, if that's okay with you.

THERAPIST: [admittedly feeling relieved that the client is interested in the 10:30 time slot, as that one is more difficult to fill, and simultaneously realizing that the client's subjugation schema is driving her choice of times and in need of further examination] If I'm remembering correctly, you're done with work around 3:00.

And there have been times when your manager has asked that you take a half day of sick leave when you have a session during work hours.

CLIENT: Oh, well, it's really okay. I have a few sick days left before the end of the year.

THERAPIST: Leslie, we're only in March. What would be the consequences if you were sick and had no sick days remaining?

CLIENT: I just wouldn't get paid that day . . . but it's really not that big of a deal.

THERAPIST: [leaning back in his chair and allowing space for the client to see the activation of her subjugation schema] What do you think is happening here, Leslie?

CLIENT: [looking sheepish] I know, I know. I'm accommodating your schedule and your other clients.

THERAPIST: What belief is associated with this accommodation in this instance?

CLIENT: I guess that the needs of the high school students on your caseload are more important than my needs. You know, it's so hard to be a high schooler these days. There is so much stress. Getting into college. Managing social media. Friend drama. You name it.

THERAPIST: It is true that the high schoolers on my caseload are experiencing a great deal of stress. However, you are really going through a lot right now as well. Help me understand how your needs are less important than theirs are.

CLIENT: [chewing on her fingernail] I don't know. I mean, I guess they aren't. But . . .

THERAPIST: [speaking gently] But what?

CLIENT: I'd just imagine that you are playing such an important role in shaping their lives, preparing them to go on to do great things. I'm a run-of-the-mill middle-aged woman who does data entry, nothing great at all. Who am I to take a prime appointment time slot?

THERAPIST: You've posed an interesting question . . . who are you to take a prime appointment time slot? One response to that question is a run-of-the-mill middle-aged woman who does data entry, nothing great at all. I'd like us to work toward crafting an alternative to that portrait, one that says that you're just as deserving as anyone because you're a human being with worth.

CLIENT: Why is it so hard for me to believe that I have as much worth as others?

THERAPIST: Although there is no definitive answer to that question, I believe that we have done some important legwork together to provide a context for that belief, as well as your behavioral tendency to subjugate your needs for the needs of others.

As an exercise in "acting as if" she has just as much importance as others, the client took the 3:30 time slot for the next week. Then, the therapist shared his case formulation with the client and invited the client to add to it and mold it in a way that fit with her lived experience of it. Throughout the remainder of the course of therapy, the therapist and client worked together to reshape fundamental beliefs that reinforced the subjugation schema, as well as to express her needs, even at times inconveniencing others, to gain practice with self-assertion and to realize that there were many more positive consequences than negative consequences in doing so. At the completion of therapy, the client laughed that her progress could be attributed to the therapist's refusal to accept her decision to have a session in the midst of a workday.

It should be acknowledged that it would have been much easier for the therapist to accept the client's offer to take the 10:30 time slot, as the therapist indeed anticipated that there would be much interest by other clients in assuming the later time slot. However, he realized that acquiescing to this suggestion would only serve to reinforce the client's maladaptive subjugation schema. By being flexible in his mindset about scheduling, the therapist implemented a pivotal intervention that helped the client seek other opportunities to live out a different way of being.

Activation of the Approval-Seeking/Recognition-Seeking Schema

Clients characterized by an approval-seeking/recognition-seeking schema often present in an opposite manner as clients characterized by a subjugation schema. Whereas clients characterized by a subjugation schema often appear timid and wish very much not to be the center of attention, clients characterized by an approval-seeking/recognition-seeking schema usually want to stand out from the crowd and be celebrated for their accomplishments and status. A core belief associated with this schema is that a person's worth is based on the approval and recognition of others. In some cases, this belief is shaped by a corresponding set of beliefs associated with low self-worth, such as a defectiveness/shame schema. In other cases, this belief is shaped by a narcissistic, entitlement/grandiosity schema. In either case, it is important for therapists to be aware of the presence of this schema so that they do not unintentionally reinforce it with positive praise, and also so that the excessive seeking of approval and recognition does not sidetrack the therapeutic work that is being pursued.

Consider the following excerpt from a first session with a male client with bipolar disorder. He presented for treatment following his divorce, and at the time of the session, he had little contact with his two young adult children. He had a history of unstable employment, jumping from one job opportunity to the next, with many of these opportunities ending abruptly after he made an impulsive and detrimental decision on the job or had a falling-out with a supervisor. However, the client truly considered himself an artist, and he took pride in the website displaying his work, as well as the feedback he received when he displayed his work at local art shows. He was eager to begin treatment in order to develop an approach to reestablishing a relationship with his adult children, repairing a relationship with a postdivorce adult girlfriend, and gathering evidence from a professional that his bipolar disorder was mild and successfully managed so that he could tell close others in his life that "nothing is wrong with him." Observe the manner in which the therapist maintains boundaries and manages the approval-seeking/recognition-seeking schema, all while balancing the development of a strong therapeutic relationship.

CLIENT: They say I have bipolar disorder. I don't really know if I do. It seems a bit extreme to me. But even if I do, that's not the root of all problems with my ex and my kids. And even my new girlfriend. They are all convinced that I am the problem . . . I don't know, maybe I am . . . but I think they blame too much on bipolar disorder, when I'm not even really sure that I have it.

THERAPIST: In light of what you just shared, what are you hoping to obtain from our work together?

CLIENT: I miss my kids, that's for sure. And I want to get my ex and my girlfriend off my back about the bipolar business. For two women who despise each other, they are really tag-teaming it and demanding that I get help that I don't think I need. Now don't get me wrong, I want to be here in therapy. But I don't think it's any sort of bipolar disorder that is the problem. I think they don't understand me. And I want to start seeing my kids more. I need help with that, Doc.

THERAPIST: It sounds to me that you'd like to focus on improving these close relationships through work in therapy.

CLIENT: Yeah, yeah definitely. And I want you to tell me once and for all if I'm bipolar. And if I'm not, my ex and my girlfriend need to hear that so that they can stop blaming all of our problems on me. Because, honestly, Doc, they have just as many problems as I do, if not more.

THERAPIST: An accurate diagnosis always helps to facilitate treatment planning, so as part of our appointment today, we can conduct a diagnostic assessment. Once we see where you fall diagnostically, we can refine our goals accordingly, and you'll have a better sense of any impact that your mental health diagnosis has on your relationships.

CLIENT: Okay, that sounds great, Doc, really great. Because I think you're going to see that I have a lot of things going for me. I told you before that I'm an artist, right? My work gets featured in major media outlets. *The Philadelphia Inquirer* did a whole story on me. Oh yeah, I told you that. Did you look up the article, like I had suggested last week when we talked on the phone? Did you look at my website? What did you think? This is going to be really important you know, so that you can really understand who I am.

THERAPIST: I'm really glad we're revisiting these requests. As I mentioned briefly on the phone, I actually do not devote time to researching my clients on the internet, especially before I have established a relationship with them. [Client looks surprised] The reason for this is to maintain appropriate professional boundaries. The foundation of our therapeutic relationship is the information that you share with me in session, and I want to give you, and all of my clients, the respect of forming opinions about your case on the basis of our back-and-forth collaboration rather than third-party information or outdated information found on the internet. This is the way that I conduct business across the board, no matter who the client is and whether or not they've received a great deal of attention in media outlets or on the internet.

CLIENT: Yeah, yeah, that makes sense, and I appreciate that. But I told you that I wanted you to check this stuff out.

THERAPIST: [noticing her muscles in her body stiffening] I do hear what you are saying, and I know how important your artwork is to you.

In fact, during the course of our work together, I'm happy for you to pick and choose images of your artwork to share with me in session as appropriate for our therapeutic goals. [using self-disclosure selectively] Personally, I very much enjoy viewing and creating art, so I'm eager to determine if there is an appropriate role for your artwork in session. But it's important that the viewing of your artwork occurs for a therapeutic purpose once we have established our therapeutic agreement and goals.

CLIENT: Huh. Well, okay. I think you're going to see, though, that you're working with someone really special. Probably much more special than the Average Joe who comes in here for therapy.

THERAPIST: [sitting back and reflecting for a moment, taking care to continue to provide warmth in the face of this bold statement, as well as by making a mild intervention to begin shaping the client's approval-seeking/recognition-seeking and entitlement/grandiosity schemas] One aspect of this job that is so fulfilling is to find and be present with the specialness in all of my clients. Each one of you has such admirable strengths and talents. And it's a true privilege, for all of you, to be able to recognize those and work them into therapy.

CLIENT: I like how you think, Doc. This is exactly what I was hoping for. I knew I wanted a strong therapist who tells it like it is. I appreciate that. I'm a tell-it-like-it-is guy, too.

The therapist in this scenario was struck by the client's persistence in making the unorthodox request for the therapist to search for his name and work on the internet. Moreover, she clearly noted the client's tendency to refer to himself as special and to assert confidence that she would come to that conclusion as well. The therapist's first reaction was to be a bit put off by his brazenness, as it reminded her of the occasional colleagues she had had throughout the years who she viewed as inappropriately self-promoting. She quickly recognized her tendency to shut down in the face of those colleagues, refraining from giving them positive feedback even when it was warranted and steering clear of them even when there would good reasons to maintain strong working relationships. On the basis of this awareness, the therapist realized that it would be detrimental to the therapeutic relationship, and inappropriate as a mental health professional, to respond in this manner. She made a mental note to call attention to this case and her reactions to her client in supervision.

In the meantime, the therapist overcame her initial reaction—her stiffening muscles, which likely would have led to a less warm and inviting stance with the client—by viewing this interaction as an opportunity to model appropriate boundary setting with someone who likely needed some help understanding boundaries and appropriate behavior. She also took care to acknowledge what seemed to be a great strength of the client's—his artistic ability—while, at the same time, gently reshaping the notion that he must be acknowledged as special and more special than the clients who she typically sees in session. She maintained a positive, strengths-based attitude to which the client readily responded. Although in this early phase of treatment, he very well might not have "caught" the subtle message that the therapist views all of her clients as special, at the end of the dialogue, there was evidence that the therapeutic relationship was developing when the client observed that they have similar styles and that her style was a match for what he was looking for in therapy.

Activation of Defectiveness/Shame Schema

The defectiveness/shame schema could be the most common maladaptive schema seen in my own clinical practice. However, the fact that it is commonly seen in clinical practice does not mean that it is associated with a mild or straightforward clinical presentation. As mentioned previously, the defectiveness/shame schema is one of the most painful schemas for clients to acknowledge, as it is often associated with a sense of worthlessness, hopelessness, and burdensomeness. In particular, the defectiveness/shame schema often characterizes clients with chronic, recurrent, and/or treatment-resistant depression.

I end this chapter with an illustration of the use of the therapeutic relationship in reshaping Sarah's defectiveness/shame schema. As mentioned previously, the seeds of this schema were planted when Sarah perceived rejection by her parents, beginning with their negative judgments about her appearance, behavior, and choice of friends and ending with them saying that she could no longer live in their household while she was still in high school. This schema was reinforced by the eventual ending of her high school romantic relationship, continued estrangement from her parents, the ending of some close female friendships, and, as her appearance became more colorful and outside the norm, strangers' negative reactions to her. The depth of this schema had reached a new level at the time she presented for treatment, when the man with whom she had been living abruptly left her to marry another woman.

The following excerpt takes place well into the course of treatment. To this point, Sarah had become proficient in cognitive restructuring to soften unhelpful thoughts that affected her emotional response in particular situations. She had become significantly more adept at social problem solving and the delivery of assertive, confident communication. Moreover, she had negotiated a sensitive situation with her husband, such that she had worked with him to finally decide to end their marriage. She had arrived at a place of acceptance that neither of these relationships had worked out. Although she was functioning much better in her daily life than she had been at the commencement of treatment and her depression and anxiety ratings were consistently down in the mild range, she continued to struggle with the shame associated with defectiveness and perceived rejection. In this dialogue, the therapist reflects on their therapeutic relationship for healing in a limited reparenting capacity.

THERAPIST: Sarah, you seem more down today than I've seen you in some time.

SARAH: No, you're right. Today is a bit of a struggle. [sighing and leaning back into the couch] Nothing really happened. If anything, things are going a lot better now. I don't know . . . it's just, just . . . this sense that something will always be wrong with me. That I will never be enough, always a disappointment. It's tough to shake.

THERAPIST: In light of our CBT work together, how can you understand that felt sense?

SARAH: That there's a reason why I feel this way. I mean, not everyone gets kicked out of their own home when they are still in high school. And I know, intellectually, that that says just as much about my parents, if not more about my parents, than it does about me. But still . . . just because we can explain it away by poor parenting doesn't mean that it did not do damage.

THERAPIST: I do appreciate that. It's a part of your history, a part that shaped your very identity, that will always be there.

SARAH: Thank you for acknowledging that. Sometimes, in the past, I've taken comments from other therapists to say that I should get over it and move on.

THERAPIST: What does it mean to you when you receive that message from other therapists?

SARAH: It's almost like they are siding with my parents. Whether or not it was a therapist I had when I was in high school, who knew my parents, or a therapist I had after high school, who did not know my parents. It's like all of them are saying, "Sarah, you're the one with the problem. You're the one who is flawed. Defective." Just like you and I pointed out as one of my core issues. Defectiveness.

THERAPIST: But your experience here has been different.

SARAH: Oh my gosh, yes. In here, I am validated as a human being. And not that you think I'm perfect. I know you don't. You've really helped me to see some areas where I could improve. But I don't feel ashamed when I tell you I messed something up. You help me with whatever I messed up, but you don't tell me that it means something bad about my character. [becoming tearful] God, if my own parents would have done that, I wouldn't have the mental health struggles that I do.

THERAPIST: Tell me the message that you get, here in therapy, when you mess up.

SARAH: That messing up is normal. Everyone does it. And instead of being something bad, it can be a learning opportunity. And that you can still be a good, decent human being even if you mess up.

THERAPIST: [pausing] How powerful those statements are, Sarah! [pausing again] I wonder what it would be like, moving forward, to operate from that mindset, rather than a mindset of defectiveness?

SARAH: [sniffing] Honestly, I think I've already started to do that. [chuckling] Don't laugh at me, but sometimes if I make a mistake, I hear your voice saying part of that.

THERAPIST: I wouldn't laugh at all, Sarah. That is the ultimate compliment about our work together. I want to be sure, though, that you give yourself credit for thinking of that all on your own when you need it, when you're not in session.

Throughout the course of their work together, the therapist took care to provide validation to Sarah, even when it appeared that she was approaching a situation with an inaccurate or an unhelpful mindset, or when she made a choice that ultimately caused difficulty for her. The main message that the therapist attempted to communicate was, "You have worth, you have strengths, and you have something to offer." From this dialogue, it appears that Sarah internalized this message. Although the negative messages that she received from her parents would not be eradicated, they are now being balanced by the validation and beneficence that she experienced in therapy.

It was hoped that Sarah would carry forward these new messages, even when she was no longer in treatment with the therapist.

CONCLUSION AND FUTURE DIRECTIONS

A strong therapeutic relationship is especially essential for schema modification for a number of reasons. First, the specific nature of a maladaptive schema takes time to discover and then modify, and its contents are often painful and associated with embarrassment and shame. A trusting therapeutic relationship will create a safe space for clients to face these schemas and ultimately consider a new way of interacting with the world. Second, most clients experience and express significant affect during schema work. Congruence between the client's affective experiencing and the therapist's ability to be present with the emotion can be a powerful experience for the client, such that they are accepted as they are even as they face their darkest beliefs about themselves and the world. Third, limited reparenting can provide a life-changing corrective learning experience that shows clients that they deserve acceptance, nurturance, and positive regard from others.

Clients and therapists alike often report significant closeness as they undergo schema modification. It is powerful work that often makes a profound difference in the client's life, and that can have implications for the therapist's life as well when it elicits therapists' own schemas or when therapists are witness to substantial change and healing. Although schema modification work can be extremely difficult—emotionally, relationally, and intellectually—many therapists and clients view it as some of the most gratifying work on which they embark in their lives.

As I have hypothesized in other chapters in this volume about other cognitive behavioral intervention strategies, I expect that the strength and quality of the therapeutic relationship would enhance outcome in schema-focused CBT. From a more specific standpoint, it would be helpful to know which specific aspects of the therapeutic relationship contribute most to the optimization of empathic confrontation and limited reparenting, two central principles of schema therapy. Moreover, given the central role of these constructs in the theoretical underpinnings of schema therapy and its subsequent clinical delivery, it is important to know the percentage of variance that each contributes to good outcome. In addition, I contend that transference and countertransference would manifest more frequently, and would play a greater role, when cognitive behavioral therapists focus on schema modification versus when they deliver some of the other strategies described in this volume. However, that is an empirical question to be tested in future research. Finally, it would be helpful to know which aspects of the therapeutic relationship account for the greatest percentage of variance in outcome as a function of the particular early maladaptive schema being treated, as knowing this would help guide cognitive behavioral therapists in their focus on therapeutic relationship development.

A focus on schema modification is often assumed after the therapist and client have firmly established a therapeutic relationship and after the client has developed a foundation of cognitive behavioral principles and strategies for addressing current stressors in their lives (Wenzel, 2012). I expect that clients who are characterized by one or more maladaptive schemas will experience the greatest change in CBT when these schemas are modified in treatment. When successful schema modification occurs, clients are often ready to move toward a reduction in the frequency of sessions or the ending of treatment. In the next chapter, I consider therapeutic relationship issues that can arise with the ending of treatment.

9

THE ENDING OF TREATMENT AND THE THERAPEUTIC RELATIONSHIP

Cognitive behavioral therapy (CBT) is a time-sensitive psychotherapy, meaning that clients understand at the commencement of treatment that it will not go on indefinitely. Indeed, many cognitive behavioral therapists observe that some of the most powerful cognitive behavioral work takes place after treatment has ended. Understandably, the ending of treatment can activate strong reactions in both clients and therapists. In the literature on supportive-expressive psychodynamic treatment, it has observed that some clients even have a temporary regression when they experience a separation from the therapist as representing a difficult separation from their past (Ben David-Sela et al., 2020; Nof et al., 2017). Such observations suggest that it would behoove cognitive behavioral therapists to be especially in tune with their clients' needs and the therapeutic relationship as the ending of treatment nears. Therapeutic relationship-focused CBT (TRF-CBT) provides a foundation for cognitive behavioral therapists to do just this. In this chapter, I provide suggestions for using aspects of the therapeutic relationship to facilitate a successful ending of treatment. In addition, I highlight issues within the therapeutic relationship that might arise when the course of therapy is coming to a close.

https://doi.org/10.1037/0000424-010
Therapeutic Relationship-Focused Cognitive Behavioral Therapy, by A. Wenzel

It is important for therapists to be mindful of the fact that the real relationship between the therapist and client can be particularly salient as treatment is nearing its end. According to Charles Gelso (2011),

> The explicit ending of a good relationship almost requires us to come forth with each other as human beings. After all, although the psychotherapy participants have played out their roles as therapist and patient throughout treatment, they are indeed two human beings whose engagement in these roles is coming to an end. Indelibly left are their humanness and their human experience of the ending of their relationship. (p. 100)

Thus, as treatment comes to a close, therapists are encouraged to be mindful of this opportunity to be especially "human" and comment on their thoughts and feelings about the client when they are genuinely moved to do so.

As shown in the chapters on clinical guidance for the practice of TRF-CBT in Part II of this volume, movement toward the ending of treatment can be handled with a lesser or a greater focus on the therapeutic relationship. In my experience, mindful attention given to the therapeutic relationship in the late stage of therapy creates an opportunity for the therapist and client to share in heartfelt, meaningful reflection on the course of therapy. Consider the differences in the following excerpts.

Excerpt 1: Less Focus on the Therapeutic Relationship

CLIENT: It's hard to believe that this is our last session. I'm in such a different place than I was when I first came to see you.

THERAPIST: You have made such a transformation. [focusing on the consolidation of learning] Tell me what take-home messages you are leaving with.

CLIENT: Well . . . it really helps to know when I am falling into one of those thinking traps, those distortions. It saves me a lot of unnecessary agita when I can slow down and look at a situation based on the facts, rather than getting so stuck in my head. And you really helped me with some of my social skills. I am much more able to speak up in meetings and bring tricky issues to the attention of my manager than I used to be.

THERAPIST: I agree that you made tremendous strides in both of those areas—the cognitive piece of CBT, as well as your capacity for interpersonal effectiveness.

CLIENT: [averting eye contact, voice wavering a bit] I don't know, though, I think I'm going to miss these sessions as well.

THERAPIST: That's a natural reaction to the ending of therapy. Just don't forget to focus on all that you have gotten from it.

CLIENT: Yeah. Yeah, you're right. There it was again, my tendency to focus on the negative.

The cognitive behavioral therapist in this excerpt was mindful of three cognitive behavioral strategies in this conversation. First, he focused on the consolidation of learning so that the client would leave the session with tangible CBT principles that will continue to serve the client after therapy has ended. Second, he normalized the client's reaction about missing therapy so that the client would not attach unnecessary negativity to this reaction. Third, the therapist reminded the client that he had gained a great deal from therapy as a way to balance the client's prediction that he would miss sessions. Although all of this constitutes "good" CBT, the therapist missed an opportunity for warmer, more mutual and heartfelt reflection on the course of therapy and the therapeutic relationship, which could have the power to be a meaningful experience that both the client and therapist could carry forward in their lives. Consider the next excerpt, in which the therapeutic relationship plays a more central role in the consolidation of learning and movement toward the end of therapy.

Excerpt 2: More Focus on the Therapeutic Relationship

CLIENT: It's hard to believe that this is our last session. I'm in such a different place than I was when I first came to see you.

THERAPIST: You have made such a transformation. [making a statement to share in the emotional experience of the ending of therapy] And I agree, it is hard to believe that this is our last session.

CLIENT: [averting eye contact, voice wavering a bit] I don't know, though, I think I'm going to miss these sessions as well.

THERAPIST: That's a natural reaction to the ending of therapy. Honestly, I'm also feeling like I will miss our weekly sessions. I have come to very much look forward to our Tuesdays at 12:30 together. [*The therapist expresses this genuine sentiment to honor the real relationship that developed between them.*]

CLIENT: [expressing a sigh of relief] I'm really glad you told me that. I was starting to wonder if I am being a bit weak here, you know, or that I can't really be this version of myself without therapy.

THERAPIST: What was it, about our work together, that has given you confidence about being this version of yourself?

CLIENT: You really armed me with a lot of knowledge, you know, knowledge about how our thinking can affect how we feel, ways to understand what traps I might be falling into, ways to negotiate tricky interpersonal situations. But, at the same time, you let me absorb that knowledge in my own way, and you listened to me and gave me space as I figured out how to make it work in my own life. [pausing] Honestly, I haven't had this sort of figure in my life before. Almost like a spirit guide. My parents, they were so controlling, they just tried to tell me how to think and what to do. Same with bosses I have had in my work life. But this . . . this just felt so much more respectful. And I was given the benefit of the doubt that I would figure it out and be okay. You had confidence in me every step of the way, which I don't think I've experienced quite like this before.

THERAPIST: And so the confidence that you felt from me contributed to your own confidence?

CLIENT: Yeah. Yeah, exactly. It was really a win-win. Either I was able to put the CBT into action, or when it didn't quite work out the way that we expected it to, there was confidence that we could learn from it and try again.

THERAPIST: And this is different than what you have experienced in other contexts before.

CLIENT: Oh definitely. I think I told you this, but it took me a long time to even convince myself to start therapy because I assumed that it would be a lot of you telling me everything I was doing wrong.

THERAPIST: [smiling warmly] Well, I'm certainly pleased to hear that you had a different experience here. [pausing] How can you carry this forward, this confidence-boosting experience you've had in therapy?

CLIENT: You have said all along that CBT is not really just doing a bunch of exercises, that instead it is a way of life. So I'm going to continue to live out that way of life so that I can keep seeing the positive effects in my life. [Therapist nods and smiles] But I also think there is something else. This whole experience has taught me that I don't have to have a bunch of toxic people in my life who are unsupportive and try to get me to live according to their agenda. I need to seek out people who are more supportive, less judgmental.

THERAPIST: And now you know what that feels like.

CLIENT: Yes! Now I know what that feels like. It's been transformative, really. And I thank you for that.

The dialogue in the second excerpt diverged from the first when the therapist normalized the client's emotional reaction to wondering if he would miss the sessions. Instead of suggesting that the client focus on all he has gotten from his therapy experience, the therapist in the second excerpt shared the experience of anticipating that he would also miss the sessions. He embraced the client's emotional reaction to a greater degree, which opened room for the client to express his doubts about his ability to maintain his gains. Not only did this conversation then lead to the consolidation of learning, but it was done so in the context of reflecting on the way in which the therapeutic relationship contributed to these gains. Through this reflection, the client realized that the therapy experience reset his expectations for the types of relationships he would like in his life. Moreover, this dialogue left space for the client and therapist to express heartfelt sentiments about the meaning that their therapeutic work held for each of them.

TIPS FOR ENDING TREATMENT THROUGH THE LENS OF THE THERAPEUTIC RELATIONSHIP

It is important to honor and respect the focused effort that clients have invested into the course of therapy, as well as the vulnerability that the client has entrusted to the therapist. Although it is important for the therapist to communicate this honor and respect throughout the course of treatment, there is the opportunity to make this message explicit as therapy comes to a close and to use it in a way that brings together the gains the client has achieved. It is hoped that the client will leave treatment with a positive view of therapy, considering it a worthwhile endeavor that was not only productive but that also provided a sense of understanding and of being heard that was curative in and of itself. Therapists are mindful of this as they address the three main components of ending therapy: (a) looking back (i.e., reflecting on what has been learned), (b) saying good-bye, and (c) looking forward (i.e., applying the learning to future relationships; Marx & Gelso, 1987). The following are five specific suggestions for minding the therapeutic relationship as the course of CBT is coming to a close.

Tip 1: Anticipate the Ending of Therapy as Therapy Commences

This suggestion—to anticipate the ending of therapy as therapy commences— might sound odd. However, it is important to keep in mind that CBT was developed as a short-term, time-limited psychotherapy so that clients could observe meaningful changes in their lives without the anticipation of participating in a seemingly endless number of sessions. Over time, the CBT community has begun to refer to CBT as being "time sensitive" rather than "time limited," to account for the fact that courses of CBT might be somewhat lengthy for complicated clinical presentations (J. S. Beck, 2021). Nevertheless, it is understood that there is an eventual end to courses of CBT. It is respectful and helpful when therapists make this aspect of CBT clear to the client, so that the client enters into the therapy contract with the overt knowledge that there will be an end to therapy and that they can anticipate it as they work through the stages of therapy. From a different standpoint, it can be said that the ending of treatment is likely to be less effective if it is introduced abruptly without time for the client to process it (Okamoto et al., 2019).

Many clients seek out CBT precisely because of its time-sensitive nature. They are hoping to find an active approach to treatment in which there is a possibility of experiencing great gains in a reasonable period of time. Psychotherapy is a great investment of time, effort, money, and sometimes other resources (e.g., childcare), so it is important for therapists to communicate respect of clients' investment and commit to bringing a level of expertise that will maximize the degree to which clients address the issues that brought them to therapy. In fact, a long-standing joke in the CBT community is that cognitive behavioral therapists want to put themselves out of business by teaching their clients how to become their own cognitive behavioral therapists. I find that sharing this sentiment with new clients brings a bit of levity to the beginning of the therapy process and demonstrates a commitment to productivity and excellence—all of which go a long way in establishing a strong therapeutic relationship.

Tip 2: Collaborate on Deciding to End Treatment

Although clients are socialized into the idea from the outset that there will be an end to therapy, unless the client is participating in a research study or an insurance plan in which a set number of sessions has been preplanned, in most cases the ending of treatment is determined as therapy progresses. Factors influencing the decision to move toward the ending of treatment include the following:

- The client supplies low quantitative ratings of symptoms during the mood check for several consecutive sessions.

- The client has demonstrated the ability to implement CBT principles and strategies in their life outside of session.
- The problems that the client had hoped to address in therapy have largely resolved, and the client has met their goals for treatment.
- The client begins to present for session with little material for the agenda.

The decision to end treatment is not simply sprung on the client at the will of the therapist. In the spirit of collaboration and respecting the client's input, when there are no external constraints determining the number of sessions that will occur, it is important for the client and therapist to make the decision to end treatment together. This approach to the ending of treatment reinforces that the client is an important member of the team and that their viewpoint, wishes, and preferences are valued.

Even when both parties agree that the client's symptoms have remitted, that the client's goals have been met, and that the principles and strategies of CBT have generalized to the client's life outside of session, therapy typically does not end abruptly in that same session. Rather, the client schedules at least one more session, often a few more sessions, perhaps further spread out over time. Between-session work can consist of reflecting on what was learned in CBT, perhaps compiled into a resource that can be consulted after therapy has ended. I once was ending therapy with a client due to an external constraint—the ending of my time at a particular organization—and he compiled an "operating" manual that summarized the CBT strategies that we had practiced in session and his view of the types of situations that would be best suited for the implementation of these strategies.

There are instances when clients meet the "criteria" listed earlier to end treatment, but they, nevertheless, express a desire to continue with therapy. Of course, it is important to detect whether there are forces at work that would be contraindicated to the continuation of treatment, such as avoidance of living life without the support of therapy and/or dependency on the therapist. Even if one of these contraindicated forces is at work, the therapist does not simply overrule the client and dictate that therapy is coming to an end. Rather, additional sessions are scheduled so that there is ample time for clients to work through these forces and apply the cognitive behavioral principles and strategies that they have learned to resolve them.

In my experience, there are two, more common reasons why clients request to continue with therapy even when they have met their goals, and they often work in concert. First, many clients come to value the therapeutic relationship and the curative factors themselves that are evident in a strong therapeutic relationship. In other words, they express a desire to continue with psychotherapy precisely because of the rich experience that the therapeutic relationship offers them. Second, many clients come to realize that there are additional goals on which they would like to focus. I have observed a phenomenon in which clients first present for treatment when things are not going well in their lives and they are not functioning as well as they typically do. During the course of CBT, they steadily approach their pretherapy baseline level of functioning. It is at that point that they wish to shift their pretherapy baseline level of functioning higher, and they view a continuation of CBT as a way to do so. In these instances, we collaboratively identify new goals for treatment, and we continue our work in the spirit of optimizing their well-being, bringing it to greater heights than they had imagined when they first sought out therapy. Thus, although CBT is generally known and conducted as a time-sensitive treatment, there are many instances in which CBT follows a longer-term course (1 year or more), and this often stems from the foundation of a strong, collaborative, and productive therapeutic relationship in which both parties are working actively toward the client's personal optimization.

Tip 3: Validate Mixed Feelings

As evidenced in the excerpts presented in the first section of this chapter, it is natural for clients to have mixed feelings about the ending of treatment. On the one hand, it is hoped that they can bask in the accomplishments that they have achieved by integrating the principles and tools of CBT into their lives, and they can look toward the future with hope, optimism, and confidence. On the other hand, they could express some trepidation about the ending of therapy due to concern about continued success without the support of therapy or to simply missing the connection that they felt with their therapist. All of these responses are natural and are commonly experienced in the late phase of CBT.

It is here that there is an opportunity for the therapist to engage with the client in the emotional experience of ending therapy in a genuine manner, putting their real relationship first and foremost. The client will see that the therapist is heartfelt in their connection with the client; as a result, the client's emotional experience will be validated, and the client will feel valued within the relationship. This serves as another important corrective learning experience, particularly for clients who report a history of abuse, bullying, rejection, and/or invalidation by close others.

Tip 4: Reflect Fondly

Along with the validation and sharing of mixed feelings about the ending of therapy is the opportunity to reflect fondly on the accomplishments and poignant moments that took place during the course of therapy. The question asked in the first excerpt earlier in this chapter can facilitate such reflection (i.e., "Tell me what take-home messages you are leaving with"). This prompt certainly facilitates the consolidation of learning, such that the client has the opportunity to put their own language onto the principles and strategies they have learned, which increases the likelihood that they can access them in times of need after therapy has ended (cf. Khattra et al., 2017; Macaulay et al., 2017). However, this question also usually leads to the client reflecting on what has been helpful and on the successes and achievements that they created for themselves during the course of therapy. Such reflection helps clients to leave treatment with a positive view of therapy and with warm feelings toward the therapeutic relationship.

This is also an opportunity for the therapist to demonstrate genuine fond reflection of the therapy process as well. It can certainly provide space to give the client credit for their accomplishments and successes. However, it can also create a space for appropriate intimacy that honors the closeness and the connection that has developed. I often share with clients what I admired about them as they applied the CBT principles and strategies, or I comment on the tremendous growth that they attained. Most clients are touched when the therapist reflects fondly in this manner, and it can serve as a gift that they can bring with them as they enter a new way of being in the world without regular psychotherapy.

Tip 5: Welcome "Tune-Ups"

The notion of the "booster session" has been a staple of CBT for decades (J. S. Beck, 2021; D. Dobson & Dobson, 2017). A booster session is scheduled awhile out after the final CBT session (e.g., 3 or 6 months later) so the client can check in and describe how they have been applying CBT principles and strategies in their lives when they are no longer attending regular psychotherapy sessions. Clients usually look forward to booster sessions in order to reconnect with their therapist, share how well they have been doing, and address any challenging issues that have arisen between sessions.

Some clients experience a recurrence or relapse of symptoms following the ending of treatment or, even in the absence of a recurrence or relapse, they encounter additional life challenges that would be appropriate to address in therapy. These clients sometimes contact their therapist to have what many of my clients have affectionately called a "tune-up" in CBT. Resumption of CBT services is not viewed as a treatment failure but rather as a treatment success, because these clients recognize the need for intervention before they are fully overcome by their symptoms or life challenges (O'Donohue & Cucciare, 2008). In fact, it has been posited that ongoing maintenance therapy (i.e., the occasional therapy session, such as monthly or bimonthly) is indicated for clients who struggle with recurrent mental health disorders (Stangier et al., 2013).

It is for these reasons that, as therapy is ending, I communicate to clients that I am always available if they would like a booster session or tune-up. Clients seem to appreciate this offer, not only for health maintenance reasons but also because it demonstrates that the therapist is interested in their well-being and in continuing a relationship with them if appropriate. On occasion, clients comment that just knowing that their therapist is available for a booster session or tune-up gives them the confidence to end therapy and practice living their lives without ongoing sessions.

THE ENDING OF TREATMENT IN THE CONTEXT OF THERAPEUTIC RELATIONSHIP ISSUES

Although the ending of treatment is built into the very fabric of CBT, there are occasions in which clients have a negative reaction to the ending of treatment. Such reactions can have a negative effect on the therapeutic relationship. Because treatment is ending, it is essential to repair the rupture in order to end the course of treatment on a hopeful, life-enhancing note. Three of the most common client reactions that can arise include worry about relapse, activation of an abandonment schema, and grief about the loss of regular contact with the therapist. Each reaction is discussed next.

Worry About Relapse

Clients with a history of anxiety and/or a low sense of self-efficacy are often concerned that they will experience a relapse if they no longer have the active support of a therapist in regularly scheduled psychotherapy sessions. It is hoped that, throughout the course of CBT, clients have demonstrated to themselves the ability to enact the principles and strategies of CBT outside of session (i.e., within the context of therapy "homework") and that these "success experiences" will instill confidence that they can handle the stressors and challenges that life throws them on their own, without the need for continued therapy. Nevertheless, the prospect of ending therapy could activate worry about relapse because clients are faced with a transition in which an important aspect of their life will now be different.

Fortunately, much can be done to prevent relapse. From a psychoeducation perspective, therapists can instill knowledge of relapse rates associated with CBT in their clients so that clients have an accurate, factual view of relapse rates after a successful course of CBT (Hollon et al., 2006). As mentioned in the previous section, the client can schedule booster sessions to monitor the maintenance of the gains made in treatment, or they can schedule a tune-up if it becomes clear that further professional help is needed. In addition, it is wise during the late stage of therapy to develop a *relapse prevention plan*. Although the precise components of a relapse prevention plan can vary depending on the client's needs and circumstances, it generally consists of the following: (a) warning signs that signal the possibility of a relapse; (b) strategies the client learned in CBT that they can implement actively to prevent relapse; (c) people who can provide support during periods of increased stress, symptomatology, and life challenges; and (d) indicators that they should contact their former therapist and schedule a tune-up (Wenzel, 2019).

Clients can also "cope ahead"—to borrow a term from Marsha Linehan's dialectical behavior therapy (Linehan, 2015)—to anticipate a relapse and walk themselves through how they would handle it. This technique is adapted from our CBT for suicide prevention approach (Wenzel et al., 2009), in which we encourage clients who have successfully acquired cognitive behavioral suicide prevention tools to imagine an event that, in the past, might have prompted a suicidal crisis and consider the ways in which they would apply what they learned in therapy to make a different choice than attempting suicide. The original technique was designed to make use of mental imagery, such that the client would describe in vivid detail both the events that were occurring in the crisis as well as the specific steps in the application of CBT tools. However, even if nonsuicidal clients are not necessarily identifying one particular event that would prompt a crisis, they can nevertheless describe in detail the CBT tools to which they would turn if they noticed an increase in symptoms or if they were in the midst of a new life challenge.

Having these sorts of precautions in place helps the client to feel confident in what has been learned in therapy as well as in the ending of treatment. Moreover, it instills the client's confidence in the therapist because the therapist is demonstrating a systematic and thorough approach to addressing the possibility of relapse. It also demonstrates that the therapist is taking seriously the client's concern about relapse and responding to their need to have a plan.

Activation of an Abandonment Schema

For some clients, it is not difficult to imagine that the abandonment/instability schema would be activated by the prospect of ending treatment, even if, logically, they know that they have been preparing for it and that their therapist will be available for tune-ups as needed. The ending of treatment can be viewed as an opportunity to put into action the wisdom cultivated from schema modification. Consider the following dialogue, in which the therapist draws on the previous work in treatment, life experience, and the client's inherent wisdom to work through the sense of abandonment prompted by the ending of treatment:

CLIENT: I'm so angry at myself! Why does this feel like abandonment? The whole purpose of CBT is to not be so reliant on therapy. I knew this! Ugh!

THERAPIST: [speaking gently] What is your best guess as to why this feels like abandonment? [*This question is aimed to help the client remember the case formulation of the way in which her abandonment schema developed.*]

CLIENT: I guess it does make sense, doesn't it? I mean, abandonment is my "thing," between my dad leaving and starting a new family, and my mom only being present some of the time due to all of her issues.

THERAPIST: Yes, exactly. [drawing on the self-compassion work they had done earlier in treatment] How could you view yourself in a more compassionate manner?

CLIENT: That is a good question. Um . . . that even though I've worked through a lot of my abandonment issues, it is natural that they would arise when an important relationship is coming to an end?

THERAPIST: [smiling warmly] That sounds like a big dose of self-compassion to me. How much do you believe it?

CLIENT: [sighing] I do believe it. A great deal. You're not abandoning me. It just feels like it because I will miss this, and when I more objectively was abandoned by others—my parents, various partners—I missed them as well.

THERAPIST: This is quite an astute insight. The feelings are similar, so it's easy to conclude that you are being abandoned.

CLIENT: [brightening] Yeah, I think it is. It's like that emotional reasoning trap that we talked about in some of our sessions.

Of course, not all clients will be as psychologically sophisticated when working through the activation of an abandonment schema—some will express anger at the therapist. In such cases, it is paramount that the therapist does not become defensive and attempt to convince the client that they are not being abandoned. A calm, reasoned stance can be particularly difficult to attain in light of the credo to which mental health providers adhere—that they will not abandon their clients. Thus, when clients accuse their therapists of abandoning them, it is conceivable that therapists will experience a host of alarms (e.g., being reported to a governing body for abandonment) as well as activation of their own schemas (e.g., failure). Therapists are encouraged to be aware of these cognitive and emotional reactions, apply cognitive restructuring and acceptance strategies for keeping these reactions in perspective and maintaining a helpful therapeutic stance, and tolerating the intensity of the emotion that the client might be expressing. Therapists who experience such a scenario can approach it as an opportunity for continued schema modification and (if necessary) rupture repair, being mindful of the research indicating that successful resolution of a rupture is associated with better outcome than had a rupture not occurred (e.g., Safran & Muran, 2000; Safran et al., 2001).

Grief Associated With the Loss of Regular Therapeutic Contact

In many instances, if there is a pronounced reaction to the end of treatment, it is not indicative of pathology or a rupture in the therapeutic alliance, but instead indicative of understandable grief associated with the loss of an important, consistent relationship. The therapeutic relationship is an indispensable relationship in the lives of many clients. Although most of these clients realize the significance of ending treatment and living their lives without the anticipation of regular therapy sessions, the ending of treatment can nevertheless evoke an emotional reaction. It is important to honor and respect the place that the therapeutic relationship holds for the client, as well as to share in the poignancy of the relationship in a genuine and authentic manner.

Sarah[1] was grappling with this issue of grief associated with loss when she came to the end of therapy. She had decided to move back to her hometown and move in with her close girlfriend from high school. She was able to get a transfer to serve as an assistant manager within the same restaurant franchise. Because Sarah had worked with the therapist in pre-COVID times, before the existence of PsyPACT (i.e., the Psychology Interjurisdictional Compact that allows the practice of telehealth and temporary face-to-face practice across state lines) that would enable them to continue their therapeutic relationship across state lines, she was unable to continue work with her therapist. The following dialogue illustrates how the therapist utilized congruence and genuineness to cultivate a heartfelt, meaningful ending to the course of therapy with Sarah.

SARAH: I can't believe it's finally here. I'm leaving in 3 days. Divorcing Carlos. Away from the friends I've made here . . . and away from therapy [becoming tearful].

---

[1]Client identity has been disguised to protect client confidentiality.

THERAPIST: [speaking in a way that demonstrates a genuine connection with Sarah] I can't tell you how meaningful it has been to see the way in which you've grown over the time we've spent together.

SARAH: [sniffing] No, I feel it too. Believe me, I'm going to take this experience with me for the rest of my life.

THERAPIST: I will take many pieces of this experience with me as well.

SARAH: I really appreciate that. I hope that my journey can somehow help others.

THERAPIST: I have no doubt that it will, Sarah. And know that our work also touched me personally, as well. [*This is a genuine statement that reflects the strength of the real relationship.*]

SARAH: [looking grateful] It did? Sometimes I wondered whether this is just a job to you . . . but when it came down to it, I knew better.

THERAPIST: [smiling warmly]

SARAH: There is so much that I got out of this experience . . . the skills, the tools. But I think the biggest thing I will take away is that I am no longer the mental patient. For most of my life, ever since middle school at least, I was told that the problem was me. That I was too eccentric, that I was too much of a troublemaker, that I didn't know how to handle stress. And you know what? I think I rose to that bar, and the bar was low. You showed me that the bar is higher. That I am not the mental patient. And that I don't have to respond like one. I can dig deep into my strengths, my skills, and the things I hold important, and I can weather the storms that come my way without self-harm, substance abuse, or anything that I was doing that was self-defeating.

Sarah was able to put words onto a significant core belief shift. She and her therapist worked with many interrelated schemas such as defectiveness/shame and rejection, and they ultimately arrived at the most apt description of the underlying belief with which Sarah presented for treatment—that she was the mental patient who was expected to respond to challenges with emotion dysregulation and self-defeating behavior. Through CBT, Sarah learned to view herself in a different manner: as someone who is resilient and who possesses many impressive strengths (but who certainly is not perfect and who does not always make good decisions), rather than as someone who is the "mental patient" (defective, dysfunctional, and without redemption).

When she began to adopt this new, more balanced schema, she began to make and enact decisions accordingly, and she made significant changes in her life after feeling stuck in her loveless marriage, in a job that she found unfulfilling, and in a location where she had always felt like an outsider. The heartfelt exchange between Sarah and the therapist in this final session solidified Sarah's gains, and it helped her to see how meaningful they were.

CONCLUSION AND FUTURE DIRECTIONS

The therapeutic relationship plays a central role in the ending of therapy for many reasons. The therapist skills described in Chapter 2 of this volume can facilitate an ending of therapy that is respectful of the myriad emotions that both clients and therapists experience as they move toward the end of their work together. Moreover, the ending of therapy can prompt therapeutic relationship-specific issues, such as the client's perception of abandonment. By this point in the course of treatment, a strong foundation of cognitive behavioral principles and strategies will have been established. The therapist can rely on that foundation to address potential ruptures in the therapeutic relationship that arise in the final sessions of treatment. It is hoped, again, as referenced throughout this volume, that if any therapeutic relationship-related issue arises, it will ultimately serve as a corrective learning experience that will have important implications for functioning in other important relationships in the client's life, outside of the therapy relationship. All of this is consistent with the primary tenets of TRF-CBT.

Most of the research on ruptures in the therapeutic alliance examines ruptures that occur in the middle phase of therapy. As has been summarized previously, that research suggests that the presence of ruptures that are successfully repaired is associated with better outcome in therapy than instances in which a rupture had never occurred. However, it would behoove researchers to confirm that this same association is evident when a rupture takes place in the late phase of treatment, as the client and therapist are moving toward the ending of treatment. In addition, it would be helpful for future research to examine what (beyond symptom reduction) constitutes a successful ending of treatment, and what aspects of the therapeutic relationship in the late phase of treatment are associated with a successful ending of treatment. Moreover, it would benefit the CBT community to identify whether there is an association between the strength of the therapeutic relationship at the end of treatment and the likelihood of returning for a booster session, as well as whether there is an association between the strength of the therapeutic relationship and usage of the strategies and tools acquired in CBT, which could, in turn, be associated with long-term outcome.

To this point in the volume, the reader has attained a sense of the setup, delivery, and ending of CBT with a focus on the therapeutic relationship. In the final chapter of this volume, the guidance for the practice of TRF-CBT is brought together, and a fresh perspective on the importance of the therapeutic relationship in CBT is presented.

CONCLUSION

A Fresh Perspective on the Therapeutic Relationship and Cognitive Behavioral Therapy

The cultivation and experiencing of connection in the therapeutic relationship is one of the most gratifying aspects of psychotherapy for clients and therapists alike. The authentic, spontaneous, and heartfelt interaction between a client and therapist is what brings the "art" to the "science" of psychotherapy. The relationship between a therapist and client is special, and I encourage therapists to honor it as such. After all, clients often share their darkest secrets, admit to their shameful moments, and display raw emotion when they are in session—and we, as therapists, are witnesses to it. From my perspective, there is no greater privilege than to be trusted with this manner of sharing and experiencing.

The main premise of this book is that the therapeutic relationship can very much play a central role in the process and outcome in cognitive behavioral therapy (CBT). I contend that the therapeutic relationship and its components play two roles in the successful delivery of CBT. First, I believe that the therapeutic relationship and its components set the stage of the delivery of specific cognitive behavioral strategies and techniques as a facilitator of change. In other words, I believe that CBT intervention strategies, such as cognitive restructuring, problem solving, exposure, schema modification,

https://doi.org/10.1037/0000424-011
Therapeutic Relationship-Focused Cognitive Behavioral Therapy, by A. Wenzel

and relapse prevention (among others), can be highly successful because clients are open to them in the context of a therapeutic relationship characterized by connection, warmth, empathy, and positive regard. Second, I believe that the therapeutic relationship and its components can serve as an agent of change in and of themselves when they are attended to and cultivated in a strategic, mindful way throughout the course of therapy. A strong therapeutic relationship can shift clients' beliefs about their worth in their interpersonal relationships, about the trustworthiness of others, and about the consequences of interpersonal vulnerability. A strong therapeutic relationship that weathers a rupture teaches clients that relationships need not end (and end badly) even when there is tension or disagreement. A strong therapeutic relationship provides the opportunity for clients to practice receiving support, encouragement, and wisdom. Moreover, a strong therapeutic relationship allows clients to practice behaviors that draw them close to others and allows others to see clients' authentic selves.

In the following sections, I consider the value of the ways in which the three components of the therapeutic relationship often referenced in the psychotherapy literature—the therapeutic alliance, transference and countertransference, and the real relationship—can enhance the practice of CBT. From this consideration, I propose a definition of the CBT therapeutic relationship. Then, I summarize the main suggestions that have emerged in this volume for conducting therapeutic relationship-focused CBT (TRF-CBT), utilizing the CBT framework within which cognitive behavioral therapists already practice and making TRF-CBT a client-centered approach to therapy. I close this chapter with some final words about the respect I hope I have shown to the power of the therapeutic relationship throughout this volume.

THE TRIPARTITE MODEL OF THE THERAPEUTIC RELATIONSHIP

The general framework I adopted in this book rests on the notion that there are three components of the therapeutic relationship—the therapeutic alliance, transference and countertransference, and the real relationship. I am far from convinced that this will be the way in which I view the therapeutic relationship in my future scholarship (e.g., see Wampold & Flückiger's [2023] innovative two-factor model that was published as I was finishing work on this volume). Nevertheless, for the purpose of this volume, I adopted this framework for two reasons. One reason was out of deference to the scholars and clinicians who dedicated their careers to the study and cultivation of the therapeutic relationship. I wanted to take special care to learn from these giants in the field of psychotherapy (e.g., Ralph Greenson, Carl Rogers, Charles Gelso, and even Sigmund Freud, himself) who advanced theory that served as the basis of scholarship and clinical practice for many decades. Second, I hoped to consider the way in which two of the constructs—transference and countertransference and the real relationship—can advance our understanding and use of the therapeutic relationship as an agent of change within CBT, as these constructs have, historically, received little attention in the CBT literature.

As mentioned throughout this volume, the therapeutic alliance is the component of the therapeutic relationship that has been considered most frequently in relation to CBT outcome. The therapeutic alliance essentially captures the essence of the collaborative working relationship between the client and therapist. In general, the strength of the therapeutic alliance correlates with post-treatment symptom reduction to a similar degree in CBT as it does in other approaches to psychotherapy. Innovative research by Webb et al. (2011), examining cognitive therapy for depression, suggests that agreement on the goals and tasks of therapy predicts outcome even when prior symptom change is controlled, whereas the therapeutic bond predicts outcome but not when prior symptom change is controlled. This intriguing pattern of results suggests that cognitive behavioral therapists should pay special attention to the agreement on the goals and tasks of therapy from the commencement of treatment, communicating (verbally and nonverbally) collaboration, respect, patience, competence, and hope. As time goes on and clients observe improvements in the issues that brought them to treatment, the bond naturally strengthens. I call on cognitive behavioral therapists to harness the power of the bond that develops as a result of early symptom change and use it as a foundation to give honest therapeutic feedback, suggest interventions that might push clients beyond their comfort zone, and experiment with creative interventions that are uniquely tailored to the client's personality, strengths, and life situation. Moreover, when a rupture in the therapeutic alliance is threatening or actually occurs, we know that its repair is associated with better outcome in CBT than would have been achieved had the rupture never occurred (Strauss et al., 2006), a pattern of results that is similar to what is obtained in the study of other types of therapy.

A strong therapeutic alliance is undoubtedly a facilitator of the successful delivery of cognitive behavioral interventions because both the client and therapist are focused on a particular goal and working in collaboration to achieve it. The goals of therapy are well-defined, and markers of progress will be clear to both parties. Moreover, being aligned in the work of therapy will build momentum and instill hope, so that specific cognitive behavioral interventions can build on one another. And yet, it can also be an agent of change, particularly in clients who struggle with collaborating with others, formulating goals, aligning those goals to tasks that would help to achieve them, and creating a bond with people with whom they are working toward the same goal. In these cases, the therapeutic alliance becomes an agent of change because it shows the client how to achieve these aims and gives them a dose of experiential learning in doing so. In other words, when clients have a deficit in their ability to engage in collaborative work to achieve goals in work or in life in general, a strong therapeutic alliance provides a game-changing corrective learning experience.

Much less is written about transference and countertransference in CBT, but as Gelso and Hayes (2007) aptly noted, these phenomena are present across all forms of psychotherapy. It is very true that the resolution of transference in clients is not a central goal in CBT. Nevertheless, I believe that transference and countertransference can play important roles in CBT and that cognitive behavioral therapists would be wise to recognize them when they occur. Take, for example, a situation in which a client acts out toward a therapist when the client perceives that the therapist is holding them to unreasonable standards, just as their parents did. A curious, nondefensive, and nonjudgmental therapist response in this case could provide a corrective, and even essential, learning experience for the client, resulting in powerful belief shifts about relationships (e.g., "I will not be punished if I act out and am not at my best." "Not everyone is as rigid as I experienced my parents as being." "When people encourage me to better myself, it is because they care and not because they expect me to meet their standard or expectation"). This learning experience would also provide a template for repairing relationships when there has been a misunderstanding. It would increase the client's awareness of their reactions toward others, outside of session, whom they believe hold them to high standards and might eventually prevent them from "blowing up" in a way that would damage the relationship. Moreover, it would provide evidence that a relationship is not necessarily "ruined" if the client has acted out in session due to false assumptions. The opportunity for this transference reaction to occur serves as a facilitator of change, and the successful working through of the client's transference serves as an agent of change that can then be applied to other important relationships in the client's life.

The real relationship—the aspect of the therapeutic relationship that captures the genuine, authentic, and human connection outside of interactions tainted by transference and countertransference—is characterized by many of the common factors described in Chapter 2 of this volume. Empathy, positive regard, genuineness, and congruence facilitate the work of therapy because they provide a safe, inviting foundation on which clients can build to take risks and practice new skills. Moreover, they serve as an agent of change because patients experience important belief shifts about relationships—about their worthiness to receive both positive regard and the trustworthiness of others in relationships—and because patients get practice in receiving positive regard and in functioning within a caring, supportive relationship.

CONTEMPORARY DEFINITIONS

I developed an interest in the therapeutic relationship in CBT in the mid-2010s after many powerful clinical experiences that made a tremendous impact on my professional and personal growth. As I continued my own scholarship on basic and innovative interventions in CBT, I began to think about basic definitions, including of CBT itself (a daunting prospect, indeed). In my 2017 book, *Innovations in Cognitive Behavioral Therapy: Strategic Interventions for Creative Practice*, I proposed a definition of *integrative CBT*, or CBT practiced in a contemporary manner with real-life clients who have an array of nuances to their clinical presentations and who would be best served by a customized treatment package that is driven by their unique case formulation. That definition read as follows:

> A strategic and customized treatment package that emerges from the case conceptualization of the individual client's clinical presentation and incorporates cognitive, behavioral, and acceptance-based strategies, balanced with the cultivation and maintenance of the therapeutic relationship. (Wenzel, 2017, p. 168)

Thus, I did and continue to advocate for the therapeutic relationship being included as a central component in the basic definition of the CBT approach.

The definitions of the therapeutic relationship that I presented in Chapter 1 of this volume, which cut across schools of psychotherapy, are all applicable to CBT. Recall that Norcross and Lambert (2019) described the therapeutic relationship as the "healing alliance between client and clinician" (p. 2); Gelso and Carter (1985) referred to the therapeutic relationship as "the feelings and attitudes that therapist and client have toward one another and the manner in which they are expressed" (p. 159); and Kazantzis et al. (2017) defined the therapeutic relationship as "an exchange between therapist and client that develops for the purpose of sharing intimate thoughts, beliefs, and emotions in an endeavor to facilitate change" (p. 17). These definitions emphasize the bidirectional nature of the interactions between the client and therapist, as well as the feelings and cognitions that emerge from those interactions, that are directed in the service of healing and promoting positive changes in the client's life. Here, I expand these definitions of the therapeutic relationship into one that is more specific to the *CBT therapeutic relationship*. On the basis of the ideas developed in this volume, I propose the following:

> The CBT therapeutic relationship is an ever-emerging alliance characterized by benevolence and positive regard that provides the foundation for the successful implementation of cognitive behavioral principles, strategies, and techniques; that advances progress toward the client's mental health and self-growth goals; and that serves as a corrective learning experience for clients who have experienced damage in past and current formative relationships with important individuals in their lives.

Recall that in their seminal book *Cognitive Therapy of Depression*, Dr. Aaron T. Beck and colleagues (1979) stated that the therapeutic relationship is "a necessary but not sufficient agent of change" (p. 59). I believe that when the CBT therapeutic relationship is conceptualized in this manner, it invokes the client-centered, relationship-focused delivery of cognitive behavioral interventions. From this perspective, the therapeutic relationship in CBT can, indeed, be a sufficient agent of change.

DELIVERING CBT THROUGH THE LENS OF THE THERAPEUTIC RELATIONSHIP

There is no question that CBT requires effort from both the therapist and the client. Therapists deliver psychoeducation about clients' mental health disorders, the cognitive behavioral model, and the rationale underlying specific cognitive behavioral strategies and techniques. Clients are called upon to think critically about their life circumstances, consider alternative viewpoints, develop plans to solve problems, and transfer the learning that they achieve in session to their daily lives. As one of my trainees aptly observed many years ago, "You can't coast in CBT."

This does not mean, however, that CBT needs to be rote, dry, lecture-y, rigid, or even boring. This is where the therapeutic relationship comes into play. By maintaining simultaneous foci on the therapeutic relationship and on cognitive behavioral strategy and technique, CBT becomes engaging, enriching, and even inspiring. This balance can be achieved by invoking the spirit of the real relationship, or by being human. My view of "being human" occurs when therapists allow their personality and genuine caring for their clients to shine through specific strategies and techniques. Moreover, when cognitive behavioral therapists are cognizant of ways that the therapeutic relationship can itself be a vehicle of change—whether that occurs by changing clients' views about relationships, giving them practice in interpersonal skills that can enhance relationships, or solving a problem that has arisen in the relationship—client experiences in CBT have the potential to be truly transformative.

It is through these insights and observations that I developed the pillars of TRF-CBT. As a recap, the central premises of TRF-CBT are as follows:

a. The therapeutic relationship is cultivated as early as during the very first contact with the client.

b. Relatively equal attention is paid to the therapeutic relationship and cognitive behavioral strategies and techniques as the course of a client's CBT progresses.

c. CBT strategies and techniques are delivered from a client-centered framework.

d. When issues arise within the therapeutic relationship, CBT strategies and techniques are applied in "real time" to repair any potential rupture to the relationship and create a corrective learning experience that can be applied to relationships in clients' lives outside of session.

e. When relevant, the therapeutic relationship is cultivated in a way that provides a fundamental learning experience for clients who have had damaging relationships with key figures, such as a parent, a significant romantic other, or another person who played an important role in their lives.

f. When relevant, the strength of the therapeutic relationship is relied upon to weather temporary plateaus and impasses that occur during the course of treatment.

g. Elements of the therapeutic relationship are used strategically, or in a way that facilitates the successful implementation of CBT strategies and techniques as well as serves as an active agent of important cognitive, emotional, and behavioral change.

Above all, the delivery of TRF-CBT involves the delivery of CBT from a stance of genuine, authentic interaction and reflection on that interaction. I encourage cognitive behavioral therapists to allow their strengths and unique features of their personalities to shine. I encourage cognitive behavioral therapists to allow themselves to truly care for their clients and to not be hesitant to communicate that care when appropriate. I encourage cognitive behavioral therapists to be aware of their own issues that might activate their own schemas and the way in which they contribute to reactions to certain types of client behaviors. When a rupture arises, I encourage cognitive behavioral therapists to focus much more on the relationship than on technique, as research shows that therapists who emphasize technique are rated especially negatively by clients (Castonguay et al., 1996; cf. Castonguay et al., 2010) and that flexible responding enhances outcome (Constantino et al., 2020). Equally so, when something positive occurs in the relationship, such as when the client expresses heartfelt appreciation for the therapist's help, I encourage cognitive behavioral therapists to bask in the moment with their client. Positive moments in the therapeutic relationship can supply every bit of an opportunity for a collective learning experience as instances of potential or actual rupture.

FUTURE RESEARCH

Our conceptualization of the therapeutic relationship is ever-evolving because of the intricate nature of this construct. In fact, members of the Third Interdivisional APA Task Force on Evidence-Based Relationships and Responsiveness used the analogy that "the therapy relationship is like a diamond—a diamond composed of multiple, interconnected facets" that is a "complex and multidimensional entity" (Norcross & Lambert, 2019, p. 4). The therapeutic relationship is bidirectional and reciprocal, with therapist perceptions and behaviors, client perceptions and behaviors, and the inter-action between the two all being relevant variables. Indeed, newcomers to the greater psychotherapy process literature on the therapeutic relationship can become quite overwhelmed with contradictory findings, complicated statistical procedures, and methodological decisions in individual studies that have important implications in the interpretations of results.

In each clinical chapter in this volume, I proposed an agenda for future research examining the intersection of the therapeutic relationship and the particular CBT strategy under consideration. In a general sense, I raised the possibility that skill in the delivery of particular CBT strategies would affect the therapeutic relationship, such that the skillful, nonrigid delivery of a CBT strategy would enhance the quality of the therapeutic relationship, whereas the less skillful, more rigid delivery of the CBT strategy would decrease the quality of the therapeutic relationship. Moreover, I suggested that future research should quantify the percentage of variance in outcome accounted by the interaction between therapist skill in using a particular strategy and the strength of the therapeutic relationship. I also encouraged researchers to isolate the particular aspects of the therapeutic relationship and outcome—not only the therapeutic alliance but also the strength of the real relationship, the ability to resolve transference and countertransference, as well as other therapist behaviors that we know are so important to the therapeutic relationship (e.g., empathy, genuineness, congruence, cultural competence, and cultural adaptation). Scholars within the CBT field are just beginning to embark on empirical research that speaks to the association among therapist competence, aspects of the therapeutic relationship, and outcome, although to date, competence is assessed for the delivery of CBT as a package rather than for its specific components (Impala et al., 2022; Weck, Grikscheit, et al., 2015).

Furthermore, I believe that qualitative research into both clients' and therapists' experiences within the therapeutic relationship will yield important and fruitful directions for future empirical research. The quantification of aspects of the therapeutic relationship can be elusive. Perhaps hearing clients' and therapists' experiences will shed light on important processes that psychotherapy researchers can then operationalize and assimilate into a measure, yielding quantitative measurement that will, in turn, shed light on the therapeutic relationship variables and processes that therapists—not only cognitive behavioral therapists—can incorporate into their work with clients to enhance outcome.

FINAL MUSINGS ON THE THERAPEUTIC RELATIONSHIP AND CBT

Even when CBT is delivered with expert strategy and technique, when asked to name the most helpful factors in treatment, clients tend to mention aspects of the therapeutic relationship (Mathews et al., 1976; Rabavilas et al., 1979). I certainly experience this in my own practice. Much more often than not, when I ask clients who are ending treatment for final feedback on the course of our work together, they tell me that what was most helpful was my positive regard for them, the space I provided for them to truly be heard, and the support that they experienced from me. Earlier in my career, I found this both to be gratifying as well as frustrating, as I did not want my clients to forget about the impressive gains they had made in their ability to enact CBT principles in their lives, as doing so would have a preventive effect against relapse or recurrence. At this stage of my career, I no longer experience the frustration piece of it. The gains that my clients have made in therapy are almost always crystal clear in each session, as evidenced by the mood ratings provided at the beginning of each session; the overt discussion of homework completed in between sessions and the learning that occurred because of it; and the deliberate application of CBT principles, strategies, and techniques applied to discussion of topics deemed to be important in each session. Instead, at this stage of my career, positive feedback on the therapeutic relationship is a warm reminder of the privilege I have of bringing the science and practice of CBT to help people I grow to care very much about achieve a state of fulfillment and actualization.

Consider the following correspondence that the therapist received from Sarah[1] approximately 2 years after therapy had ended. The message read something like this:

> Hello!
>
> I think of you often and I hope you are well! I have to tell you I am such a better version of myself here, and I have you to thank for so much of that! You were the first person to ever say out loud that my environment could be contributing to my state at the time. I want you to know, I got a new job, I bought my own house, and I am participating in my first art show which is today and tomorrow! I have been a creative powder keg and cannot stop making things! People love my works, and I cannot tell you how good it feels to hear people gush about how much they love this piece or that piece. So ultimately, I miss you and thank you so much. As cliche as it is, you had way more faith in me than I had.

Remember that Sarah had adeptly acquired a vast array of cognitive behavioral skills and tools, such as the ability to restructure her unhelpful thoughts, apply the principles of social problem solving, and recognize when maladaptive schemas were activated. Moreover, we targeted other CBT principles, skills, and tools that were not captured in this volume, such as acceptance, mindfulness, distress tolerance, and emotion regulation. Sarah was fully enacting the majority of what she learned in therapy. But that is not what stuck with her. What stuck with her was the relationship in which her therapist respected her as an equal member of the therapeutic team and even admired her for her talents and for transcending the challenges that she had faced in her life. What stuck with her was the nonjudgmental environment into which she was welcomed, which was so different than the environment that she experienced with her family-of-origin. What stuck with her were the messages "I believe you" and "I believe in you." As a result, Sarah demonstrated a strengthened sense of agency to make positive choices and enhance her quality of life.

However, despite our best efforts, and because we are human, there are times when the therapeutic relationship falls short. In the last month of finishing the writing of this volume, I had a long-standing client abruptly end treatment, saying that she had had enough. I attempted to balance a stance of respecting her autonomy and right to know what is best for herself with examining whether there was a rupture in the relationship that could be ripe for repair. Throughout our work together, this client struggled with a belief

---

[1]Client identity has been disguised to protect client confidentiality.

that she did not have enough friends and wondered what role she had played in some failed relationships in the past. Thus, my sense was that this could be a pivotal opportunity not only to address what was happening between the two of us but also to construct a template for understanding and adaptively addressing any tension in her relationships that might emerge in the future. Moreover, in the process of being honest with myself, I acknowledged that we had seen each other for quite some time, and I had the sense that our therapeutic work was becoming a bit stale. I wondered whether I had inadvertently been providing the client less empathy, positive regard, and astute attention than I do with my other clients, or less than I had at the beginning of the course of our work together. In other words, I wondered if I was "prizing" her to a lesser degree than I had in the past, and that she felt it.

Alas, it was not to be. The client was not interested in going down this route. I had the sense that something was most definitely "off" and that rupture repair was indicated. At the same time, I sensed that I was treading closely to a line that could be easily crossed into not respecting my client's wish to end treatment if I pushed an agenda of rupture repair. I eventually shifted toward a stance of relapse prevention and a hopeful summary of all of the nuggets of wisdom that she had taken from our work together.

We learn from our clients every bit as much as they learn from us. I became a better cognitive behavioral therapist because of my work with the clients who formed the inspiration for the case of Sarah, and many, many clients like her. I learned how to create a portal for clients to reach in and take hold of the positive regard I have for them and turn it into confidence and empowerment in their own lives. In addition, I would like to think that, after reflection, I became a better cognitive behavioral therapist from the abrupt ending of therapy with the long-standing client that I just described. I will be honest about the fact that I found the experience to be jarring for a number of reasons, not least of which is that I was writing a volume on the centrality of the therapeutic relationship at this time this occurred. However, after the session ended, I operationalized three therapist behaviors that contribute to "prizing" the client that I sensed might have dropped off in our interactions, and I made a renewed commitment to enact those behaviors in a genuine manner with the rest of the clients that I saw for therapy that day. As it turned out, I happened to have some of the best sessions I had had in some time, and I believe it was because I regrouped with my focus on the therapeutic relationship.

In his outstanding book on the real relationship in psychotherapy, Charles Gelso (2011) stated on many occasions that cognitive behavioral therapists show little interest in the nuances of the therapeutic relationship and, in particular, that their interest in genuineness is only "peripheral" (p. 25). The renowned Barry Farber and his colleagues remarked that cognitive behavioral therapists "tend to be more invested in the technical interventions that presumably drive treatment success, especially when compared with their psychodynamic colleagues" (Suzuki et al., 2021, p. 140). I have much, much respect for these colleagues and, simultaneously, I also believe that these notions are overstated for the many, many cognitive behavioral therapists who served as mentors to me, for those whom I view as esteemed colleagues, for the thousands of therapists I have trained and supervised, and, of course, for myself. I call upon cognitive behavioral therapists to demonstrate—scientifically and clinically—the central role that a genuine, authentic therapeutic relationship contributes significantly to the CBT experience in our clients. As I stated at the beginning of this volume, I believe that some of the best CBT occurs when cognitive behavioral principles, strategies, and techniques are applied to an issue that arises within the therapeutic relationship. This is what is encapsulated in TRF-CBT. The time is ripe to provide empirical verification for this assertion.

The therapeutic relationship is, indeed, "the heart and soul of all effective psychotherapies" (Okamoto et al., 2019, p. 113). I leave the reader here with a mantra that I have crafted based on years of reading, research, and critical thought about the therapeutic relationship that I read each morning before I start a day of clinical work. It is not uncommon for me to work with my clients in CBT to develop their own personal mantra that orients them to their strengths, values, and long-term goals that they would like to achieve. I believe that it is important for cognitive behavioral therapists to "practice what they preach" so that they have genuine credibility with their clients and can understand what it is like to implement any of the CBT suggestions that we raise. So, this mantra is much like the mantra that I encourage my clients to develop for themselves to guide the way in which they live their lives. In my case, it orients me to the honor it is to be able to enter into the intimate worlds of clients and to the difference that CBT and our therapeutic relationship has the potential to make in their lives. I encourage my clinician readers to craft a similar statement to bear in mind as they enter into each and every session with their clients and share in the gift of psychotherapy.

May I prize each client as their champion, with positive regard, kindness, empathy, and grace, knowing that they are struggling and fully, fully appreciating what a privilege it is that they have chosen me to be present with their vulnerability, pain, and growth.

References

Abramowitz, J. S., Deacon, B. J., & Whiteside, S. P. H. (2019). *Exposure therapy for anxiety: Principles and practice* (2nd ed.). Guilford Press.

Accurso, E. C., Fitzsimmons-Craft, E. E., Ciao, A., Cao, L., Crosby, R. D., Smith, T. L., Klein, M. H., Mitchell, J. E., Crow, S. J., Wonderlich, S. A., & Peterson, C. B. (2015). Therapeutic alliance in a randomized clinical trial for bulimia nervosa. *Journal of Consulting and Clinical Psychology, 83*(3), 637–642. https://doi.org/10.1037/ccp0000021

Ackerman, S. J., & Hilsenroth, M. J. (2001). A review of therapist characteristics and techniques negatively impacting the therapeutic alliance. *Psychotherapy: Theory, Research, Practice, Training, 38*(2), 171–185. https://doi.org/10.1037/0033-3204.38.2.171

Ackerman, S. J., & Hilsenroth, M. J. (2003). A review of therapist characteristics and techniques positively impacting the therapeutic alliance. *Clinical Psychology Review, 23*(1), 1–33. https://doi.org/10.1016/S0272-7358(02)00146-0

Alexander, F., & French, T. M. (1946). *Psychoanalytic therapy: Principles and application.* Ronald Press.

American Psychological Association Presidential Task Force on Evidence-Based Practice. (2006). Evidence-based practice in psychology. *American Psychologist, 61*(4), 271–285.

Arkowitz, H., Miller, W. R., & Rollnick, S. (2015). *Motivational interviewing in the treatment of psychological problems* (2nd ed.). Guilford Press.

Arnkoff, D. G. (1983). Common and specific factors in cognitive therapy. In M. J. Lambert (Ed.), *Psychotherapy process: Current issues and future directions* (pp. 85–125). Dorsey.

Arredondo, P., Toporek, R., Brown, S. P., Jones, J., Locke, D. C., Sanchez, J., & Stadler, H. (1996). Operationalization of the multicultural counseling competencies. *Journal of Multicultural Counseling and Development, 24*(1), 42–78. https://doi.org/10.1002/j.2161-1912.1996.tb00288.x

Asnaani, A., & Foa, E. B. (2014). Expanding the lens of evidence-based practice in psychotherapy to include a common factors perspective: Comment on Laska, Gurman, and Wampold. *Psychotherapy, 51*(4), 487–490. https://doi.org/10.1037/a0036891

Bachrach, H. M. (1976). Empathy: We know what we mean, but what do we measure? *Archives of General Psychiatry, 33*(1), 35–38. https://doi.org/10.1001/archpsyc.1976.01770010021003

Barber, J. P., Connolly, M. B., Crits-Christoph, P., Gladis, L., & Siqueland, L. (2000). Alliance predicts patients' outcome beyond in-treatment change in symptoms. *Journal of Consulting and Clinical Psychology, 68*(6), 1027–1032. https://doi.org/10.1037/0022-006X.68.6.1027

Barrett-Lennard, G. T. (1985). The helping relationship: Crisis and advance in theory and research. *The Counseling Psychologist, 13*, 279–294.

Beck, A. T., Brown, G., Steer, R. A., Eidelson, J. I., & Riskind, J. H. (1987). Differentiating anxiety and depression: A test of the cognitive content-specificity hypothesis. *Journal of Abnormal Psychology, 96*(3), 179–183.

Beck, A. T., Grant, P., Inverso, E., Brinen, A. P., & Perivoliotis, D. (2021). *Recovery-oriented cognitive therapy for serious mental health conditions.* Guilford Press.

Beck, A. T., Rush, A. J., Shaw, B. F., & Emery, G. (1979). *Cognitive therapy of depression.* Guilford Press.

Beck, A. T., Steer, R. A., & Brown, G. K. (1996). *The Beck Depression Inventory: Manual* (2nd ed.). Psychological Corporation.

Beck, J. S. (2021). *Cognitive behavior therapy: Basics and beyond* (3rd ed.). Guilford Press.

Bedics, J. D., Atkins, D. C., Harned, M. S., & Linehan, M. M. (2015). The therapeutic alliance as a predictor of outcome in dialectical behavior therapy versus nonbehavioral psychotherapy by experts for borderline personality disorder. *Psychotherapy, 52*(1), 67–77. https://doi.org/10.1037/a0038457

Ben David-Sela, T., Nof, A., & Zilcha-Mano, S. (2020). "We can work it out": Working through termination ruptures. *Psychotherapy, 57*(4), 491–496. https://doi.org/10.1037/pst0000297

Bernal, G., Bonilla, J., & Bellido, C. (1995). Ecological validity and cultural sensitivity for outcome research: Issues for the cultural adaptation and development of psychosocial treatments with Hispanics. *Journal of Abnormal Child Psychology, 23*(1), 67–82. https://doi.org/10.1007/BF01447045

Bieling, P. J., Blasioli, E., & Friedman-Wheeler, D. G. (2021). Cognitive case formulation. In A. Wenzel (Ed.), *Handbook of cognitive behavioral therapy* (Vol. 1, pp. 131–155). American Psychological Association. https://doi.org/10.1037/0000218-005

Björgvinsson, T., Hart, J., & Heffelfinger, S. (2007). Obsessive-compulsive disorder: Update on assessment and treatment. *Journal of Psychiatric Practice, 13*(6), 362–372. https://doi.org/10.1097/01.pra.0000300122.76322.ad

Bordin, E. S. (1979). The generalizability of the psychoanalytic concept of the working alliance. *Psychotherapy: Theory, Research, & Practice, 16*(3), 252–260. https://doi.org/10.1037/h0085885

Brewer, W. F. (2000). Bartlett's concept of the schema and its impact on theories of knowledge representation in contemporary cognitive psychology. In A. Saito (Ed.), *Bartlett, culture, and cognition* (pp. 69–89). Psychology Press.

Buchholz, J. L., & Abramowitz, J. S. (2020). The therapeutic alliance in exposure therapy for anxiety-related disorders: A critical review. *Journal of Anxiety Disorders, 70*, 102194. https://doi.org/10.1016/j.janxdis.2020.102194

Burns, D. D., & Nolen-Hoeksema, S. (1992). Therapeutic empathy and recovery from depression in cognitive-behavioral therapy: A structural equation model. *Journal of Consulting and Clinical Psychology, 60*(3), 441–449. https://doi.org/10.1037/0022-006X.60.3.441

Button, M. L., Norouzian, N., Westra, H. A., Constantino, M. J., & Antony, M. M. (2019). Client reflections on confirmation and disconfirmation of expectations in cognitive behavioral therapy for generalized anxiety disorder with and without motivational interviewing. *Psychotherapy Research, 29*(6), 723–736. https://doi.org/10.1080/10503307.2018.1425932

Cameron, S. K., Rodgers, J., & Dagnan, D. (2018). The relationship between the therapeutic alliance and clinical outcomes in cognitive behaviour therapy for adults with depression: A meta-analytic review. *Clinical Psychology & Psychotherapy, 25*(3), 446–456. https://doi.org/10.1002/cpp.2180

Carroll, L. (2010). *Alice's adventures in wonderland and through the looking-glass.* Cosimo, Inc.

Casas, J. M., Suzucki, L. A., Alexander, C. M., & Jackson, M. A. (Eds.). (2016). *Handbook of multicultural counseling.* Sage.

Castonguay, L. G., Constantino, M. J., & Holtforth, M. G. (2006). The working alliance: Where are we and where should we go? *Psychotherapy: Theory, Research, Practice, Training, 43*(3), 271–279. https://doi.org/10.1037/0033-3204.43.3.271

Castonguay, L. G., Constantino, M. J., McAleavey, A. A., & Goldfried, M. R. (2010). The therapeutic alliance in cognitive behavioral therapy. In J. C. Muran & J. P. Barber (Eds.), *The therapeutic alliance: An evidence-based guide to practice* (pp. 150–171). Guilford Press.

Castonguay, L. G., Goldfried, M. R., Wiser, S., Raue, P. J., & Hayes, A. M. (1996). Predicting the effect of cognitive therapy for depression: A study of unique and common factors. *Journal of Consulting and Clinical Psychology, 64*(3), 497–504. https://doi.org/10.1037/0022-006X.64.3.497

Chang, D. F., Dunn, J. J., & Omidi, M. (2021). A critical-cultural-relational approach to rupture resolution: A case illustration with a cross-racial dyad. *Journal of Clinical Psychology, 77*(2), 369–381. https://doi.org/10.1002/jclp.23080

Cloitre, M., Koenen, K. C., Cohen, L. R., & Han, H. (2002). Skills training in affective and interpersonal regulation followed by exposure: A phase-based treatment for PTSD related to childhood abuse. *Journal of Consulting and Clinical Psychology, 70*(5), 1067–1074. https://doi.org/10.1037/0022-006X.70.5.1067

Constantino, M. J., Castonguay, L. G., & Schut, A. J. (2002). The working alliance: A flagship for the "scientist-practitioner" model in psychotherapy. In

G. S. Tyron (Ed.), *Counseling based on process research: Applying what we know* (pp. 81–131). Allyn & Bacon.

Constantino, M. J., Coyne, A. E., & Muir, H. J. (2020). Evidence-based therapist responsivity to disruptive clinical process. *Cognitive and Behavioral Practice, 27*(4), 405–416. https://doi.org/10.1016/j.cbpra.2020.01.003

Constantino, M. J., Vîslă, A., Coyne, A. E., & Boswell, J. F. (2019). Cultivating positive outcome expectation. In J. C. Norcross & M. J. Lambert (Eds.), *Psychotherapy relationships that work: Vol. 1. Evidence based therapist contributions* (3rd ed., pp. 461–494). Oxford University Press. https://doi.org/10.1093/med-psych/9780190843953.003.0013

Constantino, M. J., Westra, H. A., Antony, M. M., & Coyne, A. E. (2019). Specific and common processes as mediators of the long-term effects of cognitive-behavioral therapy integrated with motivational interviewing for generalized anxiety disorder. *Psychotherapy Research, 29*(2), 213–225. https://doi.org/10.1080/10503307.2017.1332794

Couch, A. S. (1999). Therapeutic functions of the real relationship in psychoanalysis. *The Psychoanalytic Study of the Child, 54*(1), 130–168. https://doi.org/10.1080/00797308.1999.11822499

Craske, M. G., Kircanski, K., Zelikowsky, M., Mystkowski, J., Chowdhury, N., & Baker, A. (2008). Optimizing inhibitory learning during exposure therapy. *Behaviour Research and Therapy, 46*(1), 5–27. https://doi.org/10.1016/j.brat.2007.10.003

Craske, M. G., Treanor, M., Conway, C. C., Zbozinek, T., & Vervliet, B. (2014). Maximizing exposure therapy: An inhibitory learning approach. *Behaviour Research and Therapy, 58*, 10–23. https://doi.org/10.1016/j.brat.2014.04.006

Crits-Christoph, P., Crits-Christoph, K., & Connolly Gibbons, M. B. (2010). Training in alliance-fostering techniques. In J. C. Muran & J. P. Barber (Eds.), *The therapeutic alliance: An evidence-based guide to practice* (pp. 304–319). Guilford Press.

Crits-Christoph, P., Siqueland, L., Chittams, J., Barber, J. P., Beck, A. T., Frank, A., Liese, B., Luborsky, L., Mark, D., Mercer, D., Onken, L. S., Najavits, L. M., Thase, M. E., & Woody, G. (1998). Training in cognitive, supportive-expressive, and drug counseling therapies for cocaine dependence. *Journal of Consulting and Clinical Psychology, 66*(3), 484–492. https://doi.org/10.1037/0022-006X.66.3.484

de Felice, G., Giuliani, A., Halfon, S., Andreassi, S., Paoloni, G., & Orsucci, F. F. (2019). The misleading Dodo Bird verdict. How much of the outcome variance is explained by common and specific factors? *New Ideas in Psychology, 54*, 50–55. https://doi.org/10.1016/j.newideapsych.2019.01.006

DeRubeis, R. J., & Feeley, M. (1990). Determinants of change in cognitive therapy for depression. *Cognitive Therapy and Research, 14*(5), 469–482. https://doi.org/10.1007/BF01172968

Dobson, D., & Dobson, K. S. (2017). *Evidence-based practice of cognitive behavioral therapy* (2nd ed.). Guilford Press.

Dobson, K. S. (2022). Therapeutic relationship. *Cognitive and Behavioral Practice,* *29*(3), 541–544. https://doi.org/10.1016/j.cbpra.2022.02.006

Doran, J. M. (2016). The working alliance: Where have we been, where are we going? *Psychotherapy Research, 26*(2), 146–163. https://doi.org/10.1080/10503307.2014.954153

D'Zurilla, T. J., & Nezu, A. M. (2007). *Problem-solving therapy: A positive approach to clinical intervention* (3rd ed.). Springer.

Eames, V., & Roth, A. (2000). Patient attachment orientation and the early working alliance–a study of patient and therapist reports of alliance quality and ruptures. *Psychotherapy Research, 10*(4), 421–434. https://doi.org/10.1093/ptr/10.4.421

Elliot, R., Bohart, J. C., Watson, D., & Murphy, D. (2019). Empathy. In J. C. Norcross & M. J. Lambert (Eds.), *Psychotherapy relationships that work. Vol. 1. Evidence based therapist contributions* (3rd ed., pp. 245–287). Oxford University Press. https://doi.org/10.1093/med-psych/9780190843953.003.0007

Eubanks, C. F., & Goldfried, M. R. (2019). A principle-based approach to psychotherapy integration. In J. C. Norcross & M. R. Goldfried (Eds.), *Handbook of psychotherapy integration* (3rd ed., pp. 88–104). Oxford University Press. https://doi.org/10.1093/med-psych/9780190690465.003.0004

Eubanks, C. F., Muran, J. C., & Safran, J. D. (2018). Alliance rupture repair: A meta-analysis. *Psychotherapy, 55*(4), 508–519. https://doi.org/10.1037/pst0000185

Eubanks-Carter, C., Muran, J. C., & Safran, J. D. (2010). Alliance ruptures and resolution. In J. C. Muran & J. P. Barber (Eds.), *The therapeutic alliance: An evidence-based guide to practice* (pp. 74–95). Guilford Press.

Falkenström, F., Ekeblad, A., & Holmqvist, R. (2016). Improvement of the working alliance in one treatment session predicts improvement of depressive symptoms by the next session. *Journal of Consulting and Clinical Psychology, 84*(8), 738–751. https://doi.org/10.1037/ccp0000119

Farber, B. A., Suzuki, J. Y., & Lynch, D. A. (2019). Positive regard and affirmation. In J. C. Norcross & M. J. Lambert (Eds.), *Psychotherapy relationships that work* (3rd ed., pp. 168–186). Oxford University Press. https://doi.org/10.1093/med-psych/9780190843953.003.0008

Farber, B. A., Suzuki, J. Y., & Ort, D. (2022). *Understanding and enhancing positive regard in psychotherapy: Carl Rogers and beyond.* American Psychological Association. https://doi.org/10.1037/0000312-000

Feeley, M., DeRubeis, R. J., & Gelfand, L. A. (1999). The temporal relation of adherence and alliance to symptom change in cognitive therapy for depression. *Journal of Consulting and Clinical Psychology, 67*(4), 578–582. https://doi.org/10.1037/0022-006X.67.4.578

Feeny, N., Hembree, E., & Zoellner, L. (2003). Myths regarding exposure therapy for PTSD. *Cognitive and Behavioral Practice, 10*(1), 85–90. https://doi.org/10.1016/S1077-7229(03)80011-1

Flückiger, C., Del Re, A. C., Wampold, B. E., & Horvath, A. O. (2018). The alliance in adult psychotherapy: A meta-analytic synthesis. *Psychotherapy, 55*(4), 316–340. https://doi.org/10.1037/pst0000172

Flückiger, C., Rubel, J., Del Re, A. C., Horvath, A. O., Wampold, B. E., Crits-Christoph, P., Atzil-Slonim, D., Compare, A., Falkenström, F., Ekeblad, A., Errázuriz, P., Fisher, H., Hoffart, A., Huppert, J. D., Kivity, Y., Kumar, M., Lutz, W., Muran, J. C., Strunk, D. R., & Barber, J. P. (2020). The reciprocal relationship between alliance and early treatment symptoms: A two-stage individual participant data meta-analysis. *Journal of Consulting and Clinical Psychology, 88*(9), 829–843. https://doi.org/10.1037/ccp0000594

Foa, E. B., Zoellner, L. A., Feeny, N. C., Hembree, E. A., & Alvarez-Conrad, J. (2002). Does imaginal exposure exacerbate PTSD symptoms? *Journal of Consulting and Clinical Psychology, 70*(4), 1022–1028. https://doi.org/10.1037/0022-006X.70.4.1022

Frank, J. D. (1961). *Persuasion and healing: A comparative study of psychotherapy.* Johns Hopkins University Press.

Fuertes, J. N., Mislowack, A., Brown, S., Gur-Arie, S., Wilkinson, S., & Gelso, C. J. (2007). Correlates of the real relationship in psychotherapy: A study of dyads. *Psychotherapy Research, 17*(4), 423–430. https://doi.org/10.1080/10503300600789189

Gaines, A. N., Goldfried, M. R., & Constantino, M. J. (2021). Revived call for consensus in the future of psychotherapy. *BMJ Mental Health, 24*(1), 2–4. https://doi.org/10.1136/ebmental-2020-300208

Gaston, L. (1990). The concept of the alliance and its role in psychotherapy: Theoretical and empirical considerations. *Psychotherapy: Theory, Research, Practice, Training, 27*(2), 143–153. https://doi.org/10.1037/0033-3204.27.2.143

Gelso, C. (2014). A tripartite model of the therapeutic relationship: Theory, research, and practice. *Psychotherapy Research, 24*(2), 117–131. https://doi.org/10.1080/10503307.2013.845920

Gelso, C. J. (2002). Real relationship: The "something more" of psychotherapy. *Journal of Contemporary Psychotherapy, 32*(1), 35–40. https://doi.org/10.1023/A:1015531228504

Gelso, C. J. (2011). *The real relationship in psychotherapy: The hidden foundation of change.* American Psychological Association. https://doi.org/10.1037/12349-000

Gelso, C. J. (2019). *The therapeutic relationship in psychotherapy practice: An integrative approach.* Routledge.

Gelso, C. J., & Bhatia, A. (2012). Crossing theoretical lines: The role and effect of transference in nonanalytic psychotherapies. *Psychotherapy, 49*(3), 384–390. https://doi.org/10.1037/a0028802

Gelso, C. J., & Carter, J. A. (1985). The relationship in counseling and psychotherapy. *The Counseling Psychologist, 13*(2), 155–243. https://doi.org/10.1177/0011000085132001

Gelso, C. J., & Carter, J. A. (1994). Components of the psychotherapy relationship: Their interaction and unfolding during treatment. *Journal of Counseling Psychology, 41*(3), 296–306. https://doi.org/10.1037/0022-0167.41.3.296

Gelso, C. J., Fassinger, R. E., Gomez, M. J., & Latts, M. J. (1995). Countertransference reactions to lesbian clients: The role of homophobia, counselor gender, and countertransference management. *Journal of Counseling Psychology, 42*(3), 356–364. https://doi.org/10.1037/0022-0167.42.3.356

Gelso, C. J., & Hayes, J. A. (1998). *The psychotherapy relationship: Theory, research, and practice.* Wiley.

Gelso, C. J., & Hayes, J. A. (2007). *Countertransference and the therapist's inner experience: Perils and possibilities.* Lawrence Erlbaum Associates, Inc. https://doi.org/10.4324/9780203936979

Gelso, C. J., Kelley, F. A., Fuertes, J. N., Marmarosh, C., Holmes, S. E., Costa, C., & Hancock, G. R. (2005). Measuring the real relationship in psychotherapy: Initial validation of the therapist form. *Journal of Counseling Psychology, 52*(4), 640–649. https://doi.org/10.1037/0022-0167.52.4.640

Gelso, C. J., Kivlighan, D. M., & Markin, R. D. (2018). The real relationship and its role in psychotherapy outcome: A meta-analysis. *Psychotherapy, 55*(4), 434–444. https://doi.org/10.1037/pst0000183

Gelso, C. J., & Kline, K. V. (2019). The sister concepts of the working alliance and the real relationship: On their development, rupture, and repair. *Research in Psychotherapy, 22*(2), 373. https://doi.org/10.4081/ripppo.2019.373

Gelso, C. J., & Samstag, L. W. (2008). A tripartite model of the therapeutic relationship. In S. Brown & R. Lent (Eds.), *Handbook of counseling psychology* (pp. 267–283). Wiley.

Gilbert, P., & Leahy, R. L. (Eds.). (2007). *The therapeutic relationship in cognitive behavioral psychotherapies.* Routledge. https://doi.org/10.4324/9780203099995

Goldfried, M. R. (2003). Cognitive behavior therapy: Reflections on the evolution of a therapeutic orientation. *Cognitive Therapy and Research, 27*(1), 53–69. https://doi.org/10.1023/A:1022586629843

Goldfried, M. R. (2013). Evidence-based treatment and cognitive-affective-relational-behavior-therapy. *Psychotherapy, 50*(3), 376–380. https://doi.org/10.1037/a0032158

Goldfried, M. R., Burckell, L. A., & Eubanks-Carter, C. (2003). Therapist self-disclosure in cognitive-behavior therapy. *Journal of Clinical Psychology, 59*(5), 555–568. https://doi.org/10.1002/jclp.10159

Goldfried, M. R., & Davila, J. (2005). The role of relationship and technique in therapeutic change. *Psychotherapy: Theory, Research, Practice, Training, 42*(4), 421–430. https://doi.org/10.1037/0033-3204.42.4.421

Goldfried, M. R., & Davison, G. C. (1976). *Clinical behavior therapy: Expanded edition.* John Wiley & Sons.

Goodwin, B. J., Coyne, A. E., & Constantino, M. J. (2018). Extending the context-responsive psychotherapy integration framework to cultural processes in psychotherapy. *Psychotherapy, 55*(1), 3–8. https://doi.org/10.1037/pst0000143

Grayson, J. B., Foa, E. B., & Steketee, G. (1982). Habituation during exposure treatment: Distraction vs attention-focusing. *Behaviour Research and Therapy, 20*(4), 323–328. https://doi.org/10.1016/0005-7967(82)90091-2

Greenberg, L. S. (2002). *Emotion-focused therapy: Coaching clients to work through their feelings*. American Psychological Association. https://doi.org/10.1037/10447-000

Greenberger, D., & Padesky, C. A. (2016). *Mind over mood: Change how you feel by changing the way you think* (2nd ed.). Guilford Press.

Greenson, R. R. (1965). The working alliance and the transference neurosis. *The Psychoanalytic Quarterly, 34*(2), 155–181. https://doi.org/10.1080/21674086.1965.11926343

Greenson, R. R. (1967). *The technique and practice of psychoanalysis* (Vol. 1). International Universities Press.

Greenson, R. R. (1978). *Explorations in psychoanalysis*. International Universities Press.

Gülüm, I. V., & Soygüt, G. (2022). Limited reparenting as a corrective emotional experience in schema therapy: A preliminary task analysis. *Psychotherapy Research, 32*(2), 263–276. https://doi.org/10.1080/10503307.2021.1921301

Hara, K. M., Aviram, A., Constantino, M. J., Westra, H. A., & Antony, M. M. (2017). Therapist empathy, homework compliance, and outcome in cognitive behavioral therapy for generalized anxiety disorder: Partitioning within- and between-therapist effects. *Cognitive Behaviour Therapy, 46*(5), 375–390. https://doi.org/10.1080/16506073.2016.1253605

Hara, K. M., Westra, H. A., Aviram, A., Button, M. L., Constantino, M. J., & Antony, M. M. (2015). Therapist awareness of client resistance in cognitive behavioral therapy for generalized anxiety disorder. *Cognitive Behaviour Therapy, 44*(2), 162–174. https://doi.org/10.1080/16506073.2014.998705

Hara, K. M., Westra, H. A., Constantino, M. J., & Antony, M. M. (2018). The impact of resistance on empathy in CBT for generalized anxiety disorder. *Psychotherapy Research, 28*(4), 606–615. https://doi.org/10.1080/10503307.2016.1244616

Hara, K. M., Westra, H. A., Coyne, A. E., Di Bartolomeo, A. A., Constantino, M. J., & Antony, M. M. (2022). Therapist affiliation and hostility in cognitive-behavioral therapy with and without motivational interviewing for severe generalized anxiety disorder. *Psychotherapy Research, 32*(5), 598–610. https://doi.org/10.1080/10503307.2021.2001069

Hatcher, R. L. (2010). Alliance theory and measurement. In J. C. Muran & J. P. Barber (Eds.), *The therapeutic alliance: An evidence-based guide to practice* (pp. 7–27). Guilford Press.

Hatcher, R. L., & Gillaspy, J. A. (2006). Development and validation of a revised short version of the Working Alliance Inventory. *Psychotherapy Research, 16*(1), 12–25. https://doi.org/10.1080/10503300500352500

Haugen, P. T., Werth, A. S., Foster, A. L., & Owen, J. (2017). Are rupture–repair episodes related to outcome in the treatment of trauma-exposed World Trade Center responders? *Counselling & Psychotherapy Research, 17*(4), 276–282. https://doi.org/10.1002/capr.12138

Hayes, J. A., & Gelso, C. J. (1993). Male counselors' discomfort with gay and HIV-infected clients. *Journal of Counseling Psychology, 40*(1), 86–93. https://doi.org/10.1037/0022-0167.40.1.86

Hayes, J. A., McCracken, J. E., McClanahan, M. K., Hill, C. E., Harp, J. S., & Carozzoni, P. (1998). Therapist perspectives on countertransference: Qualitative data in search of a theory. *Journal of Counseling Psychology, 45*, 468–482.

Hayes, S. C., Strosahl, K. D., & Wilson, K. G. (1999). *Acceptance and commitment therapy: An experiential approach to behavior change.* Guilford Press.

Hayes, S. C., Strosahl, K. D., & Wilson, K. G. (2012). *Acceptance and commitment therapy: The process and practice of mindful change* (2nd ed.). Guilford Press.

Hays, P. A. (2008). *Addressing cultural complexities in practice: Assessment, diagnosis, and therapy* (2nd ed.). American Psychological Association. https://doi.org/10.1037/11650-000

Hays, P. A. (2009). Integrating evidence-based practice, cognitive-behavior therapy, and multicultural therapy: Ten steps for culturally competent practice. *Professional Psychology: Research and Practice, 40*(4), 354–360. https://doi.org/10.1037/a0016250

Hembree, E. A., Foa, E. B., Dorfan, N. M., Street, G. P., Kowalski, J., & Tu, X. (2003). Do patients drop out prematurely from exposure therapy for PTSD? *Journal of Traumatic Stress, 16*(6), 555–562. https://doi.org/10.1023/B:JOTS.0000004078.93012.7d

Hill, C. E. (2010). Qualitative studies of negative experiences in psychotherapy. In J. C. Muran & J. P. Barber (Eds.), *The therapeutic alliance: An evidence-based guide to practice* (pp. 63–73). Guilford Press.

Hinton, D. E., & Jalal, B. (2019). Dimensions of culturally sensitive CBT: Application to Southeast Asian populations. *American Journal of Orthopsychiatry, 89*(4), 493–507. https://doi.org/10.1037/ort0000392

Hinton, D. E., & Patel, A. (2017). Cultural adaptations of cognitive behavioral therapy. *Psychiatric Clinics of North America, 40*(4), 701–714. https://doi.org/10.1016/j.psc.2017.08.006

Hoffart, A., Borge, F. M., Sexton, H., & Clark, D. M. (2009). The role of common factors in residential cognitive and interpersonal therapy for social phobia: A process-outcome study. *Psychotherapy Research, 19*(1), 54–67. https://doi.org/10.1080/10503300802369343

Hoffart, A., & Sexton, H. (2002). The role of optimism in the process of schema-focused cognitive therapy of personality problems. *Behaviour Research and Therapy, 40*(6), 611–623. https://doi.org/10.1016/S0005-7967(01)00027-4

Hofmann, S. G., Asnaani, A., Vonk, I. J. J., Sawyer, A. T., & Fang, A. (2012). The efficacy of cognitive behavioral therapy: A review of meta-analyses. *Cognitive Therapy and Research, 36*(5), 427–440. https://doi.org/10.1007/s10608-012-9476-1

Hofmann, S. G., & Barlow, D. H. (2014). Evidence-based psychological interventions and the common factors approach: The beginnings of a rapprochement? *Psychotherapy, 51*(4), 510–513. https://doi.org/10.1037/a0037045

Hollon, S. D., Stewart, M. O., & Strunk, D. (2006). Enduring effects for cognitive behavior therapy in the treatment of depression and anxiety. *Annual Review of Psychology, 57*(1), 285–315. https://doi.org/10.1146/annurev.psych.57.102904.190044

Horvath, A. O. (1994). Empirical validation of Bordin's pantheoretical model of the alliance: The Working Alliance Inventory perspective. In A. O. Horvath & L. S. Greenberg (Eds.), *The working alliance: Theory, research, and practice* (pp. 109–128). Wiley.

Horvath, A. O., Del Re, A. C., Flückiger, C., & Symonds, D. (2011). Alliance in individual psychotherapy. *Psychotherapy, 48*(1), 9–16. https://doi.org/10.1037/a0022186

Horvath, A. O., & Luborsky, L. (1993). The role of the therapeutic alliance in psychotherapy. *Journal of Consulting and Clinical Psychology, 61*(4), 561–573. https://doi.org/10.1037/0022-006X.61.4.561

Horvath, A. O., & Symonds, B. D. (1991). Relation between working alliance and outcome in psychotherapy: A meta-analysis. *Journal of Consulting and Clinical Psychology, 61*(4), 561–573. https://doi.org/10.1037/0022-006X.61.4.561

Huppert, J. D., Kivity, Y., Barlow, D. H., Gorman, J. M., Shear, M. K., & Woods, S. W. (2014). Therapist effects and the outcome–alliance correlation in cognitive behavioral therapy for panic disorder with agoraphobia. *Behaviour Research and Therapy, 52*, 26–34. https://doi.org/10.1016/j.brat.2013.11.001

Impala, T., Dobson, K. S., & Kazantzis, N. (2022). Does the working alliance mediate the therapist competence-outcome relationship in cognitive behavior therapy for depression? *Psychotherapy Research, 32*(1), 126–138. https://doi.org/10.1080/10503307.2021.1946195

Jacoby, R. J., & Abramowitz, J. S. (2016). Inhibitory learning approaches to exposure therapy: A critical review and translation to obsessive-compulsive disorder. *Clinical Psychology Review, 49*, 28–40. https://doi.org/10.1016/j.cpr.2016.07.001

Jung, E., Wiesjahn, M., Rief, W., & Lincoln, T. M. (2015). Perceived therapist genuineness predicts therapeutic alliance in cognitive behavioural therapy for psychosis. *British Journal of Clinical Psychology, 54*(1), 34–48. https://doi.org/10.1111/bjc.12059

Kaczkurkin, A. N., & Foa, E. B. (2015). Cognitive-behavioral therapy for anxiety disorders: An update on the empirical evidence. *Dialogues in Clinical Neuroscience, 17*(3), 337–346. https://doi.org/10.31887/DCNS.2015.17.3/akaczkurkin

Karlin, B. E., Brown, G. K., Trockel, M., Cunning, D., Zeiss, A. M., & Taylor, C. B. (2012). National dissemination of cognitive behavioral therapy for depression in the Department of Veterans Affairs health care system: Therapist and patient-level outcomes. *Journal of Consulting and Clinical Psychology, 80*(5), 707–718. https://doi.org/10.1037/a0029328

Kazantzis, N., Beck, J. S., Clark, D. A., Dobson, K. S., Hofmann, S. G., Leahy, R. L., & Wong, C. W. (2018). Socratic dialogue and guided discovery in cognitive behavioral therapy: A modified Delphi panel. *International Journal of Cognitive Therapy, 11*(2), 140–157. https://doi.org/10.1007/s41811-018-0012-2

Kazantzis, N., Cronin, T. J., Norton, P. J., Lai, J., & Hofmann, S. G. (2015). Reservations about the conclusions of the Interdivisional (APA Divisions 12 & 29) Task Force on Evidence-Based Therapy Relationships: What do we know, what don't we know? *Journal of Clinical Psychology, 71*(5), 423–427. https://doi.org/10.1002/jclp.22178

Kazantzis, N., Dattilio, F. M., & Dobson, K. S. (2017). *The therapeutic relationship in cognitive behavioral therapy: A clinician's guide.* Guilford Press.

Kazantzis, N., Dattilio, F. M., McGinn, L. K., Newman, C. F., Persons, J. B., & Radomsky, A. S. (2018). Defining the role and function of the therapeutic relationship in cognitive behavioral therapy: A modified Delphi panel. *International Journal of Cognitive Therapy, 11*(2), 158–183. https://doi.org/10.1007/s41811-018-0014-0

Kazantzis, N., Fairburn, C. G., Padesky, C. A., Reinecke, M., & Teesson, M. (2014). Unresolved issues regarding the research and practice of cognitive behavior therapy: The case of guided discovery using Socratic questioning. *Behaviour Change, 31*(1), 1–17. https://doi.org/10.1017/bec.2013.29

Kazantzis, N., Whittington, C., Zelencich, L., Kyrios, M., Norton, P. J., & Hofmann, S. G. (2016). Quantity and quality of homework compliance: A meta-analysis of relations with outcome in cognitive behavior therapy. *Behavior Therapy, 47*(5), 755–772. https://doi.org/10.1016/j.beth.2016.05.002

Kazdin, A. E., & Krouse, R. (1983). The impact of variations in treatment rationales on expectancies for therapeutic change. *Behavior Therapy, 14*(5), 657–671. https://doi.org/10.1016/S0005-7894(83)80058-6

Kelley, F. A., Gelso, C. J., Fuertes, J. N., Marmarosh, C., & Lanier, S. H. (2010). The real relationship inventory: Development and psychometric investigation of the client form. *Psychotherapy: Theory, Research, Practice, Training, 47*(4), 540–553. https://doi.org/10.1037/a0022082

Kessler, R. C., Chiu, W. T., Demler, O., Merikangas, K. R., & Walters, E. E. (2005). Prevalence, severity, and comorbidity of 12-month *DSM-IV* disorders in the National Comorbidity Survey Replication. *Archives of General Psychiatry, 62*(6), 617–627. https://doi.org/10.1001/archpsyc.62.6.617

Khattra, J., Angus, L., Westra, H., Macaulay, C., Moertl, K., & Constantino, M. (2017). Client perceptions of corrective experiences in cognitive behavioral therapy and motivational interviewing for generalized anxiety disorder: An exploratory pilot study. *Journal of Psychotherapy Integration, 27*(1), 23–34. https://doi.org/10.1037/int0000053

Kivity, Y., Strauss, A. Y., Elizur, J., Weiss, M., Cohen, L., & Huppert, J. D. (2021). The alliance mediates outcome in cognitive-behavioral therapy for social anxiety

disorder, but not in attention bias modification. *Psychotherapy Research,*
31(5), 589–603. https://doi.org/10.1080/10503307.2020.1836423

Klein, D. N., Schwartz, J. E., Santiago, N. J., Vivian, D., Vocisano, C., Castonguay,
L. G., Arnow, B., Blalock, J. A., Manber, R., Markowitz, J. C., Riso, L. P.,
Rothbaum, B., McCullough, J. P., Thase, M. E., Borian, F. E., Miller, I. W.,
& Keller, M. B. (2003). Therapeutic alliance in depression treatment: Controlling for prior change and patient characteristics. *Journal of Consulting*
and Clinical Psychology, 71(6), 997–1006. https://doi.org/10.1037/0022-
006X.71.6.997

Kohlenberg, R., & Tsai, M. (1991). *Functional analytic psychotherapy: Creat-*
ing intense and curative therapeutic relationships. Springer. https://doi.org/
10.1007/978-0-387-70855-3

Kolden, G. G., Chia-Chiang, W., Austin, S. B., & Klein, M. B. (2019). Congruence/
genuineness. In J. C. Norcross & M. J. Lambert (Eds.), *Psychotherapy relation-*
ships that work (3rd ed., pp. 323–350). Oxford University Press.

Kuyken, W., Padesky, C. A., & Dudley, R. (2006). *Collaborative case conceptualiza-*
tion: Working effectively with clients in cognitive behavioral therapy. Guilford
Press.

Lambert, M. J., Whipple, J. L., Hawkins, E. J., Vermeersch, D. A., Nielsen, S. L.,
& Smart, D. W. (2003). Is it time for clinicians to routinely track client outcome?
A meta-analysis. *Clinical Psychology: Science and Practice, 10*(3), 288–301.
https://doi.org/10.1093/clipsy.bpg025

Lambert, M. J., Whipple, J. L., & Kleinstäuber, M. (2019). Collecting and delivering client feedback. In J. C. Norcross & M. J. Lambert (Eds.), *Psychotherapy*
relationships that work: Vol 1: Evidence-based therapist contributions (3rd ed.,
pp. 580–630). Oxford University Press. https://doi.org/10.1093/med-psych/
9780190843953.003.0017

Lang, A. J., & Craske, M. G. (2000). Manipulations of exposure-based therapy to
reduce return of fear: A replication. *Behaviour Research and Therapy, 38*(1),
1–12. https://doi.org/10.1016/S0005-7967(99)00031-5

La Roche, M., & Christopher, M. S. (2008). Culture and empirically supported
treatments: On the road to a collision? *Culture and Psychology, 14*(3), 333–356.
https://doi.org/10.1177/1354067X08092637

Laska, K. M., Gurman, A. S., & Wampold, B. E. (2014). Expanding the lens of
evidence-based practice in psychotherapy: A common factors perspective.
Psychotherapy, 51(4), 467–481. https://doi.org/10.1037/a0034332

Leahy, R. L. (2012). *Overcoming resistance in cognitive therapy.* Guilford Press.

Lejuez, C. W., Hopko, D. R., Levine, S., Gholkar, R., & Collins, L. M. (2005). The
therapeutic alliance in behavior therapy. *Psychotherapy: Theory, Research, Prac-*
tice, Training, 42(4), 456–468. https://doi.org/10.1037/0033-3204.42.4.456

Linehan, M. M. (2015). *DBT skills training manual* (2nd ed.). Guilford Press.

Lorenzo-Luaces, L., DeRubeis, R. J., & Webb, C. A. (2014). Client characteristics
as moderators of the relation between the therapeutic alliance and outcome in

cognitive therapy for depression. *Journal of Consulting and Clinical Psychology,* *82*(2), 368–373. https://doi.org/10.1037/a0035994

Lorenzo-Luaces, L., Driessen, E., DeRubeis, R. J., Van, H. L., Keefe, J. R., Hendriksen, M., & Dekker, J. (2017). Moderation of the alliance-outcome association by prior depressive episodes: Differential effects in cognitive behavioral therapy and short-term psychodynamic supportive therapy. *Behavior Therapy,* *48*(5), 581–595. https://doi.org/10.1016/j.beth.2016.11.011

Luborsky, L. (1984). *Principles of psychoanalytic psychotherapy: A manual for supportive-expressive treatment.* Basic Books.

Luong, H. K., Drummond, S. P. A., & Norton, P. J. (2020). Elements of the therapeutic relationship in CBT for anxiety disorders: A systematic review. *Journal of Anxiety Disorders,* *76*, 102322. https://doi.org/10.1016/j.janxdis.2020.102322

Macaulay, C., Angus, L., Khattra, J., Westra, H., & Ip, J. (2017). Client retrospective accounts of corrective experiences in motivational interviewing integrated with cognitive behavioral therapy for generalized anxiety disorder. *Journal of Clinical Psychology: In Session,* *73*(2), 168–181. https://doi.org/10.1002/jclp.22430

Maher, M. J., Wang, Y., Zuckoff, A., Wall, M. M., Franklin, M., Foa, E. B., & Simpson, H. B. (2012). Predictors of patient adherence to cognitive-behavioral therapy for obsessive-compulsive disorder. *Psychotherapy and Psychosomatics,* *81*(2), 124–126. https://doi.org/10.1159/000330214

Marmarosh, C. L., Gelso, C. J., Markin, R. D., Majors, R., Mallery, C., & Choi, J. (2009). The real relationship in psychotherapy: Relationships to adult attachment, working alliance, transference, and therapy outcome. *Journal of Counseling Psychology,* *56*(3), 337–350. https://doi.org/10.1037/a0015169

Martin, D. J., Garske, J. P., & Davis, M. K. (2000). Relation of the therapeutic alliance with outcome and other variables: A meta-analytic review. *Journal of Consulting and Clinical Psychology,* *68*(3), 438–450. https://doi.org/10.1037/0022-006X.68.3.438

Marx, J. A., & Gelso, C. J. (1987). Termination of individual counseling in a university counseling center. *Journal of Counseling Psychology,* *34*(1), 3–9. https://doi.org/10.1037/0022-0167.34.1.3

Mathews, A. M., Johnston, D. W., Lancashire, M., Munby, M., Shaw, P. M., & Gelder, M. G. (1976). Imaginal flooding and exposure to real phobic situations: Treatment outcome with agoraphobic patients. *The British Journal of Psychiatry,* *129*(4), 361–371. https://doi.org/10.1192/bjp.129.4.361

Mearns, D., & Cooper, M. (2018). *Working at relational depth in counseling & psychotherapy* (2nd ed.). Sage.

Meissner, W. W. (2007). Therapeutic alliance: Themes and variations. *Psychoanalytic Psychology,* *24*(2), 231–254. https://doi.org/10.1037/0736-9735.24.2.231

Miller, G. A. (1956). The magical number seven plus or minus two: Some limits on our capacity for processing information. *Psychological Review,* *63*(2), 81–97. https://doi.org/10.1037/h0043158

Miller, W. R., & Rollnick, S. (2013). *Motivational interviewing: Helping people change* (3rd ed.). Guilford Press.

Muñoz, R. F., Ippen, C. G., Rao, S., Le, H.-N., & Dwyer, E. V. (2000). *Manual for group cognitive-behavioral therapy of major depression: A reality management approach.* https://i4health.paloaltou.edu/downloads/CBT_Instructor_English.pdf

Muran, J. C., & Eubanks, C. F. (2020). *Therapist performance under pressure: Negotiating emotion, difference, and rupture.* American Psychological Association. https://doi.org/10.1037/0000182-000

Muran, J. C., Safran, J. D., & Eubanks-Carter, C. (2010). Developing therapist abilities to negotiate alliance ruptures. In J. C. Muran & J. P. Barber (Eds.), *The therapeutic alliance: An evidence-based guide to practice* (pp. 320–340). Guilford Press.

Muran, J. C., Safran, J. D., Gorman, B. S., Samstag, L. W., Eubanks-Carter, C., & Winston, A. (2009). The relationship of early alliance ruptures and their resolution to process and outcome in three time-limited psychotherapies for personality disorders. *Psychotherapy: Theory, Research, Practice, Training, 46*(2), 233–248. https://doi.org/10.1037/a0016085

Murphy, R. T., Thompson, K. E., Murray, M., Rainey, Q., & Uddo, M. M. (2009). Effect of a motivation enhancement intervention on veterans' engagement in PTSD treatment. *Psychological Services, 6*(4), 264–278. https://doi.org/10.1037/a0017577

Murphy, S. T., Garcia, R. A., Cheavens, J. S., & Strunk, D. R. (2022). The therapeutic alliance and dropout in cognitive behavioral therapy of depression. *Psychotherapy Research, 32*(8), 995–1002. https://doi.org/10.1080/10503307.2021.2025277

Myers, S. A. (2003). Relational healing: To be understood and to understand. *Journal of Humanistic Psychology, 43*(1), 86–104. https://doi.org/10.1177/0022167802238815

Myers, S. A., & White, C. M. (2010). The abiding nature of empathic connections: A 10-year followup study. *Journal of Humanistic Psychology, 50*(1), 77–95. https://doi.org/10.1177/0022167809337475

Nezu, A. M., & Nezu, C. M. (2019). *Emotion-centered problem-solving therapy: Treatment guidelines.* Springer.

Nof, A., Leibovich, L., & Zilcha-Mano, S. (2017). Supportive-expressive interventions in working through treatment termination. *Psychotherapy, 54*(1), 29–36. https://doi.org/10.1037/pst0000094

Norcross, J. C. (2002). *Psychotherapy relationships that work: Therapist contributions and responsiveness to patient needs.* Oxford University Press.

Norcross, J. C. (2011). *Psychotherapy relationships that work* (2nd ed.). Oxford University Press.

Norcross, J. C., & Lambert, M. J. (2018). Psychotherapy relationships that work III. *Psychotherapy, 55*(4), 303–315. https://doi.org/10.1037/pst0000193

Norcross, J. C., & Lambert, M. J. (2019). *Psychotherapy relationships that work: Volume 1: Evidence-based therapist contributions.* Oxford University Press.

Norcross, J. C., & Wampold, B. E. (2019). *Psychotherapy relationships that work: Volume 2: Evidence-based therapist responsiveness.* Oxford University Press.

Norouzian, N., Westra, H. A., Button, M. L., Constantino, M. J., & Antony, M. M. (2021). Ambivalence and the working alliance in variants of cognitive behavioural therapy for generalised anxiety disorder. *Counselling & Psychotherapy Research, 21*(3), 587–596. https://doi.org/10.1002/capr.12332

O'Donohue, W. T., & Cucciare, M. A. (Eds.). (2008). *Terminating psychotherapy: A clinician's guide.* Routledge.

Okamoto, A., Dattilio, F. M., Dobson, K. S., & Kazantzis, N. (2019). The therapeutic relationship in cognitive behavioral therapy: Essential features and common challenges. *Practice Innovations, 4*(2), 112–123. https://doi.org/10.1037/pri0000088

Okamoto, A., & Kazantzis, N. (2021). Alliance ruptures in cognitive-behavioral therapy: A cognitive conceptualization. *Journal of Clinical Psychology, 77*(2), 384–397. https://doi.org/10.1002/jclp.23116

Olatunji, B. O., Cisler, J. M., & Deacon, B. J. (2010). Efficacy of cognitive behavioral therapy for anxiety disorders: A review of meta-analytic findings. *Psychiatric Clinics of North America, 33*(3), 557–577. https://doi.org/10.1016/j.psc.2010.04.002

Olatunji, B. O., Deacon, B. J., & Abramowitz, J. S. (2009). The cruelest cure? Ethical issues in the implementation of exposure-based treatments. *Cognitive and Behavioral Practice, 16*(2), 172–180. https://doi.org/10.1016/j.cbpra.2008.07.003

Orlinsky, D. E., Grawe, K., & Parks, B. K. (1994). Process and outcome in psychotherapy. In A. E. Bergin & S. L. Garfield (Eds.), *Handbook of psychotherapy and behavior change* (4th ed., pp. 270–376). Wiley.

Pan, D., Huey, S. J., Jr., & Hernandez, D. (2011). Culturally adapted versus standard exposure treatment for phobic Asian Americans: Treatment efficacy, moderators, and predictors. *Cultural Diversity and Ethnic Minority Psychology, 17*(1), 11–22. https://doi.org/10.1037/a0022534

Pennington, D. C. (2000). *Social cognition.* Routledge.

Persons, J. B. (2008). *The case formulation approach to cognitive behavior therapy.* Guilford Press.

Piaget, J. (1952). *The origins of intelligence in children.* W. W. Norton & Co. https://doi.org/10.1037/11494-000

Piper, W. E., Ogrodniczuk, J. S., Joyce, A. S., McCallum, M., Rosie, J. S., O'Kelly, J. G., & Steinberg, P. I. (1999). Prediction of dropping out in time-limited, interpretive individual psychotherapy. *Psychotherapy: Theory, Research, Practice, Training, 36*(2), 114–122. https://doi.org/10.1037/h0087787

Prochaska, J. O., & DiClemente, C. C. (1982). Transtheoretical therapy: Toward a more integrative model of change. *Psychotherapy: Theory, Research, & Practice, 19*(3), 276–288. https://doi.org/10.1037/h0088437

Prochaska, J. O., & Norcross, J. C. (2011). Stages of change. *Psychotherapy: Theory, Research, Practice, Training, 38*(4), 443–448. https://doi.org/10.1037/0033-3204.38.4.443

Rabavilas, A. D., Boulougouris, J. C., & Perissaki, C. (1979). Therapist qualities related to outcome with exposure in vivo in neurotic patients. *Journal of Behavior Therapy and Experimental Psychiatry, 10*(4), 293–294. https://doi.org/10.1016/0005-7916(79)90005-3

Rathod, S., Phiri, P., & Naeem, F. (2019). An evidence-based framework to culturally adapt cognitive behaviour therapy. *The Cognitive Behaviour Therapist, 12*, e10. https://doi.org/10.1017/S1754470X18000247

Raue, P. J., & Goldfried, M. R. (1994). The therapeutic alliance in cognitive behavior therapy. In A. O. Horvath & L. S. Greenberg (Eds.), *The working alliance: Theory, research, and practice* (pp. 131–152). Wiley.

Reich, A. (1951). On counter-transference. *The International Journal of Psychoanalysis, 32*, 25–31.

Rhodes, R., Hill, C. E., Thompson, B. J., & Elliott, R. (1994). Client retrospective recall of resolved and unresolved misunderstanding events. *Journal of Counseling Psychology, 41*(4), 473–483. https://doi.org/10.1037/0022-0167.41.4.473

Rogers, C. R. (1957). The necessary and sufficient conditions of therapeutic personality change. *Journal of Consulting Psychology, 21*(2), 95–103. https://doi.org/10.1037/h0045357

Rogers, C. R. (1959). A theory of therapy, personality, and interpersonal relationships as developed in the client-centered framework. In S. Koch (Ed.), *Psychology: A study of science. Study 1, Volume 3: Formulations of the person and the social context* (pp. 184–256). McGraw-Hill.

Rosenzweig, S. (1936). Some implicit common factors in diverse methods of psychotherapy. *American Journal of Orthopsychiatry, 6*(3), 412–415. https://doi.org/10.1111/j.1939-0025.1936.tb05248.x

Safran, J., & Segal, Z. (1990). *Interpersonal processes in cognitive therapy.* Basic Books.

Safran, J. D., Crocker, P., McMain, S., & Murray, P. (1990). Therapeutic alliance rupture as a therapy event for empirical investigation. *Psychotherapy: Theory, Research, Practice, Training, 27*(2), 154–165. https://doi.org/10.1037/0033-3204.27.2.154

Safran, J. D., & Kraus, J. (2014). Alliance ruptures, impasses, and enactments: A relational perspective. *Psychotherapy, 51*(3), 381–387. https://doi.org/10.1037/a0036815

Safran, J. D., & Muran, J. C. (1996). The resolution of ruptures in the therapeutic alliance. *Journal of Consulting and Clinical Psychology, 64*(3), 447–458. https://doi.org/10.1037/0022-006X.64.3.447

Safran, J. D., & Muran, J. C. (2000). *Negotiating the therapeutic alliance: A relational treatment guide.* Guilford Press.

Safran, J. D., Muran, J. C., & Eubanks-Carter, C. (2011). Repairing alliance ruptures. *Psychotherapy, 48*(1), 80–87. https://doi.org/10.1037/a0022140

Safran, J. D., Muran, J. C., Samstag, L. W., & Stevens, C. (2001). Repairing alliance ruptures. *Psychotherapy: Theory, Research, Practice, Training, 38*(4), 406–412. https://doi.org/10.1037/0033-3204.38.4.406

Salkovskis, P. M., Atha, C., & Storer, D. (1990). Cognitive-behavioral problem solving in the treatment of patients who repeatedly attempt suicide: A controlled trial. *The British Journal of Psychiatry, 157*(6), 871–876. https://doi.org/10.1192/bjp.157.6.871

Schwartz, C., Hilbert, S., Schlegl, S., Diedrich, A., & Voderholzer, U. (2018). Common change factors and mediation of the alliance–outcome link during treatment of depression. *Journal of Consulting and Clinical Psychology, 86*(7), 584–592. https://doi.org/10.1037/ccp0000302

Sharf, J., Primavera, L. H., & Diener, M. J. (2010). Dropout and therapeutic alliance: A meta-analysis of adult individual psychotherapy. *Psychotherapy: Theory, Research, Practice, Training, 47*(4), 637–645. https://doi.org/10.1037/a0021175

Shedler, J. (2010). The efficacy of psychodynamic psychotherapy. *American Psychologist, 65*(2), 98–109. https://doi.org/10.1037/a0018378

Simpson, H. B., Maher, M. J., Wang, Y., Bao, Y., Foa, E. B., & Franklin, M. (2011). Patient adherence predicts outcome from cognitive behavioral therapy in obsessive-compulsive disorder. *Journal of Consulting and Clinical Psychology, 79*(2), 247–252. https://doi.org/10.1037/a0022659

Soto, A., Smith, T. B., Griner, D., Rodríguez, M. C., & Bernal, G. (2019). Cultural adaptations and multicultural competence. In J. C. Norcross & B. E. Wampold (Eds.), *Psychotherapy relationships that work: Vol 2. Evidence-based therapist responsiveness* (pp. 86–132). Oxford University Press. https://doi.org/10.1093/med-psych/9780190843960.003.0004

Sotsky, S. M., Glass, D. R., Shea, M. T., Pilkonis, P. A., Collins, J. F., Elkin, I., Watkins, J. T., Imber, S. D., Leber, W. R., Moyer, J., & Oliveri, M. E. (1991). Patient predictors of response to psychotherapy and pharmacotherapy: Findings in the NIMH Treatment of Depression Collaborative Research Program. *The American Journal of Psychiatry, 148*(8), 997–1008. https://doi.org/10.1176/ajp.148.8.997

Stangier, U., Hilling, C., Heidenreich, T., Risch, A. K., Barocka, A., Schlösser, R., Kronfeld, K., Ruckes, C., Berger, H., Röschke, J., Weck, F., Volk, S., Hambrecht, M., Serfling, R., Erkwoh, R., Stirn, A., Sobanski, T., & Hautzinger, M. (2013). Maintenance cognitive-behavioral therapy and manualized psychoeducation in the treatment of recurrent depression: A multicenter prospective randomized controlled trial. *The American Journal of Psychiatry, 170*(6), 624–632. https://doi.org/10.1176/appi.ajp.2013.12060734

Stiles, W. B., Honos-Webb, L., & Surko, M. (1998). Responsiveness in psychotherapy. *Clinical Psychology: Science and Practice, 5*(4), 439–458.

Strauss, J. L., Hayes, A. M., Johnson, S. L., Newman, C. F., Brown, G. K., Barber, J. P., Laurenceau, J.-P., & Beck, A. T. (2006). Early alliance, alliance ruptures, and symptom change in a nonrandomized trial of cognitive therapy for avoidant and obsessive-compulsive personality disorders. *Journal of Consulting and Clinical Psychology, 74*(2), 337–345. https://doi.org/10.1037/0022-006X.74.2.337

Strunk, D. R., Cooper, A. A., Ryan, E. T., DeRubeis, R. J., & Hollon, S. D. (2012). The process of change in cognitive therapy for depression when combined with antidepressant medication: Predictors of early intersession symptom gains. *Journal of Consulting and Clinical Psychology, 80*(5), 730–738. https://doi.org/10.1037/a0029281

Sue, S. (1998). In search of cultural competence in psychotherapy and counseling. *American Psychologist, 53*(4), 440–448. https://doi.org/10.1037/0003-066X.53.4.440

Suzuki, J. Y., & Farber, B. A. (2016). Towards greater specificity of the concept of positive regard. *Person-Centered and Experiential Psychotherapies, 15*(4), 263–284. https://doi.org/10.1080/14779757.2016.1204941

Suzuki, J. Y., Mandavia, A., & Farber, B. A. (2021). Clients' perceptions of positive regard across four therapeutic orientations. *Journal of Psychotherapy Integration, 31*(2), 129–145. https://doi.org/10.1037/int0000186

Taylor, A., Tallon, D., Kessler, D., Peters, T. J., Shafran, R., Williams, C., & Wiles, N. (2020). An expert consensus on the most effective components of cognitive behavioural therapy for adults with depression: A modified Delphi study. *Cognitive Behaviour Therapy, 49*(3), 242–255. https://doi.org/10.1080/16506073.2019.1641146

Tee, J., & Kazantzis, N. (2011). Collaborative empiricism in cognitive therapy: A definition and theory for relationship construct. *Clinical Psychology: Science and Practice, 18*(1), 47–62. https://doi.org/10.1111/j.1468-2850.2010.01234.x

Thwaites, R., & Bennett-Levy, J. (2007). Conceptualizing empathy in cognitive behavior therapy: Making the implicit explicit. *Behavioural and Cognitive Psychotherapy, 35*(5), 591–612. https://doi.org/10.1017/S1352465807003785

Tishby, O., & Wiseman, H. (2022). Countertransference types and their relation to rupture and repair in the alliance. *Psychotherapy Research, 32*(1), 16–31. https://doi.org/10.1080/10503307.2020.1862934

Tryon, G. S., & Winograd, G. (2011). Goal consensus and collaboration. *Psychotherapy, 48*(1), 50–57. https://doi.org/10.1037/a0022061

Tsai, M., Kohlenberg, R. J., & Kanter, J. W. (2010). A functional analytic psychotherapy (FAP) approach to the therapeutic alliance. In J. C. Muran & J. P. Barber (Eds.), *The therapeutic alliance: An evidence-based guide to practice* (pp. 172–190). Guilford Press.

Tschacher, W., Junghan, U. M., & Pfammatter, M. (2014). Towards a taxonomy of common factors in psychotherapy-results of an expert survey. *Clinical Psychology & Psychotherapy, 21*(1), 82–96. https://doi.org/10.1002/cpp.1822

Tursi, M. M., & Cochran, J. L. (2006). Cognitive behavioral tasks accomplished in a person-centered relational framework. *Journal of Counseling & Development, 84*(4), 387–396. https://doi.org/10.1002/j.1556-6678.2006.tb00421.x

Van Horn, D. H. A., Wenzel, A., & Britton, P. C. (2021). Motivational interviewing. In A. Wenzel (Ed.), *Handbook of cognitive behavioral therapy, Vol 1: Overview and approaches* (pp. 313–347). American Psychological Association. https://doi.org/10.1037/0000218-011

Vîslă, A., Constantino, M. J., Newkirk, K., Ogrodniczuk, J. S., & Söchting, I. (2018). The relation between outcome expectation, therapeutic alliance, and outcome among depressed patients in group cognitive-behavioral therapy. *Psychotherapy Research, 28*(3), 446–456. https://doi.org/10.1080/10503307.2016.1218089

Wampold, B. E., & Flückiger, C. (2023). The alliance in mental health care: Conceptualization, evidence and clinical applications. *World Psychiatry, 22*(1), 25–41. https://doi.org/10.1002/wps.21035

Wampold, B. E., & Imel, Z. E. (2015). *The great psychotherapy debate: The evidence for what makes psychotherapy work* (2nd ed.). Routledge. https://doi.org/10.4324/9780203582015

Watson, J. C., & Kalogerakos, F. (2010). The therapeutic alliance in humanistic psychotherapy. In J. C. Muran & J. P. Barber (Eds.), *The therapeutic alliance: An evidence-based guide to practice* (pp. 191–209). Guilford Press.

Watson, J. C., Steckley, P. L., & McMullen, E. J. (2014). The role of empathy in promoting change. *Psychotherapy Research, 24*(3), 286–298. https://doi.org/10.1080/10503307.2013.802823

Webb, C. A., DeRubeis, R. J., Amsterdam, J. D., Shelton, R. C., Hollon, S. D., & Dimidjian, S. (2011). Two aspects of the therapeutic alliance: Differential relations with depressive symptom change. *Journal of Consulting and Clinical Psychology, 79*(3), 279–283. https://doi.org/10.1037/a0023252

Weck, F., Grikscheit, F., Jakob, M., Höfling, V., & Stangier, U. (2015). Treatment failure in cognitive-behavioural therapy: Therapeutic alliance as a precondition for an adherent and competent implementation of techniques. *British Journal of Clinical Psychology, 54*(1), 91–108. https://doi.org/10.1111/bjc.12063

Weck, F., Richtberg, S., Jakob, M., Neng, J. M. B., & Höfling, V. (2015). Therapist competence and therapeutic alliance are important in the treatment of health anxiety (hypochondriasis). *Psychiatry Research, 228*(1), 53–58. https://doi.org/10.1016/j.psychres.2015.03.042

Wenzel, A. (2012). Modification of core beliefs in cognitive therapy. In I. R. de Oliveira (Ed.), *Cognitive behavioral therapy* (pp. 17–34). Intech.

Wenzel, A. (2013). *Strategic decision making in cognitive behavioral therapy.* American Psychological Association. https://doi.org/10.1037/14188-000

Wenzel, A. (2017). *Innovations in cognitive behavioral therapy: Strategic interventions for creative practice.* Routledge. https://doi.org/10.4324/9781315771021

Wenzel, A. (2019). *Cognitive behavioral therapy for beginners: An experiential approach.* Routledge. https://doi.org/10.4324/9781315651958

Wenzel, A., Brown, G. K., & Beck, A. T. (2009). *Cognitive therapy for suicidal patients: Scientific and clinical applications.* American Psychological Association. https://doi.org/10.1037/11862-000

Wenzel, A., Dobson, K. S., & Hays, P. (2016). *Cognitive behavioral therapy techniques and strategies*. American Psychological Association. https://doi.org/10.1037/14936-000

Wenzel, A., Jeglic, E. L., Levy-Mack, H. J., Beck, A. T., & Brown, G. K. (2008). Treatment attitude and therapy outcome in patients with borderline personality disorder. *Journal of Cognitive Psychotherapy, 22*(3), 250–257. https://doi.org/10.1891/0889-8391.22.3.250

Westra, H. A. (2012). *Motivational interviewing in the treatment of anxiety*. Guilford Press.

Westra, H. A., Arkowitz, H., & Dozois, D. J. A. (2009). Adding a motivational interviewing pretreatment to cognitive behavioral therapy for generalized anxiety disorder: A preliminary randomized controlled trial. *Journal of Anxiety Disorders, 23*(8), 1106–1117. https://doi.org/10.1016/j.janxdis.2009.07.014

Westra, H. A., & Aviram, A. (2015). Integrating motivational interviewing into the treatment of anxiety. In H. Arkowitz, W. R. Miller, & S. Rollnick (Eds.), *Motivational interviewing in the treatment of psychological problems* (2nd ed., pp. 83–109). Guilford Press.

Westra, H. A., Aviram, A., Connors, L., Kertes, A., & Ahmed, M. (2012). Therapist emotional reactions and client resistance in cognitive behavioral therapy. *Psychotherapy, 49*(2), 163–172. https://doi.org/10.1037/a0023200

Westra, H. A., Constantino, M. J., & Antony, M. M. (2016). Integrating motivational interviewing with cognitive-behavioral therapy for severe generalized anxiety disorder: An allegiance-controlled randomized clinical trial. *Journal of Consulting and Clinical Psychology, 84*(9), 768–782. https://doi.org/10.1037/ccp0000098

Westra, H. A., Constantino, M. J., Arkowitz, H., & Dozois, D. J. A. (2011). Therapist differences in cognitive-behavioral psychotherapy for generalized anxiety disorder: A pilot study. *Psychotherapy, 48*(3), 283–292. https://doi.org/10.1037/a0022011

Whelen, M. L., Murphy, S. T., & Strunk, D. R. (2021). Reevaluating the alliance-outcome relationship in the early sessions of cognitive behavioral therapy for depression. *Clinical Psychological Science, 9*(3), 515–523. https://doi.org/10.1177/2167702620959352

Whisman, M. A. (1993). Mediators and moderators of change in cognitive therapy of depression. *Psychological Bulletin, 114*(2), 248–265. https://doi.org/10.1037/0033-2909.114.2.248

Williams, G. C., McGregor, H. A., Sharp, D., Levesque, C., Kouides, R. W., Ryan, R. M., & Deci, E. L. (2006). Testing a self-determination theory intervention for motivating tobacco cessation: Supporting autonomy and competence in a clinical trial. *Health Psychology, 25*(1), 91–101. https://doi.org/10.1037/0278-6133.25.1.91

Wilson, G. T., & Evans, I. M. (1977). The therapist-client relationship in behavior therapy. In A. S. Gurman & A. M. Razin (Eds.), *Effective psychotherapy: A handbook of research* (pp. 309–330). Pergamon Press.

Winnicott, D. W. (1955). Metapsychological and clinical aspects of regression within the psycho-analytical set-up. *The International Journal of Psychoanalysis, 36*(1), 16–26.

Winnicott, D. W. (1963). *The maturational processes and the facilitating environment.* Hogarth Press and the Institute of Psychoanalysis.

Wolfe, B. E., & Goldfried, M. R. (1988). Research on psychotherapy integration: Recommendations and conclusions from an NIMH workshop. *Journal of Consulting and Clinical Psychology, 56*(3), 448–451. https://doi.org/10.1037/0022-006X.56.3.448

Wolitzky-Taylor, K. B., Horowitz, J. D., Powers, M. B., & Telch, M. J. (2008). Psychological approaches in the treatment of specific phobias: A meta-analysis. *Clinical Psychology Review, 28*(6), 1021–1037. https://doi.org/10.1016/j.cpr.2008.02.007

World Health Organization. (1993). *WHOQoL study protocol* (Report No. MNH7 PSF/93.9).

Young, J. E., Klosko, J. S., & Weishaar, M. E. (2003). *Schema therapy: A practitioner's guide.* Guilford Press.

Zayfert, C., DeViva, J. C., Becker, C. B., Pile, J. L., Gillock, K. L., & Hayes, S. A. (2005). Exposure utilization and completion of cognitive behavioral therapy for PTSD in a "real world" clinical practice. *Journal of Traumatic Stress, 18*(6), 637–645. https://doi.org/10.1002/jts.20072

Zilcha-Mano, S. (2017). Is the alliance really therapeutic? Revisiting this question in light of recent methodological advances. *American Psychologist, 72*(4), 311–325. https://doi.org/10.1037/a0040435

Zilcha-Mano, S. (2021). Toward personalized psychotherapy: The importance of the trait-like/state-like distinction for understanding therapeutic change. *American Psychologist, 76*(3), 516–528. https://doi.org/10.1037/amp0000629

Zilcha-Mano, S., Eubanks, C. F., & Muran, J. C. (2019). Sudden gains in the alliance in cognitive behavioral therapy versus brief relational therapy. *Journal of Consulting and Clinical Psychology, 87*(6), 501–509. https://doi.org/10.1037/ccp0000397

Zilcha-Mano, S., McCarthy, K. S., Dinger, U., & Barber, J. P. (2014). To what extent is alliance affected by transference? An empirical exploration. *Psychotherapy, 51*(3), 424–433. https://doi.org/10.1037/a0036566

Zuroff, D. C., & Blatt, S. J. (2006). The therapeutic relationship in the brief treatment of depression: Contributions to clinical improvement and enhanced adaptive capacities. *Journal of Consulting and Clinical Psychology, 74*(1), 130–140. https://doi.org/10.1037/0022-006X.74.1.130

Index

About the Author

Amy Wenzel, PhD, ABPP, is a clinical psychologist who specializes in cognitive behavioral therapy (CBT). She is author or editor of over 25 books and treatment manuals, including the American Psychological Association's two-volume set, *Handbook of Cognitive Behavioral Therapy*. In addition, she founded the Main Line Center for Evidence-Based Psychotherapy, a CBT-based treatment center in the Philadelphia suburbs. She lectures internationally on CBT and has trained and supervised over 1,000 clinicians to achieve competency in CBT. She has adapted CBT for unique clinical presentations such as perinatal mental health disorders and menopausal distress.

Dr. Wenzel received her PhD from the University of Iowa in 2000 and completed her clinical psychology residency at the University of Wisconsin School of Medicine. She has held faculty positions at the University of Pennsylvania School of Medicine, the University of North Dakota, and the American College of Norway. While at the University of Pennsylvania, she collaborated with Dr. Aaron T. Beck, often regarded as the "father" of CBT, on CBT protocols for suicidal clients. Dr. Wenzel has also served as adjunct faculty at the Beck Institute for Cognitive Behavior Therapy and is a certified trainer-consultant with the Academy of Cognitive Behavioral Therapies.

Dr. Wenzel has authored over 100 peer-reviewed journal articles and book chapters. Her research has been funded by the National Institute of Mental Health, the American Foundation for Suicide Prevention, and the National Alliance for Research on Schizophrenia and Depression (now the Brain and Behavior Research Foundation). She has served on the scientific advisory board of the American Foundation for Suicide Prevention and has held leadership positions in the Association for Behavioral and Cognitive

Therapies. She is currently on the editorial boards of *Cognitive and Behavioral Practice*, *Cognitive Behaviour Therapy*, and the *Journal of Rational-Emotive and Cognitive-Behavior Therapy*. She has been featured in numerous video demonstrations of CBT published by the American Psychological Association. Dr. Wenzel currently divides her time between clinical practice, scholarship, and training and supervision.